Analysing Families

While families continue to be a key topic in social policy, much of the literature is simply concerned with describing the dramatic changes that are taking place. By contrast, *Analysing Families* directly addresses the social processes responsible for these changes and focuses on how government policy interacts with what families actually do. Topics covered include:

- the relationship between morality and rationality in family processes;
- the variety of contemporary family forms;
- the purposes and assumptions of government intervention in family life;
- divorce and post-divorce arrangements;
- lone parenthood and step-parenting;
- the decision to have children; and
- the economic approach to understanding family decision-making.

Including chapters on family policy in Britain, Europe and the USA, *Analysing Families* provides a new understanding of familial behaviour on which to base the policy process.

Alan Carling is Senior Lecturer in Sociology, University of Bradford; **Simon Duncan** is Professor of Comparative Social Policy, University of Bradford; and **Rosalind Edwards** is Professor of Social Policy, South Bank University.

Analysing Families

Morality and rationality in policy and practice

Edited by Alan Carling, Simon Duncan and Rosalind Edwards

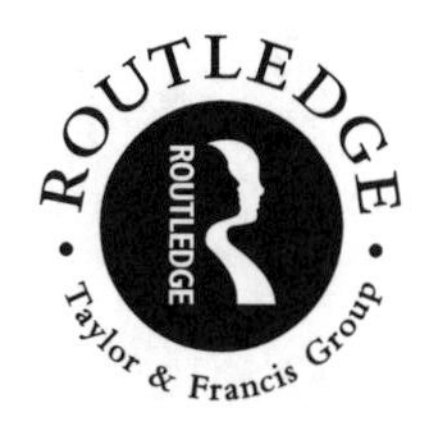

London and New York

First published 2002
by Routledge
11 New Fetter Lane, London EC4P 4EE

Simultaneously published in the USA and Canada
by Routledge
29 West 35th Street, New York, NY 10001

Routledge is an imprint of the Taylor & Francis Group

Typeset in Times by Taylor & Francis Books Ltd
Printed and bound in Great Britain by The Cromwell Press, Trowbridge, Wiltshire

British Library Cataloguing in Publication Data
A catalogue record for this book is available from the British Library

Library of Congress Cataloging-in-Publication Data
Analysing families : morality and rationality in policy and practice / edited by Alan Carling, Simon Duncan and Rosalind Edwards.
p. cm.
Includes bibliographical references and index.
1. Family–Great Britain. 2. Family–Europe. 3. Family policy–Great Britain. 4. Family policy–Europe. I. Title: Analysing families. II. Carling, Alan. III. Duncan, Simon. IV. Edwards, Rosalind.
HQ614 .A679 2002
306.85–dc21

2001045712

ISBN 0–415–25039–0 (hbk)
ISBN 0–415–25040–4 (pbk)

Contents

Illustrations

Figures

Tables

Contributors

Anne Barlow is a Senior Lecturer in Law at the University of Wales, Aberystwyth, UK. She has a particular interest in family policy and family law, especially the law relating to cohabitants, which is the main focus of her research. Her publications include *Cohabitants and the Law* (Butterworths, 1997) and *Advising Gay and Lesbian Clients: A Guide for Lawyers* (with M. Bowley QC *et al.*, Butterworths, 1999). In addition to her ongoing research into the 'common law marriage myth' in England and Wales, she is currently undertaking comparative research into the varying legal responses to the phenomenon of cohabitation in Europe.

Ulla Björnberg is Professor of Sociology, Gender and Family at the Department of Sociology, Göteborg University, Sweden. She has been engaged in several international projects on family policy and family life in Eastern and Western Europe. Her studies focus on the reconciliation of employment and family life, with perspectives on gender and class, lone motherhood and employment. She is currently leading a research programme on 'Family relations in modern society: development of theory and methods in sociological research on families', studying the subsistence strategies of lone mothers and negotiations about the distribution of money, time and domestic work in dual-earner couples. She is the author of many publications on these topics, including 'Equality and backlash: family, gender and social policy in Sweden' (in L. Hass and P. Hwang (eds), *Organisational Change and Gender Equity*, Sage, 2000) and 'Family change and family policy in Sweden' (in M. Alestalo and P. Flor (eds), *Family Change and Family Policy in the Scandinavian Welfare States*, Oxford University Press, 2001).

Alan Carling is a Senior Lecturer in Sociology at the University of Bradford, UK. He has published extensively in social theory, political philosophy and the theory of history. An especial interest is in the application of the rational choice approach to sociological topics, including families and households. He is author of *Social Divisions* (Verso, 1991) and founding editor of *Imprints: A Journal of Analytical Socialism*.

Edmund Chattoe works in the Department of Sociology at the University of Oxford, UK. He began his career as an economist and has remained interested in both decision making and the structure of markets but has lost enthusiasm for the extreme abstractions of rational choice. Computer simulation appears to offer one way of reconciling the richness of sociological data (such as interviews) with a realistic measure of formality. He has applied these ideas to family budgeting strategies and adaptation, time use, diffusion of innovation, social mobility and second-hand markets. He has been sole and co-author of papers in the journal *Sociology*.

Lynda Clarke is a Senior Lecturer in the Centre for Population Studies at the London School of Hygiene and Tropical Medicine, UK. She has undertaken research into family issues for twenty years and specialises in family demography, health and family policy. Her interest progressed through children's experiences, women's issues, lone motherhood and fathers. She published the seminal *Fathers and Fatherhood in Britain* in 1997, which included the first demographic analysis of fatherhood in Britain. Her recent research projects include 'Choosing childlessness', 'Kin beyond the household', 'The changing home: outcomes for children', 'Fatherhood in the new millennium' and 'Grandparenthood: its meaning and contribution to the quality of older people's lives'. She is also academic adviser to several UK government publications, including *Social Focus on Men* and *The Health of Our Children*.

Graham Crow is Reader in Sociology at the University of Southampton, UK, where he has worked since 1983. His research interests include the sociology of families, households and communities; comparative sociology; and sociological theory. His recent publications include *Comparative Sociology and Social Theory* (Macmillan, 1997), *Social Solidarities* (Open University Press, 2001) and *Families, Households and Society* (with Graham Allen, Palgrave, 2001). He is currently co-editor (together with Larry Ray) of the journal *Sociological Research On-line*.

Alan Deacon is Professor of Social Policy and a member of the Economic and Social Research Council Research Group on 'Care, Values and the Future of Welfare' at the University of Leeds, UK. He has written widely on the debate about welfare reform in Britain and the United States, most recently in *Political Quarterly* (1998), *Journal of Social Policy* (1999) and *Policy and Politics* (2000). His latest book, *Perspectives on Welfare*, will be published by Open University Press in 2002.

Simon Duncan is Professor in Comparative Social Policy at the University of Bradford, UK. He has published widely on gender inequality; families, welfare and employment; the local state; and housing provision. From 1994 to 1999 he was chair of the European Science Foundation network *Gender Inequality and the European Regions*. Recent publications include

Lone Mothers, Paid Work and Gendered Moral Rationalities (with R. Edwards, Macmillan, 1999) and *Gender, Economy and Culture in the EU* (co-edited with B. Pfau-Effinger, Routledge, 2001). He is currently working on a major research programme, 'Care, values and the future of the welfare state'.

Rosalind Edwards is Professor in Social Policy at South Bank University, UK, and Director of the ESRC-funded Families and Social Capital Research Group. She has carried out research on a variety of family issues, including mothers and education; lone and partnered mothers; employment, childcare and family relationships; step-families; and children's understandings of parental involvement in education. Recent publications include *Feminist Dilemmas in Qualitative Research* (co-edited with J. Ribbens, Sage, 1998), *Lone Mothers, Paid Work and Gendered Moral Rationalities* (with S. Duncan, Macmillan, 1999), *Risk and Citizenship: Key Issues in Welfare* (co-edited with J. Glover, RoutledgeFalmer, 2001) and *Children, Home and School: Regulation, Autonomy or Connection?* (ed., RoutledgeFalmer, 2001). She co-edits (with J. Brannen) *The International Journal of Social Research Methodology: Theory and Practice*.

Lluís Flaquer is Reader in Sociology at the Universitat Autònoma de Barcelona, Spain, where he was Head of the Sociology Department (1993–95). He took a BA in political science at the Institut d'Études Politiques (University of Paris), read sociology and anthropology at the universities of Lancaster and East Anglia, and took a PhD in law at the Universitat Autònoma de Barcelona. His current research topics include the changing structure of the Spanish family, new family forms, family policy and individualisation. His recent publications include several books in Spanish: *El distino de la familia* (*The Destiny of the Family*, 1998), *La estrella menguante del padre* (*The Fading Father*, 2000) and *Las políticas familiars en una perspectiva comparada* (*Family Policy in a Comparative Perspective*, 2000).

Birgit Geissler is Professor of Social Sciences at the University of Bielefeld, situated at the University of Bremen, Germany. She has published widely in the fields of social inequality, the sociology of labour markets, the sociology of social policies, family sociology and gender studies, including *FrauenArbeitsMarkt* (co-editor, Sigma, 1998), *Die ungleiche Gleichheit. Junge Frauen und der Wandel im Geschlechterverhältnis* (co-editor, Leske und Budrich, 1998), 'Zeitordnungen des erwerbssystems und biographiche bindungen an andere' (in Born and Krüger (eds), *Individualisierung und Verflechtung*, Juventa, 2001) and 'Die (un-)abhägigkeit in der ehe und das bürgerecht auf care. Überlegungen zur gender-gerechtigkeit im wohlfahrtsstaat' (in Gottschall and Pfau-Effinger (eds), *Zunkunft der Arbeit und Geschlecht*, Leske und Budrich, 2001).

Judith Glover is Reader in Social Policy at the University of Surrey, Roehampton, UK. Her research interests focus on women's employment, studied in both the UK and cross-nationally, and she has a particular interest in women's scientific education and employment. She has published in journals such as *Work, Employment and Society*, *Gender, Work and Organisations* and *Sociétés Contemporaines*. She is the author of *Women in Scientific Employment* (Macmillan, 2000).

María José González-López is a researcher at the Centre of Demographic Studies, Universitat Autònoma de Barcelona, Spain, and is currently participating in a European Commission Fifth Framework Programme research project on 'Female employment in national institutional contexts'. Her main areas of interest are the sociology of the family, gender and demographic analysis. Her recent publications include 'Households and families: changing living arrangements and gender relations' (with M. Solsona, in S. Duncan and B. Pfau-Effinger (eds), *Gender, Economy and Culture in the EU*, Routledge, 2001) and 'Who marries whom? Educational homogamy in Spain' (in H.-P. Blossfeld and A. Timm (eds), *Who Marries Whom? Educational Systems as Marriage Markets in Modern Societies*, Oxford University Press, 2002).

Susan Himmelweit teaches economics at the Open University, UK. Her research interests include the economics of caring, the gender implications of economic policy and the gender analysis of budgets. She is currently engaged on a research project examining how mothers of small children make decisions about employment and childcare. She is chair of the Women's Budget Group (an economic think tank that advises the Treasury on gender mainstreaming) and an associate editor of *Feminist Economics*. Recent publications include *Inside the Household: From Labour to Care* (Macmillan, 2000), a special issue of *Feminist Economics* on children and family policy (6: 1, 2000, jointly guest edited with Nancy Folbre) and 'Caring labor' (*Annals of the American Academy of Political and Social Sciences*, 1999).

Adrian James is Professor of Applied Social Sciences at the University of Bradford, UK. He worked as a probation officer before becoming an academic over twenty years ago. He has researched and published widely in the area of family court welfare officers and has recently completed an evaluation of the introduction of publicly funded mediation. He is currently looking at the work of family court welfare officers and guardians *ad litem* in the context of the new Children and Family Courts Advisory and Support Service. Recent major publications include *Helping Families After Divorce* (with L. Sturgeon-Adams, Polity Press/Joseph Rowntree Foundation, 1999), *Monitoring Publicly Funded Family Mediation: Report to the Legal Services Commission* (Bevan *et al.*, Legal Services Commission, 2000) and *The Child Protection Handbook* (co-edited with K. Wilson, Ballière-Tindall, 2001).

Grace James received her PhD from the University of Wales, Aberystwyth, UK, where she is currently a research fellow in the Law Department. Her research interests include labour law, family-friendly initiatives and feminist legal theory. Most recently (2001), she has published an article, 'Work and parents: competitiveness and choice'; and a report, 'Pregnancy-related unfair dismissal litigation at employment tribunals in England and Wales'.

Jane Lewis is Barnett Professor of Social Policy at the University of Oxford, UK. Her recent publications include *Lone Motherhood in Twentieth Century Britain* (with Kathleen Kiernan and Hilary Land, 1998), *Lone Mothers and European Welfare Regimes* (ed., 1998), *Gender, Social Care and Welfare State Restructuring in Europe* (ed., 1999) and *The End of Marriage? Individualism and Intimate Relationships* (2001).

Mavis Maclean is Director of the Oxford Centre for Family Law and Policy, UK, which draws together researchers from law and social policy to consider the regulation of obligations arising from personal relationships. Recent books include *Family Lawyers and The Parental Obligation*, co-authored with John Eekelaar (published by Hart). She is academic adviser to the Lord Chancellor's Department, and she served as a panel member on the recent Bristol Royal Infirmary Inquiry.

Jane Ribbens McCarthy is a Lecturer in Qualitative Methods at the Open University, UK. Her research interests centre on family lives, especially parents and children, theorising public and private, and qualitative research methods, including (auto)biographical and feminist approaches. Recent research topics have included parenting and step-parenting, and the 'family' lives of young people aged 16–18. Major publications include *Mothers and Their Children: A Feminist Sociology of Childrearing* (Sage, 1994), *Mothers and Education: Inside Out?* (with M. David, R. Edwards and M. Hughes, Macmillan, 1993), *Mothers' Intuition: Choosing Secondary Schools* (with M. David and A. West, Falmer, 1994), *Feminist Dilemmas in Qualitative Research* (co-edited with R. Edwards, Sage, 1998) and 'Pulling together, pulling apart: the family lives of young people' (with V. Gillies and J. Holland, JRF/FPSC, 2001).

David Morgan has recently retired from Manchester University, where he has taught and researched for around thirty-five years. He still holds a part-time professorial appointment at NTNU, Trondheim. His main interests include family theory and the study of gender, especially masculinities. He is currently studying the process of leaving the parental home in Britain, Spain and Norway with Clare Holdsworth. Recent publications include *Family Connections* (Polity Press, 1996) and 'Risk and family practices: accounting for change and fluidity in family life' (in E.B. Silva and C. Smart (eds), *The New Family?* (Sage, 1999).

Bren Neale is senior research fellow at the Centre for Research on Family, Kinship and Childhood, University of Leeds, UK. As a family sociologist, she has a particular interest in life course processes, parenthood, childhood, family values and family change. Her recent publications include *Family Fragments?* (with Carol Smart, Polity Press, 1999) and *The Changing Experience of Childhood: Families and Divorce* (with Carol Smart and Amanda Wade, Polity Press, 2001). She is currently researching cultures of divorce in a diversity of ethnic and religious contexts and is exploring young people's biographies in post-divorce families.

Birgit Pfau-Effinger is Professor of Sociology at the University of Jena, situated at the University of Bremen, Germany. She has published widely in the fields of comparative sociology, social inequality, sociology of labour markets, sociology of welfare states, family sociology and gender studies, including 'Gender cultures and the gender arrangement – a theoretical framework for cross-national comparisons on gender' (*Innovation*, 2, 1997), 'Change of family policies in the socio-cultural context of European societies' (*Comparative Social Research*, 18, 1999), *Kultur und Frauenerwerbstätigkeit im europäischen Vergleich* (Leske und Budrich, 2000) and *Gender, Work and Culture in the European Union* (co-editor, Routledge, 2000).

Tracey Reynolds is a research fellow at South Bank University, UK. She was awarded her PhD in 1999 and is now working on a book-length manuscript of her thesis, which examined Black mothering and family in Britain. She has published several articles that centre on the Black family, issues around race and gender and Black community groups in Britain. Her publications include '(Mis)representing the Black (super)woman' (in H. Mirza (ed.), *Black British Feminism*, 1997) and 'Black fathers in family lives' (in. H. Goulbourne (ed.), *Caribbean Families in a Transatlantic World*, 2001). She is currently working on a research project funded by the Joseph Rowntree Foundation that explores the work–family life balance for working mothers. She also teaches qualitative research methods to undergraduate students at South Bank University.

Ceridwen Roberts was Director of the UK Family Policies Centre, an independent research and policy centre that studied the interplay between pubic policy for, and the changing nature of, families, from 1992 to 2001. She was responsible for leading the centre's work analysing family policies, on families and the labour market and parenting, and she was the UK expert on the European Observatory on National Family Matters. Her areas of interest have included all aspects of women's employment and unemployment and subsequently labour market flexibility and atypical work. Her key publication in this area is *Women and Employment – A Lifetime Perspective* (with J. Martin, 1994). Her current research interests are fathers and fatherhood, grandparents, attitudes to teenage parents and international perspectives on adoption.

Selma Sevenhuijsen is Professor of the Ethics and Politics of Care at Utrecht University, the Netherlands, and is also visiting professor at the University of Leeds and the University of the Western Cape. She was previously a professor in women's studies at the Faculty of Social Sciences at Utrecht University. Her recent work is aimed at further developing the philosophical groundwork and practical applications of the ethic of care for social policy and citizenship. She investigates this for (health)care policies, family politics, psychiatry and equal opportunities politics. Her key publication on this topic is *Citizenship and the Ethics of Care* (Routledge, 1999). She also works as a consultant.

Carol Smart has been Professor of Sociology at the University of Leeds, UK since 1992 and is the founding Director of the University's Centre for Research on Family, Kinship and Childhood. She is Deputy Director of the ESRC research group on 'Care, Values and the Future of Welfare' (CAVA) at Leeds. In addition, she currently holds a number of grants for research into aspects of family life and childhood and has recently completed two projects on children's experiences of post-divorce family life. Her recent publications include *Family Fragments?* (with B. Neale, Polity Press, 1999), *The New Family?* (co-edited with E. Silva, Sage, 1999), 'Objects of concern? – Children and divorce' in *Child and Family Law Quarterly* (with A. Wade and B. Neale, 1999), *Cohabitation Breakdown* (with P. Stevens, Family Policy Studies Centre, 1999) and *The Changing Experience of Childhood: Families and Divorce* (with B. Neale and A. Wade, Polity Press, 2001).

Jeffrey Weeks is Professor of Sociology and Dean of Humanities and Social Science at South Bank University, UK. He is the author of many articles and books on the social organisation of sexuality. His latest books include *Making Sexual History* (Polity Press, 2000) and *Same Sex Intimacies: Families of Choice and Other Life Experiments* (with Brian Heaphy and Catherine Donovan, Routledge, 2001).

Preface

How to use this book

Purpose of the book

The aim of this book is to take the debate on family change and social policy on to a new level through a focus on the moralities and rationalities that underlay how families work. Most of the existing literature catalogues and describes changes, with at most a speculative engagement about origins and effects. Similarly, government intervention focuses on family forms (e.g. marriage versus cohabitation) rather than responding to what people actually do in families. In contrast, this book analyses the social processes responsible for the current changes in family life. This focus allows the book to mount a more productive analysis of policy change.

Within families especially, human behaviour is not simply a matter of economically rational responses to changing incentives; the normative and moral dimensions of motivation and behaviour must always be taken into account. But government policies often seem to depend on oversimplified assumptions about the way in which family members will respond to policy changes. If governments wish to encourage a certain social outcome in terms of family forms or family practices, simply rigging the costs and benefits in the desired direction can mean that the policy initiative fails. This is because people's reactions to the changing incentives will be mediated by a range of normative conceptions, including their understandings of what is expected of them as a particular family member. There is no universal rationality that mandates the same response to the same policy initiatives among all social groups, at all times or in all places. This is why a deeper analysis of people's understandings and behaviour as part of families needs to inform the policy process. It is this deeper type of analysis that the book provides.

Structure of the book

Each chapter is written by a specialist in that area, drawn from a variety of disciplinary and national backgrounds. The book itself is organised into five parts, which follow a developmental logic while providing a free-standing thematic treatment of successive topics. Each chapter, and each section, can therefore be read separately or used as part of the wider consideration put forward in the book as a whole.

The Introduction sets the scene by examining the relationship between morality and rationality in the family context (Chapter 1), and the empirical variety of contemporary family forms in Western societies (Chapter 2).

Part II, 'Perspectives on family policy', analyses the purposes and assumptions of government intervention in family life in Britain (Chapter 3) and in other Western countries, where Germany, Spain, Sweden and the USA are chosen as 'type cases' of different welfare state regimes and gender cultures (Chapter 4), the rationality mistake made by policy planners (Chapter 5), and 'Third Way' thinking on families (Chapter 6).

Part III, 'Family practices', examines actual family practices and family change, looking at sociological perspectives on families (Chapter 7), fathers and grandparents (Chapter 8), children, parents and divorce (Chapter 9), mothers and children (Chapter 10) and the 'elective families' of non-heterosexual relationships (Chapter 11).

Part IV on 'Modelling families' takes a more economic approach, exploring the limitations of rational choice as an explanation of family life (Chapter 12), the balancing of life and work in families (Chapter 13) and how to model family behaviour (Chapter 14).

The Conclusion (Chapter 15) returns to the question of moralities, rationalities and state policy.

Part I

Introduction

1 Family policy, social theory and the state

Alan Carling

This volume is concerned with two related questions. First, how do those interested in family life understand the action going on under that heading, whether as academics, policy makers or family members themselves? Second, to what extent can and should the state intervene to shape family life and intimate relationships, either as goals of policy in their own right or in pursuit of other goals, such as fiscal saving, moral development, social cohesion or economic growth?

The contributors to the book are all professional social scientists or lawyers, and although they espouse a variety of views on these two questions, a series of common themes and concerns emerges from the chapters below, sufficient perhaps to speak in terms of a common response.

The varieties of family life

The first point of agreement is that any discussion of contemporary family life must begin from the lived experience of actually existing families, whose hallmark is variety and change. For several decades past, people have been voting with their feet, and other parts of their anatomy, against the received forms of conventional marriage. The result has been a plethora of new forms involving serial monogamy, cohabitation, open lesbian and gay partnerships, living apart together ('LAT'), step-parenthood and/or lone parenthood. And these changes in form have been cut across by changes of role within the various relationships, including a tendency for married women to enter the labour force and for some (albeit slow) increase in the caring activities undertaken by men, which perhaps indicates that a more egalitarian construction of gender roles is taking place. As Lynda Clarke and Ceridwen Roberts remind us in Chapter 8, the claims of fathers and grandparents are also receiving a new and welcome emphasis, in the academic and critical literature at least.

But it would be a mistake to think that in this process of change conventional marriage has been replaced by some new dominant form, such as egalitarian partnership.[1] It would be more accurate to say that the various elements that conventional marriage insists belong together within a unitary legal status – copulation, co-residence and co-parenthood – have tended to become dissociated in the lives of individuals, especially over the life course, without their becoming recombined into some dominant alternative form. Yet even this statement belies the complexity that had developed in family relationships by the turn of the millennium. It is not so much that the newer forms have displaced the longer-established forms. Rather, they have added to them, as if society's repertoire of permissible family types has been expanding continuously as people respond creatively to the challenges of everyday living in contexts where some of the older cultural and institutional constraints have lost their bite (Moen and Wethington 1992). And this process has had an uneven incidence, so that the balance between the older and the emergent forms varies a good deal between countries, regions, communities and indeed sexualities.

As Jeffrey Weeks shows in Chapter 11, for example, the language and emotional tenor of 'family', which has historically carried hefty homophobic baggage, has begun to be reappropriated for use in a range of non-heterosexual contexts. Within the heterosexual world itself, Ulla Björnberg in Chapter 4.3 emphasises that in Sweden the dual-earner family with cohabiting parents has become the norm, whereas in Spain, according to Lluis Flaquer (Chapter 4.2), the 'traditional' family can still encompass younger women in full-time work, and patterns of LAT. A fascinating insight into the balance of factors creating international diversity is offered by Birgit Pfau-Effinger's account in Chapter 4.1 of family developments after German reunification, which provided a kind of natural experiment into the social forces at work. A uniform welfare policy and bureaucracy has been imposed on the whole country since unification, inherited from West Germany rather than the East. It might be expected that this new common structure of welfare provision would lead to greater uniformity in family arrangements between the two regions. This does not appear to have happened, because the application of the new systems in the former GDR has encountered a strong cultural legacy from the Communist period, which includes among other emphases a disdain for the traditional housewife role as demeaning to a modern woman. Far from dying out since 1989, this cultural orientation has tended to be preserved, as part of a self-definition of the East that resists total subsumption within the culture of the West. The preliminary conclusion is that welfare systems and cultural inheritance are joint determinants of family relationships, so that the effect of the former will always depend on the characteristics of the latter.

This view is supported by Tracey Reynolds' portrait of the Black Caribbean family in Britain (Chapter 3.4), in which she traces family characteristics not just to a uniform 'Caribbean' heritage but also to the differentiation of family tradition between different Caribbean islands, and between socio-economic strata within them. Thus, the prevalence of female-headed households is greater in Jamaica than in Barbados and Antigua, and the social interpretation of female-headed households (not to mention their statistical frequency) is affected in any case by patterns of 'visiting' relationships by male partners that have been transmitted from the Caribbean and adapted to the UK. Couples in the Black community move up and down the scales of mutual commitment, just as they do in every other community, but the significance can be lost to an outside observer because the social markers of commitment are subject to cultural variation.

Black women are sometimes head of household by circumstance and sometimes by choice, the latter often for good feminist reasons. But not all, and perhaps not even a majority, of Black families are female-headed, and the Black community as a whole is subject to external stereotyping in the anti-norm, such that the conventional married family tends to be seen as deeply unconventional in the Black context.

Concentrating more on demographic patterns than on specific cultural variables, María-José González-López in Chapter 2 provides an extensive survey of the variations in family patterns among European and North American women. Using the large data sets available for international comparisons from the UN Fertility and Family Survey, she reports a discernible tendency for women's experience to be differentiated between 'northern European' and 'southern European' models (with Canada and the USA counted for this purpose as part of northern Europe!). The northern model incorporates a larger proportion of partnerships without children (especially among younger couples) and of consensual unions (as opposed to marriages), earlier departure from the parental home, higher age of the mother at the birth of her first child and more frequent lone motherhood. The southern model, by contrast, suggests a greater prevalence of a more traditional pattern in which women remain within the parental home until marriage and have children within marriage relatively quickly thereafter.

But these are broad correlations at best, with many countervailing tendencies. Belgium is an example of a 'northern' country that is more like a 'southern' country on most dimensions of family demography. Almost a quarter of Portuguese women gave birth to their first child outside a marital union, and the proportion of lone mothers in Portugal (at first birth) is actually higher than in Sweden – the icon nation of 'the north'. Total period fertility rates crossed during the 1990s, so that Sweden's and Canada's are now among the highest, with Italy's and Spain's among the lowest. The pattern of LAT also defies easy stereotyping, in that 'southern' Italy and 'northern' Germany both show a high incidence, whereas Spain and Austria score relatively low (although there is some evidence that this status is more a matter of circumstance than choice in the southern context).

It must also be remembered that the most decisive variable remains age, so that a woman's age is typically a better predictor of her family circumstances than her national location, and marked international variations in younger cohorts tend to give way to greater uniformity in older ones. Education also emerges as an important factor in nearly every country, and 'the pressure of the "biological clock" may be felt particularly by women in higher education'

(Chapter 2, page 39). Women may therefore have more experiences in common with others in their educational stratum in every country than they have with women in different educational strata in their own.

Taking all this variation into account, it might be tempting to regard the newer forms as the more egalitarian in whichever cultural context or segment of the population they occur. This is in pursuit of what Weeks describes as 'a new norm, the quest for individual fulfilment in the context of freely chosen egalitarian relationships' (Chapter 11, page 224). This temptation to an easy optimism should nevertheless be resisted, since almost everywhere there is stubborn resistance from the viewpoint of ideal egalitarian progress. Weeks points to evidence suggesting that the egalitarian model remains an aspiration as often as an achievement in non-heterosexual communities, even apart from the persistent effects of the surrounding homophobia. Turning to the heterosexual world, it is an arresting fact that while the proportion of UK married women in paid employment has increased enormously since 1951, the proportion in *full-time* employment has hardly changed at all (Chapter 3.1, page 53). The rise in the frequency of lone parenthood has occurred without any change in the ratio of lone mothers to lone fathers, which remains remarkably constant at roughly nine to one (Duncan and Edwards 1999). The GDR model of the family, which was as we have seen very advanced in relation to women's paid employment, also revolved around 'Mutti' when mother was at home (Chapter 4.1, page 80). And it is salutary to recall that, despite the rising incidence of divorce, the average duration of marriage (in the UK at least) has changed very little in a hundred years. The obvious inference is that separation and divorce have simply replaced death as a cause of partnerships coming to an end.

The policy makers' plight

The second point on which the contributors would agree is that policy makers will err if their proposals fail to address this variety of lived experience, and the consequent range of family relationships. But it is nevertheless possible to sympathise with the policy makers' plight. On the one hand, it would be difficult to draw up a policy proposal without having in mind some conception of the type of social arrangement to which it might apply. On the other hand, it will be difficult to know which kind of social arrangement to bear in mind, given the diversity of the lived experience. Two broad approaches can then be distinguished. The attempt might be made to draw up a policy that was neutral with respect to social arrangements, even-handed between, say, marriage, cohabitation and lone parenthood; and agnostic about sexual orientation. Or the policy might be designed to favour one kind (or kinds) of imagined social arrangement rather than another (Duncan and Edwards 1999).

In the pages that follow, much forensic effort is devoted to the different family models that underlie various policy proposals, either explicitly or, more often, implicitly. In some cases, these models act simply as background assumptions against which the operation of particular policies is judged to take place. In other cases, it is the declared or undeclared purpose of the policy to *promote* particular forms of family life, or particular varieties of interpersonal conduct. In the celebrated case of the UK government's 1998 Green Paper, *Supporting Families*, the intention seems to have been to have one's cake and eat it by promoting marriage while allegedly retaining equal respect for other forms of family life.[2] Mavis Maclean's contribution in Chapter 3.3 is devoted to these problems, with a conclusion not entirely unfavourable to the New Labour record. Anne Barlow, Simon Duncan and Grace James enter a more negative verdict on the same question in Chapter 5.

It is the essence of the 'should' question whether, or in what circumstances, states are ever entitled to depart from neutrality in their family policies, thereby giving an explicit public content to their interventions in private life. And there are variations in this aspect too: by country, where French policy, for example, has been more neutral than the British; and by historical phase, in which the pendulum swings back and forth in one country between neutrality and partiality. In the UK, for example:

> … traditionally family law was directive, providing clear legal incentives to marry and legal disincentives to form families outside marriage. This was followed by a period from the mid-1970s through to the end of the 1980s when family law was regarded as 'neutral' on the issue of family structure. However, the 1990s have witnessed a return to far more directive legislative intervention in the family context.
>
> Barlow 1999: 1

One might add that the pendulum may also be stuck in different positions in different policy fields in the same country, so that in the UK, for example, policies on taxes and benefits have shown greater neutrality in recent years than family law itself.

Although the natural alignment of family policy with political ideology sets the liberalism of the Left against the moralism of the Right, a fuller account will inevitably disturb the straightforwardness of the correlation. Feminists and others on the Left would tend to be at least as interventionist as the Right on matters such as domestic violence and child abuse. There has always been a strain of social conventionalism on the Left, not entirely unrelated to the cultural conservatism of some sections of its historical labour base. And there is plenty of evidence that Old Labour tended to act on gender issues only when it was pushed (Perrigo 1996, 1999). But Jane Lewis, in her contribution, shows that New Labour welfare policy is also predicated on a strong conception of the desirable norm in family life, which has replaced the old assumptions concerning the male breadwinner with the 'adult worker' model. This presumes that both adults in any pair bond are willing and able – indeed eager – to enter the paid labour force.

This theme is taken up in a slightly different context by Barlow, Duncan and James, whose contribution speaks of the 'morality mistake' made by governments when they attribute certain normative positions to their citizens that the citizens do not in fact share. Thus, lone parents should be as anxious as their partnered peers to enter the labour force, according to the preferred New Labour model. But there is very good evidence that lone mothers in particular tend to place their role as mothers, and consequently the interests of their children, above all other considerations. Paid employment is likely to conflict with these priorities for a range of perfectly understandable practical and emotional reasons. The attempt to force lone mothers into paid employment on the basis of the 'morality mistake' is not therefore morally neutral. It involves a real brutality, in forcing lone parents to override their consciences as parents in order to obtain the wherewithal for child support.

This point about the application of policy connects with some important theoretical issues. Whether or not it is correct to see Anthony Giddens as the chief intellectual architect of the 'Third Way' on a world scale (Carling 1999), his views on the democratic family have proved influential, and a number of contributors take Giddens' work as a point of reference.

In particular, Selma Sevenhuijsen in Chapter 6 criticises one of his main contentions, that 'access to paid work is ... the primary dimension of social inclusion' (page 136). She contrasts this new version of the work ethic, which rather ironically has strong overtones of an erstwhile Communist orthodoxy, with an alternative 'ethic of care' developed from the writings of Carol Gilligan (1987) and Berenice Fisher and Joan Tronto (1990), among others. Jane Ribbens-McCarthy and Rosalind Edwards focus on another aspect of Giddens' work – the concern for intimacy – which is also echoed in related work by Beck and Beck-Gernsheim (1995). They make the telling point that, although this concern is welcome because it enriches the academic discourse on relationships and opens it to a variety of feminist insights, it ultimately tends to generate its own one-sidedness. This is because intimacy is addressed principally in its privatised and adults-only manifestations, as experienced within a series of quasi-contractual bilateral relationships between grown-ups. This approach encourages the equation of intimacy with sexual possibility. The positive revaluation of the sphere of intimate relations thus has the paradoxical effect of marginalising once again the typical experience of women, who frequently find themselves acting in multiply connected, care-laden social networks bursting with children, aged parents and sundry dependent others. With little time, one might think, for sex.

Graham Crow in our Conclusion also takes issue with the Giddens–Beck–Gernsheim conception, locating it within the intellectual history of family sociology and the broader theme of contemporary individualisation. The main problem he identifies is once again that the attempt to confine the lived experience of family life within a uniform trend of individualised and democratised existence falls foul of the empirical evidence and fails to do justice to all the countervailing forces, including values, solidarities and material circumstances.

Perhaps it is understandable that debate at the current moment is dominated by proposals from the centre Left. But this volume does peer from time to time over the other side of the political fence. Deacon's contribution (Chapter 4.4) analyses the divisions of the Republican Right in the USA on welfare policy 'along one of the oldest fault lines in political thought, that between libertarianism and paternalism' (page 103). He goes on to note one way in which this tension has been resolved, equally time-honoured, in which libertarianism is deemed best for the family life of one section of the population and paternalism for another, which is identified as an appropriate target by poverty, race, welfare need or supposed moral and intellectual deficiency. It is good to see that the Victorian distinction between the deserving and the undeserving poor is alive and well in Washington, DC, not to mention Whitehall, SW1.

Policy and social theory

But 'should' implies 'can'. There will be no point in the state or a political party formulating elaborate plans for the transformation of family life if states or parties are practically incapable of delivering the intended changes with the instruments at their disposal. In the standard policy story, people are assumed to act in a certain way, such that they will *react* in some predictable fashion to the policy initiatives of the policy maker, thereby creating the social outcome the policy maker desires. A third point of agreement between the contributors to this volume is the need to subject stories of this kind to detailed critical scrutiny and a certain degree of healthy scepticism. Policy proposals often rest on assumptions about the character and motivations of individuals, which are usually tacit and often partial or controversial when brought into the light of day.

One such example arises from Adrian James' analysis of the pilot tests for divorce law reform in the UK (Chapter 3.2), which seem to be predicated on the assumption that in the fraught conditions of marital break-up, all parties will be keen to seek a negotiated and peaceful settlement. But the most pervasive example of this phenomenon is what Barlow, Duncan and James (Chapter 5) term 'the rationality mistake', which is the erroneous assumption that people will act principally in accordance with an optimising calculation that focuses on a narrowly defined range of material incentives. This assumption is close to the heart of rational choice theory, and of mainstream economics as an explanatory discipline. The rational choice conception crosses the threshold between theory and practice when those with plenty of the relevant resources, such as state officials, envisage the use of those resources to change the incentives facing individuals within their jurisdiction, thereby changing the latter's behavioural responses. The thought, to put it at its crudest, is that money backed by prison can always achieve the outcome the planner/official requires.[3]

This is not to say that money and the threat of punishment are irrelevant to behaviour. Rather, it is to point out that changed incentives are but one element in a more complex motivational picture, which also includes norms prescribing right conduct, convictions about what goes to make healthy personal relationships, role expectations, and a range of possible emotional responses to conflicting social pressures. For example, it is clear that mothers' behaviour is strongly conditioned by their conceptions of 'good motherhood', which may or may not be consistent with being in full-time paid work. The response to changed incentives regarding such work will then depend *inter alia* on the precise conception of motherhood that a particular mother entertains, and this will vary by social group and social context (Barlow 1999: 9; Barlow, Duncan and James, Chapter 5).

Judith Glover in Chapter 13 makes the related argument that the way in which a person responds to a given incentive for an action may depend not only on the value of the incentive in itself but also on the (negative or positive) contribution that the contemplated action will make to the overall balance of the actor's interpersonal relationships. Thus, an action that appears irrational at first sight will seem perfectly reasonable once it is understood that the balance of a person's commitments is an independent criterion of decision. And since it is women who may be differentially involved in such juggling of commitments, it is women's experience that is most distorted by the failure of standard theory to take it into account.

However, these points about the operative norms cut deeper. David Morgan argues in Chapter 7 that the very existence of 'the family' as a distinct social domain, and therefore a distinct object of enquiry, depends on dense networks of normative understanding that give generic terms like 'mother' and 'father' determinate local content. Any male parent who has been driven in exasperation to exclaim with Morgan 'because I'm your father' will know exactly what he means (and no longer 'Dad' in the apocryphal quotation, the reader will notice, as in 'Daaaad…'). Morgan fleshes out the insight with a novel application of Everett Hughes' concepts of 'license' and 'mandate', which give family members limits of permission in their dealings with each other and the outside world, and corresponding degrees of latitude.

Ribbens McCarthy and Edwards plough a parallel furrow in their analysis in Chapter 10 of the contemporary usages of the terms 'public' and 'private', which are intrinsic to the normative architecture of both the state and the family sphere. They point out that the contrast between the public and the private can be worked both ways. On the one hand, the public domain can be presented as the centre of collective political endeavour, and therefore of discourse, value and meaning, by favourable contrast with the residual category of the merely private and personal. This is the sense in which, when one 'declares a personal interest' in a public debate, one thereby volunteers oneself out of the debate.

On the other hand, the private domain, or at any rate the family domain, can be represented as the 'heart of a heartless world', and the privileged site of a supportive network of caring and intimate relationships, by favourable contrast with the individualised and materialistic arenas of public life. Margaret Thatcher's notorious assertion that 'there is no such thing as society' made this contrast explicit in its subordinate clause – 'only individuals and their families' – since the family is by implication the only place where 'society' exists at all.[4]

Pursuing their critique of the Giddens–Beck–Gernsheim line, they suggest that the terms 'public' and 'private' be reserved for *social* relationships within the respective domains, so that a third term – 'the personal' – can be applied to the inward dimensions of personal experience in both domains. Such personal experience may be socially caused or even socially constructed, but a valid distinction nevertheless exists between 'a set of practices and orientations that are shared within social settings and interactions' on the one hand and 'interior experience' on the other (Chapter 10, page 209). A hard-pressed mother managing her children may well be acting in private even if her audience is large, but her feelings about the situation are personal. The founding slogan of second-wave feminism appears to require revision, or rather bifurcation, in the light of the proposed vocabulary. The primary message is now expressed by the thought that the private is political. But the personal will still remain political, to the extent that our inner experiences, including our experiences of intimacy, are conditioned by the workings of social power.

Regardless of the precise ways in which these usages pan out, the underlying contrasts are deeply gendered. If the public domain is valued positively as the place where the serious business of the world goes on, then this is man's business in a man's world. If the private sphere is valued, this is where, or this is because it is the place where, the wife and mother presides, or at least resides, as angel of the hearth. As James Brown's splendidly sentimental anthem reads, 'this is a man's world', or as it is sung, 'a maaaaan's world', before adding, as if by way of compensation, 'but it ain't nothing without a wooomaaan'.

Sociology and economics

The normative vantage point adopted by Morgan and by Ribbens McCarthy and Edwards invites three general observations relevant to the disciplinary contrast between sociology and economics, a contrast also captured in our subtitle's reference to the '*morality* and *rationality* of family life'.

First, whenever the state ventures into the family arena as an actor with normative ambitions, it is entering a crowded field, already structured – indeed already constituted – by the normative perceptions recurrently enacted by family members in areas of their daily lives to which they are liable to attach great significance. This fact alone is almost guaranteed to make family policy a site of acute ideological and political struggle.

Second, 'the economics of the family' is strictly speaking a contradiction in terms, since economics – at least in the conventional sense, which equates it with rational choice – knows no norms, and therefore knows no internal geography of the social domain. So there is an important sense in which policies predicated on rational choice have missed the point about families from the very beginning.

Susan Himmelweit's critique of family economics in Chapter 12 powerfully reinforces this judgement. She sets out from the standard assumptions of mainstream economics, that persons act according to the consequences of their actions, in the light of preferences that are (1) fixed by factors beyond the scope of economic analysis, (2) self-interested, and (3) oriented solely towards the 'consumption of purchased goods and services' (page 233). She then allows rational choice its maximum hope of success by asking if an appropriate 'economics of care' can be generated by relaxing these assumptions step by step, thus expanding the explanatory scope of the theory step by step.

Her conclusion is that no such relaxation will do the job required, since the central task of parenthood – the assumption of responsibility for childcare – cannot be undertaken in the instrumental spirit of economics ('What's in it for me?') but must be seen as a moral obligation. This represents a final break with the rational choice paradigm, however generously it is interpreted, since the corresponding behaviour of parents is not calculating and outcome-oriented but is 'much more like the adoption of an internally imposed rule' (*ibid.*: page 240). So if Himmelweit begins in the mainstream of economics, the upshot of her closely argued *démarche* on the economics of childhood is to take her beyond the viewpoint dominant in her profession. There is a notable critical convergence here with Sevenhuijsen's advocacy of an ethics of care, which arises from a similar critique of ideas prevailing in her discipline of political theory.

Edmund Chattoe (Chapter 14) places rational choice under the microscope from the methodological angle. The task here is to show that fruitful quantitative methods in social science are not confined to the rational choice paradigm, and Chattoe argues that computer simulation, in particular, can offer an attractive alternative. Simulation techniques model social processes as unfolding sequences of interaction, as opposed to the equilibrium solutions of pay-off structures, which is the stock-in-trade of rational choice analysis. As such, simulation offers a greater potential variety of behavioural microfoundations than rational choice. And these variations can in principle accommodate the kind of critique levelled at rational choice by Himmelweit and others in this book. As an example, Chattoe puts forward a simple simulation model of the family based on the insights of Barlow, Duncan, Edwards and James. This application is inspired by the admirable thought that 'it is one thing to deconstruct rational choice theory, but another to have a technique that allows model building for the new assumptions.'[5]

However, the critique of rational choice is not confined to these contributions: it runs throughout this book like lettering in seaside rock. The various critiques differ in their detail and their emphases, with some contributors inevitably more friendly than others towards the rational choice paradigm, but all would recognise with Himmelweit the need to engage seriously with the explanatory paradigm that mainstream economic theory provides. This might serve to distinguish members of our authors' collective from some other groups of sociologists and political scientists, who tend to respond to the economist's typical disdain with an equal and opposite distaste.

The minimum ground for such an engagement is the recognition that economic theory is driving many aspects of contemporary policy, sometimes explicitly but more often implicitly. This creates the need to understand the applications of the theory, if only to understand the source of the social damage that is being done. A more substantial ground would hold that economic concepts of rationality pick out one strand of human motivation, but that we need to extend our theoretical vocabulary a good deal before we can begin to cope with the diversity of the lived experience.

Bren Neale and Carol Smart's contribution in Chapter 9 presents an object lesson in this viewpoint. Their detailed study into the adjustments made by divorcing heterosexual parents shows that a kind of bargaining does take place, and that instrumental considerations are often not far from the surface, but that the character of the bargaining is much richer than is acknowledged by the abstract tenets of economic theory. The mothers in the study do indeed tend to start from an orientation to care, while the fathers start from an orientation to career, and this stereotypical contrast is alive in much of what follows. But there is considerable variation from the stereotypes, including at least one case in the sample of role reversal and variation of the extent to which instrumental attitudes prevail. Perhaps most importantly, there are very few 'pure' cases of role differentiation, and most parents – both fathers and mothers – are concerned to maintain both care and career, in different guises and contexts: 'counterposing the idea of the "atomistic economic" father with that of "caring mother" would be far too simplistic' (Chapter 9, pages 195–6).

The negotiations on divorce thus bring to the table not just history and resources but also demands for access against issues of time, old commitments against new possibilities, and material arrangements against status and meaning. In the argot of management speak, divorce is not just a threat but also an opportunity and, however its effects are evaluated, a potential catalyst for change.

The thought that mothers and fathers who have lived in the same house have been living to some extent in different social universes raises the third main issue in the relationship between sociology and economics. If the geography of the social world is pre-structured by norms, there may be regions of that world whose norms permit, or even encourage – 'licence' – the kinds of behaviour, and the kinds of person, theorised by rational choice. This is one way of understanding the existence, and also the boundaries, of market relationships and the market domain, being the centre of the realm in which this form of behaviour, and type of person, is licensed to perform. For example, Deacon's discussion of US policy in Chapter 4.4 suggests that an incentive-based approach has been more successful in some areas of application (e.g. welfare to work) than in others (e.g. planned parenthood). A related point is that since individuals are moving between the various social domains, the same person will tend to adopt in turn the different personae appropriate to the respective domains. As Ribbens McCarthy and Edwards emphasise in Chapter 10, the ground rules of behaviour differ, for example between the private and public domains, with differing *degrees* of 'individualisation', which also read into the gender stereotypes. Certain kinds of self-seeking behaviour that are acceptable, indeed praiseworthy, in public life are less so within the confines of the home.

But this idea throws a new light on the policy process too. Policy predicated on rational choice assumptions may now be understood as an attempt in part to transform its target domain in a manner that makes the theory applicable within that domain. This is more ambitious than the attempt to change behaviour. It is the attempt to recreate persons and make over the subjects of policy in the image of economics. If this attempt is successful, and the target domain entirely rationalised, there would be a corresponding closure of the circle: policy would work, its assumptions would be vindicated, and economics would emerge in triumph as a genuine explanatory science.

Enough has been sketched in this Introduction to show how unfortunate such an outcome would be. It would represent an ethical disaster, in cutting off one whole side of human conduct and deliberation – the side summed up in Sevenhuijsen's 'ethic of care'. It would mistake the fundamental character of any activity, such as childcare or adult intimacy, based on the acceptance of responsibility for the welfare of others. And it would cut across the freedoms people enjoy to weigh their own motives and improvise their own solutions in their own lives.

It has already been noted that Barlow, Duncan and James (Chapter 5) have added the 'morality mistake' to the 'rationality mistake' in the litany of potential sins they see committed by governments. How are we to understand the connection between the two? It is certainly possible to make the case that they are conceptually distinct. The Humean line of thought posits a radical separation between the means and ends of action. Reason then becomes a purely instrumental phenomenon: it concerns the choice of the appropriate means to ends that are given beyond the determination of reason itself.

From this perspective, the rationality mistake would involve a false assumption concerning the procedures adopted by agents for linking means with ends. Thus a policy maker might follow standard rational choice theory in assuming that mothers facing decisions on childcare optimise a convex utility function containing arguments such as job satisfaction, leisure time, net family income and the welfare of the child. In fact, as the evidence presented in this volume suggests, mothers are more likely to place the welfare of the child above all other considerations and adopt a lexicographic decision-making procedure: first the welfare of the child, *then* leisure time, *then* job satisfaction, and so on. The policy maker's rationality mistake is to misattribute *the form of reasoning* adopted by a given class of agents (in this case, mothers). A nice variant of this procedural misconception would be the 'irrationality mistake', in which policy makers falsely attribute lack of rationality to agents. A case in point might be Lawrence Mead's view that the long-term poor are, in Alan Deacon's précis, 'not competent, functioning individuals who act rationally to further their interests' (Chapter 4.4, page 103). The 'morality mistake' would then figure as a distinct error, namely the false attribution of ends or values to the agents in question, such as the false assumption that mothers are pure carers who are not motivated at all by the satisfaction of paid employment.

The theoretical position outlined in the previous paragraph is a coherent one, but it will not be advocated here. First, the idea that the ends of action are in general beyond the scope of reason is not very persuasive. As Elster (1989) has argued, rational considerations such as consistency and autonomy impinge on the kingdom of ends. Second, it is in any case very difficult to sustain a radical distinction between the forms and the ends of reasoning. In the hypothetical example given above, the shift from an aggregative to a lexicographic decision-making procedure involved a change in values as much as a change in the method of calculation: a reordering of preferences by the mother who placed the child's interests first.

The fundamental point here is that the rational actor cannot be conceived of merely as an amoral behavioural technician, choosing the best alternative from an exogenously determined opportunity set. To be a rational actor is to inhabit a subject position that is normatively constructed, in a manner that embraces both ends and means. For example, monetary incentives work (when they do) not just because a given payment tips the balance between net loss and net gain (the instrumental aspect) but also because money figures as a motivating factor (the ends aspect). So to expect monetary incentives to work is to imagine that people are of the kind that regards money as a relevant value in the relevant domain. This mental operation presupposes certain ends, and their contextual social legitimacy, as well as positing a certain (optimising) relationship between means and ends.

This argument suggests that the rationality mistake is an instance of the morality mistake, with the rider that the mistake has two aspects (the false attribution of forms of reasoning, and the false attribution of values). In terms of the evolution of the intellectual project initiated by Duncan and Edwards (1999), this implies that the unveiling in this book of the 'morality mistake' is not the addition of a new dimension but rather a *generalisation* of the previous line of attack: an embedding of the rationality mistake in a larger solecism.

Suppose that this argument about the mistakenly simplified complexity of social agents is conjoined with the earlier points about the mistakenly simplified variety of social context. The conjunction suggests that policy formulation is generally subject to a double distortion, according to which the policy maker's impoverished imagination places diminished kinds of people in fictitious circumstances. The real individuals who are the intended subjects of a policy may not be moved in the official ways, and they may not place the official construction on themselves or their relationships. And if this is the case, it can hardly be a surprise if the policy fails to achieve its official objectives.

The contractual model of the family

But what is to be done? Several considerations suggest that it will be irresponsible to throw up one's hands at the complexity of it all, mumble something ironic about our postmodern world and stand aside. First, governments are going to go on formulating policy willy nilly, and it is presumably better than not that this is informed by social theory and evidence, to the extent that such is possible. Second, it is difficult to imagine circumstances in which the family (whatever that means precisely) is not regulated to some degree by social policy and law, and it is a requirement of reason in its cognitive aspect that this regulation should aspire to consistency. Third, it is in any case a demand of elementary equity that different persons should be placed in similar social positions in respect of their ability to live together, form intimate relationships, raise children and so forth. But how, or at what level, can this consistency be achieved, given the variety of preferences and circumstances under review?

One superficially attractive model is the contractual family: that is, a model in which the family members draw up a legally binding partnership agreement (or perhaps a series of bilateral contracts) specifying a schedule of their rights and obligations with respect to each other. The attractions of the proposal are first that it tracks, and thereby has some chance of regulating, the dissociation of family life that is happening in any case, and it responds to the supposed individualisation of family relationships. A significant example of this trend already evident in the UK would be the provisions of the 1989 Children Act, which in effect decouple the mother–child and father–child relationships from the relationship between the parents themselves. Divorce is seen as a disruption of the latter but not a disruption of the former (at least in principle), since the parent–child relationships continue for life (Giddens 1998).

Second, the contractual model permits a range of variation within a common form, since it is up to the partners to design their own family and specify their own schedule of commitments. Any distinction between heterosexual and non-heterosexual unions, for example, would lapse. This is one important feature of the French PACS initiative (Pacte Civile de Solidarité), which moves in the direction of the contractual family (Chapter 5). The contractual proposal thus promises to square the circle between the demands of legal uniformity and the facts of social variety.

Third, legal software ripe for adaptation to the family context already exists, in the shape of the current law of contract. Indeed, in a long enough historical perspective one could see the proposal as the final culmination of the transition from status to contract in the field of personal relationships. The traditional marriage tie may take the form of a contract, but its content negates its form. The tie is indissoluble, inequitable in the distinctions it makes between husbands and wives, and it lays unconditional obligations on the parties, some of which are apparently impossible to fulfil unconditionally: can one love the unlovable and honour the dishonourable? The contractual model of the family can then be seen by contrast as the completion of the work of ages, in which the promise of a marriage contract is finally made real, through the latitude available to individuals to specify their own conditions. And since those conditions are freely chosen, it would be reasonable to expect the parties to live up to them. The match between law and enforcement could then be restored, and the state could act as guarantor of last resort for personal relationships, to the benefit and security of all.

If these are some of the attractions of the contractual model, I will conclude with the opposing features that render these attractions superficial in my view. First, the notion of contract depends upon a certain legal fiction: the normative construction of the individual self as an independent agent who then enters (and leaves) relationships by legal agreement (Barlow 1999). This conception is immediately subject to the Sevenhuijsen critique and vulnerable to the alternative perspective, which sees the self as an entity already constituted by the web of relationships in which it stands. And if Sevenhuijsen is correct in her ethical conclusions, the contractual model of the family will be thoroughly biased against an ethic of responsibility and care.

Second, just as economics finds difficulty in recognising children as rational agents, so the law will have difficulty in recognising them as legal subjects. How do we assign children between contractual family units? Who writes the conditions in the contract on behalf of the child? In line with the main critical thrust of Ribbens McCarthy and Edwards in Chapter 10, it seems unwise to support a proposal on the reorganisation of family life whose basic ground plan finds no place for children.

Third, economics itself has recently woken up to the difficulties caused by the fact that it is impossible to write a perfectly specified and costlessly enforceable contract.[6] If the motive in writing an explicit contract is to substitute legal controls for trust as the means by which people live up to their mutual obligations, the inevitable imperfections of the contract process will lead to the same problem reappearing in a new guise. For if one ultimately has to rely on trust to secure compliance with the letter and the spirit of the contract, it appears that the existence of the contract has not resolved any problems caused by lack of trust but merely displaced them from the substantive underlying issues to the details of contract compliance. This is not to say that contracts are necessarily a useless distraction, but it underlines that they are likely to serve better as a constitutional reference point and statement of basic principles than as a blueprint for day-to-day activities.

The fourth, and perhaps most serious, reservation about the contract model is usefully introduced by returning to Jeffrey Weeks' new norm of personal conduct: 'the quest for individual fulfilment in the context of freely chosen egalitarian relationships'. The contract model may ensure that relationships are freely chosen. Indeed, its merit may consist chiefly in the way it institutionalises freedom of choice. But will this make the consequent relationships egalitarian? I am not sure what clauses the pre-nuptial agreements of Hollywood stars contain, but my guess is that they reflect the respective box-office receipts of the parties' latest films.

In general, the terms of a contract reflect the bargaining positions of the parties, which may be highly unequal.[7] After all, it would be very difficult to draw any legal distinction between contracts of prostitution and other family agreements under the conditions envisaged, where two parties freely negotiate an exchange of benefits and services. Would polygamy be allowed, as long as it was freely entered into? Would indissoluble marriage be an option and women thus enabled to sign away freely some of their current freedoms? What limits would exist for First World men contracting for Third World brides?

All these considerations suggest that, while there may well be a place for some movement of the law in the contractual direction, the contractual family cannot be a self-sufficient ideal. Its possible forms would need to be circumscribed by values, and the experience of it would still depend on the distribution of material resources. Egalitarian families would not arise by contract in an inegalitarian society. The cultural ethos of the society would be an important independent variable too, and the culture of 'care as a democratic practice' outlined by Sevenhuijsen at the conclusion of her chapter offers an intriguing recipe for a balanced family life. Susan Himmelweit's conclusion lies in a similar direction, with a careful analysis of the ways in which egalitarian norms might evolve to replace the former expectations of gendered social roles. But do these conclusions imply that one cannot escape some specification, at some level, of what it is to be a 'normal family'?

The contributors to this book end with no specific recommendations, but they do invite the reader to join them in exploring the issues. We are united in the hope that the reader will find the experience both worthwhile and enjoyable.

Notes

1 Subsequent history would therefore lead us to reject the Whiggism of Young and Wilmott's *The Symmetrical Family* (1973), according to which families throughout the industrialised West were in the process of converging towards a new norm of equal marriage partnership.

2 This tension in the Green Paper rises to the level of palpable contradiction in paragraphs 4.3 and 4.4:

> 4.3: This Government believes that marriage provides a strong foundation for stable relationships. This does not mean trying to make people marry, or criticising or penalising those who choose not to. We do not believe the Government should interfere in people's lives in that way. But we do share the belief of the majority of people that marriage provides the most reliable framework for raising children.
>
> 4.4: We are therefore proposing: measures to strengthen the institution of marriage, including an enhanced role for marriage registrars; support for all families, including better advice on adult relationships.
>
> *Supporting Families*, HMSO 1998: p.30

It is difficult to see how one can strengthen marriage as a specific form of family relationship, thereby leaving other forms out of account, while remaining true to the ringing declaration of the neutrality principle in the previous paragraph: 'we do not believe that Governments …'.

3 And governments can be fairly crude. Here is an example drawn almost at random from the news:

> the government … is keen to be seen acting strongly following the case of Alan and Judith Kilshaw, who bought baby twins Beverley and Kimberley from a Californian adoption broker they found on the internet … [it has] announced that parents who adopted from abroad without undergoing the proper checks would face up to three months in prison and a fine of £600.
>
> *The Guardian*, 22 Jan 2001.

4 The public/private contrast offers a first approximation at best to a complex set of distinctions. The next approximation would isolate civil society as a third domain that is external to both the state and the family, being 'private' with respect to the former and 'public' with respect to the latter.

5 Edmund Chattoe, personal communication.

6 See Bowles and Gintis (1998) for an interesting exploration of these issues in the context of the principal-agent problem in economic theory.

7 This is the founding insight for the theories of social class arising from Roemer (1982).

References

Barlow, A. (1999) 'Mothers and family restructuring: legal rationality and moral discourses', ESRC seminar, South Bank University.

Beck, U. and Beck-Gernsheim, E. (1995) *The Normal Chaos of Love*, Cambridge: Polity Press.

Bowles, S. and Gintis, H. (1998) *Recasting Egalitarianism: New Rules for Communities, States and Markets*, edited by E.O. Wright. London: Verso.

Carling, A. (1999) 'New Labour's polity: Tony Giddens and the "Third Way"', *Imprints* 3(3): 214–42.

Duncan, S. and Edwards, R. (1999) *Lone Mothers, Paid Work and Gendered Rationalities*, London: Macmillan.

Elster, J. (1989) *Nuts and Bolts for the Social Sciences*, Cambridge: Cambridge University Press.

Fisher, B. and Tronto, J. (1990) 'Towards a feminist theory of caring', in E.K. Abel and M.K. Nelson (eds) *Circles of Care: Work and Identity in Women's Lives*, New York: State University of New York Press.

Giddens, A. (1998) *The Third Way*, Cambridge: Polity Press.

Gilligan, C. (1987) 'Moral orientation and moral development', in E. Feder Kitay and D.T. Meyers (eds) *Women and Moral Theory*, Totowa, NJ: Rowman & Littlefield.

Moen, P. and Wethington, E. (1992) 'The concept of family adaptive strategies', *Review of Sociology* 18: 233–51.

Perrigo, S. (1996) 'Women and change in the Labour Party 1979–1995', in J. Lovenduski and P. Norris (eds) *Women in Politics*, Oxford: Oxford University Press.

—— (1999) 'Women, gender and New Labour', in G.R. Taylor (ed.) *The Impact of New Labour*, Basingstoke: Macmillan.

Roemer, J.E. (1982) *A General Theory of Exploitation and Class*, Cambridge, Mass.: Harvard University Press.

Supporting Families: A Consultation Document (1998), Home Office: HMSO.

Young, M. and Wilmott, P. (1973) *The Symmetrical Family*, Harmondsworth: Penguin.

2 A portrait of Western families

New models of intimate relationships and the timing of life events

María José González-López

Introduction

The turn of the millennium has witnessed a fruitful literature on family change (see, for example, Boh *et al.* 1989; Kuijsten 1996; Kaufmann *et al.* 1997). This is no coincidence but a response to evidence that the traditional family model, and traditional patterns of family formation, are gradually losing their hegemony in most Western countries. By the *traditional family model*, I refer to the nuclear family in which married spouses have a rigid gender division of labour, with the wife predominantly responsible for unpaid homemaking and caring and the husband focusing on a breadwinning role. Traditional family formation refers to the timing and progression of successive life events, such as leaving the parental home in the late teenage years to directly enter a marital union, followed by a series of births within that marriage.

Some authors has interpreted these ongoing changes as evidence of family decline (e.g. Popenoe 1993), but in reality most of the changes simply reflect the emergence of alternative living arrangements and more complex ways of organising the individual life cycle. The monolithic image of the traditional married nuclear family is progressively vanishing to give rise to a richer variety of families, which are present to a greater or lesser extent in Western countries. Every day there are more young adults who choose to cohabit outside marriage either as a permanent arrangement or as a prelude to a marital union; more women who have children outside marriage; more young people who experience long periods living alone or sharing a household with friends before entering a partnership; more homosexual partners who openly claim their rights to be recognised in law as married couples, and so on. There are also noticeable changes in the duration and time at which life events occur. The clearest examples are the progressive postponement of motherhood and fatherhood, the increasing number of childless women and the shortened duration of partnerships as individuals can more easily exit unwanted relationships. These are just some examples of ever more common change in contemporary Western families.

The aim of this chapter is to provide an overall picture of current living arrangements and family patterns in Western countries. It is based mainly upon the fertility and family surveys (hereafter FFS) that were carried out in the 1990s by the United Nations Economic Commission for Europe (UN-ECE) and coordinated by the Population Activity Unit. The main goal of the surveys was the production of comparable data in ECE member countries for the study of fertility and family change. By the end of the project, twenty-four selected member states of the UN-ECE had participated in the FFS. However, only twelve countries have been included in this chapter: Austria, Belgium, Canada, Finland, France, Germany, Italy, Norway, Portugal, Spain, Sweden and the United States.[1] These were selected to cover a full range of both different welfare state regimes and gender cultures (see Duncan 1995).

The potentially large scale of the comparison requires a compromise concerning the population and indicators used here, if only for reasons of space. First, I have chosen to limit the analysis to the female population. This is not an arbitrary choice. FFS questionnaires have collected more extensive and detailed information for the female population, and this allows further data transformation and cross-tabulation without losing statistical reliability. Second, some aspects of family life, such as union dissolution, remarriage, step-families, homosexual partnerships and voluntary childlessness, have not been examined. Instead, particular indicators are more deeply analysed, with special emphasis on behavioural differences associated with age and educational differences. Educational attainment is not just an important background variable, it is especially relevant when the most educated individuals often pioneer the transformation of family life. For some family events, such as the timing and prevalence of childbearing, educational level is a central explanatory variable in most Western countries. Finally, the chapter focuses on the early phases of the family formation processes while neglecting later stages of the individual life course such as the 'empty nest' stage, retirement and widowhood.

The transformation of family life and family formation patterns: obstacles and incentives for emerging trends

We need to understand the processes that instigate family change to be able to detect, as well as to predict, trends in living arrangements and family formation patterns. In this way, social policy makers should be able to adapt their legislation to the real needs of the population. This simple premise does not always apply, however, as social policy tends to lag behind the rhythm of change marked by individuals' lives. In some cases, social policy not only ignores or intentionally neglects emerging patterns but even encourages the prescription of certain normative behaviour. This happens, for instance, when married couples are given preference in adoption to homosexual partnerships or to single individuals not living with a partner, or when consensual unions are given fewer social rights than marital unions (see Chapters 3 and 5 for the case of Britain).

After the Second World War, most Western countries assumed the model of the housewife marriage, which presupposed clear gendered norms and expectations in the organisation of the individual life cycle and of intimate relationships. In this model, the woman directly became the main unpaid carer, and hence also family dependent, upon marriage, whereas the man became the main wage earner or family provider. This presumed that women left the parental home to build a new family based on married co-residence in the nuclear or extended family, with a rigid gender division of labour. These families also had to retain a monopoly over intimate relationships (including sexuality) as well as reproduction, because they were the only legitimate and socially accepted spheres for motherhood and fatherhood. This model, which might have existed as such only in the social imagination of the state, shaped and influenced social policy and social behaviour until recently in most Western countries.[2]

The fact is that the housewife marriage represents an outdated model, or at least a model that most young women now reject. Indeed, the image of this model rather portrays the *bourgeois* family, since working-class women have always had to engage in some form of paid labour to help to sustain their families in most industrialised countries (Lewis 1992). Furthermore, we cannot be certain from the FFS survey data that there are not remainders of this old family model in current non-traditional relationships, such as gender inequalities in the allocation of time to do unpaid and caring work; certainly, qualitative evidence suggests that this is the case (e.g. Hufton and Kravaritou 1998). However, we can clearly see in the FFS data the progressive emergence of new living arrangements such as the formation of consensual unions; the formation of intimate relationships with those living in separate households (normally known as living apart together: LAT); having a child outside marriage or without a partner; the formation of reconstituted partnerships; voluntary childlessness, and so on. In brief, the map of living arrangements and the individual life cycle become more complex and difficult to predict.

The first demographic trend that marked the transformation of families in Western countries was the reduction in fertility since at least the mid-1960s, although starting some years later in southern European states (see Figure 2.1). Today, the total fertility rate continues to be low in most Western countries.[3] This is partly explained by the postponement of child-bearing to 25–30 years of age and even beyond in most Western countries, together with the postponement of marriage and the increase in consensual unions (which usually have lower fertility than marital unions). The question is what causes these trends, and I shall follow this question up throughout the chapter.

Declining fertility has caused a major debate around the issue of an ageing population, and of how to guarantee the level needed for the replacement of generations (2.1 children per woman) in order to sustain future economic development as well as national systems of social protection such

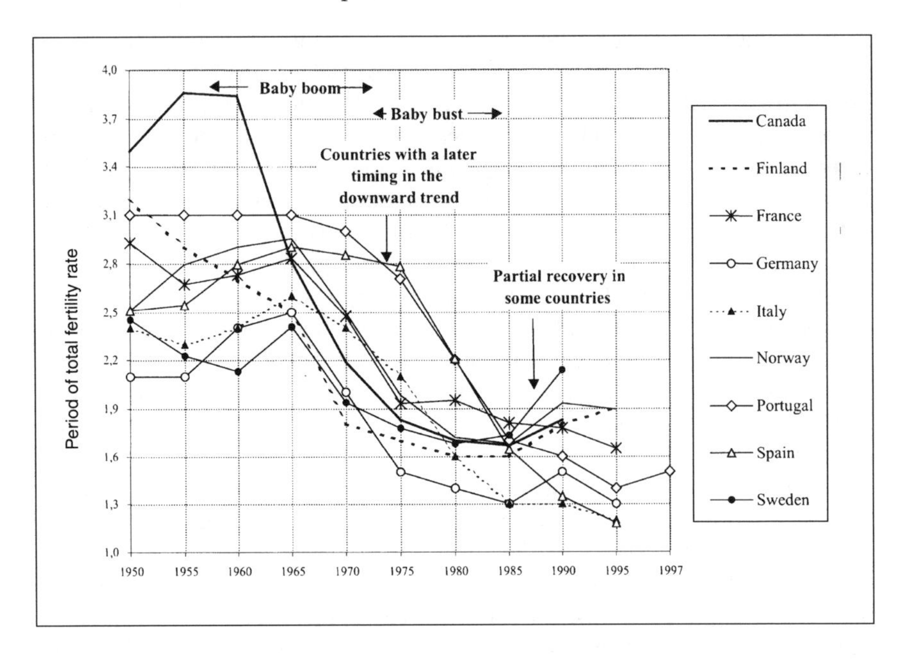

Figure 2.1 Total period fertility rate: selected Western countries, 1950–97

Source: FFS Country Reports.

as pensions. However, this is mainly a socio-economic concern, which does not necessarily capture women's personal concerns, such as how to fit their fertility desires, normally above the current levels of fertility, with their occupational prospects. As argued by McDonald (2000: 438),

> very low fertility rates will persist unless gender equity within family-oriented institutions rises to much higher levels than today. In a context of high gender equity in individual-oriented institutions, higher gender equity in family-oriented institutions will tend to raise fertility.

This argument seems to be supported by the fact that the 'women-friendly' welfare state regimes in Scandinavia – with considerable state support for parenting and for mothers continuing in long hours of employment – have higher fertility rates, while fertility rates in Italy and Spain – with negligible support – have among the lowest fertility rates in the world (see Chapter 4.2 for Spain).

As many authors have argued, one of the major instigators of family change (which includes current low levels of fertility and childbirth timing adjustments) is the new role of women in society, together with the redefinition of more egalitarian gender relations (see, for instance, González and Solsona 2000; Oppenheim-Mason and Jensen 1995). While influential economic theories have attempted to include the new role of women in their explanatory framework, they have used a very restricted approach based purely on cost–benefit rationality. This is the case for Becker (1993) and other neo-classical economists. They argue that the increase in women's earning power, which arises from their higher investment in human capital and labour force participation, discourages them from marriage and raises the relative cost of children. The higher cost of children would also reduce demand for them. However, authors such as Blossfield (1995) argue that marriage and fertility are currently postponed, rather than avoided, in most countries and that this is parallel to the increase in women's educational attainment. The evidence is that most women end up married or living with a partner irrespective of their level of education, and therefore lower fertility is not a matter of women's lack of interest in marriage associated with the increased opportunity costs of motherhood.

Oppenheimer (1996), who does not work within the neo-classical rational choice tradition, does not predict a reduced interest in marriage by women. She defines marriage as a social relationship that typically involves a 'multi-dimensional package of mutual interdependencies' (*ibid.*: 239). In this conceptualisation of partnership, the contribution by the husband and wife to the marriage goes beyond income and unpaid care. It also involves companionship over a sustained period of time and a varied and large set of rewards, mutual support and obligations. This definition would most adequately fit within the context of post-industrial societies, where housewife marriage is replaced by a 'newly integrated family autonomy model' (Crouch 1999). This model is characterised by a low level of female domesticity, a higher age at marriage, higher female education levels, more career-oriented individuals and careful mate selection processes. The post-industrial context thus opens a large array of living arrangements and different sequences of events over the life course. The next section describes the extent to which these new living arrangements and family formation patterns are diffused across countries in contemporary Western societies.

Differences in living arrangements: Western countries in the 1990s

This section provides information on women's living arrangements using a cross-sectional perspective across countries. The statistics provided here are comparable because the same age groups have been taken as a reference for each country. However, the FFS fieldwork was carried out in different years (*c.* early 1990s), which means that women were interviewed at slightly different times.

Household composition in the early phases of the family life course

This section begins by presenting a portrait of women's position in the household at different ages, generally for the age range 20–44, in all the countries analysed here. Figure 2.2 shows the prevalence of four main

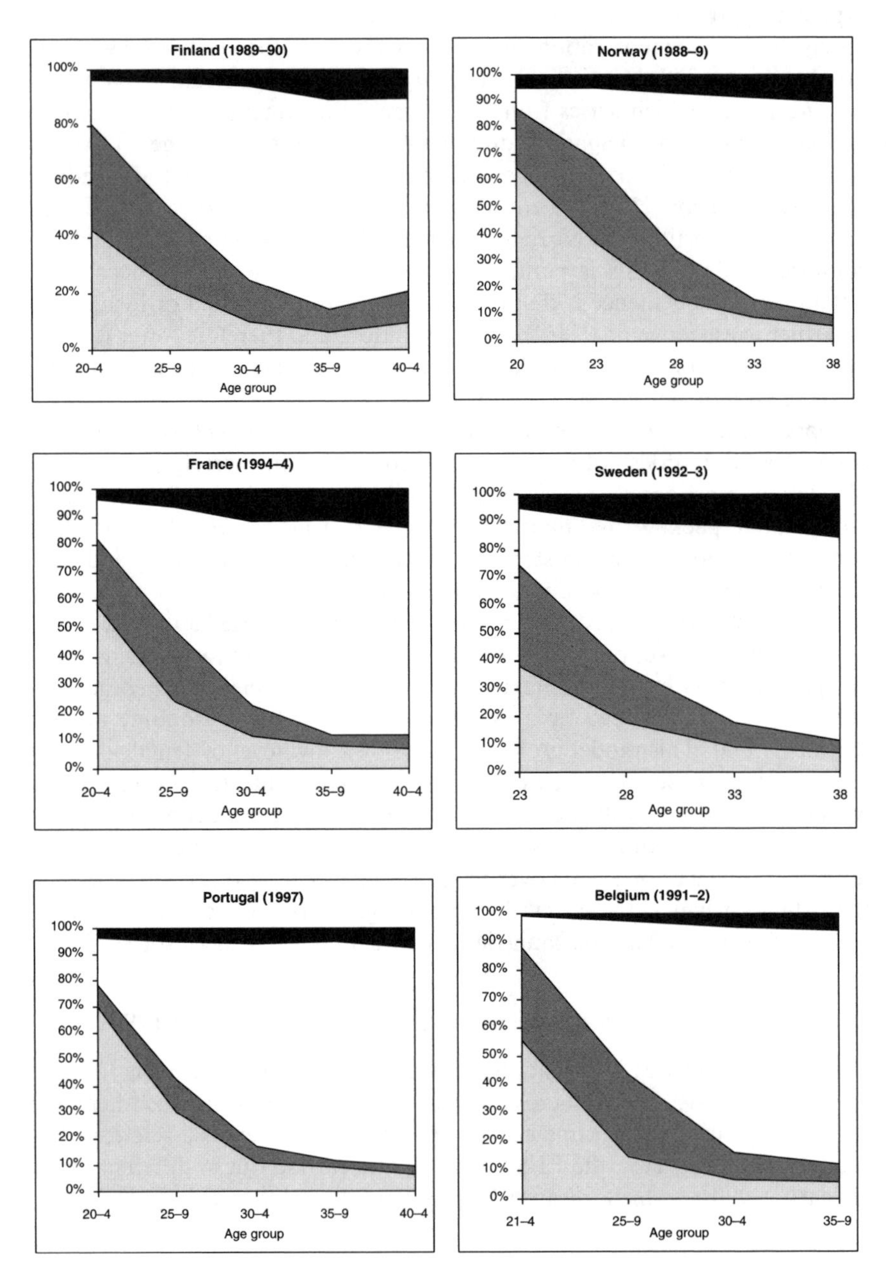

Figure 2.2 Women's household composition by age: selected Western countries, early 1990s

Source: FFS Standard Country Reports and Standard Record Files (US, Germany and Finland).

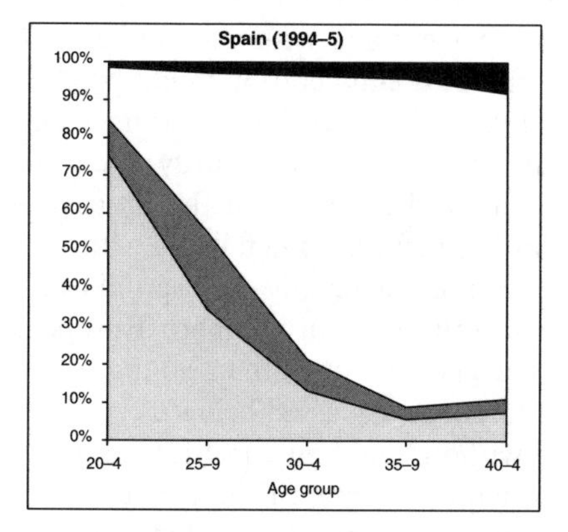

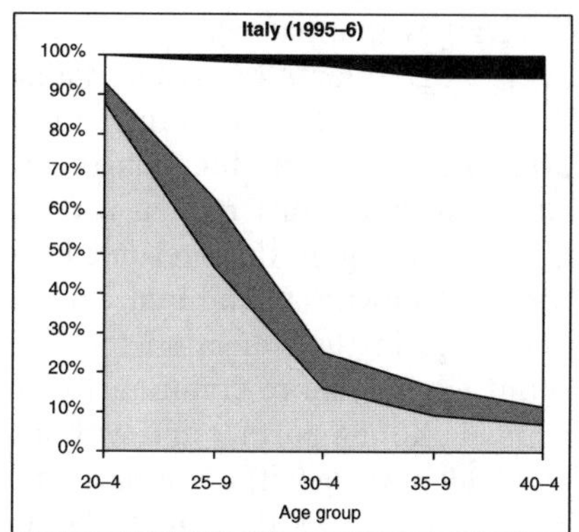

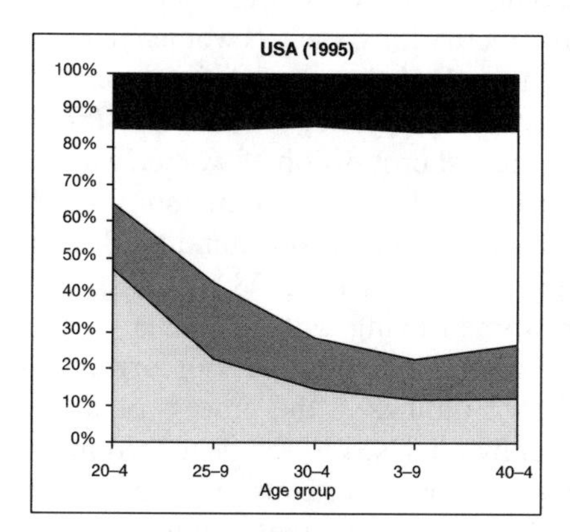

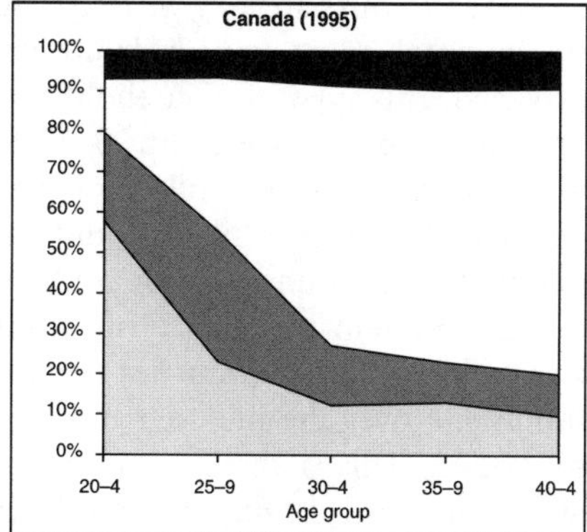

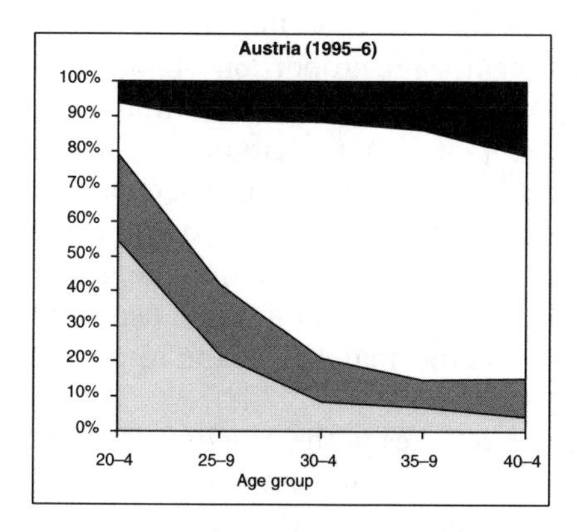

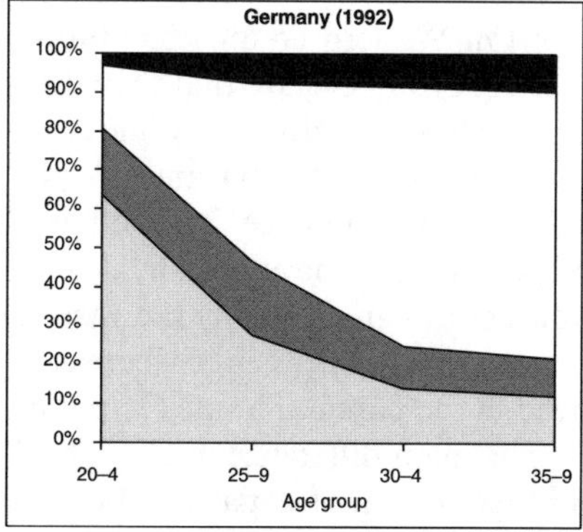

Without children or partner
Without children, with partner
With children and partner
With children, without partner

types of living arrangement: (1) living without a partner and without children; (2) living with a partner; (3) living with a partner and with children; and (4) living with children but without a partner.[4] This enumeration might produce the impression that we assume a normative sequence of living arrangements over the individual life course. Today, this is not necessarily the case, although there must remain a certain standard sequence in the process of family building. In this presumed standard sequence, women living without a partner and without children, for instance, might generally correspond to the first stage in the transition to adulthood (although in southern European countries it is more common to find old people rather than young adults living without a partner and without children, as discussed below).

Women living without a partner and without children constitute an interesting category as they might be, in principle, excepted from strong family responsibilities and might also have chosen to remain in that position. However, in this category we find a mix of situations, such as women living in the parental home, women living with friends and women living alone. As expected, this type of household mostly involves young women (see Figure 2.2). In the specific age group 20–24, the highest proportion of women without a partner and without children is found in southern European countries (70 per cent or above), while in countries such as Finland, Belgium and Sweden many of these young women are living with a partner (30–38 per cent).

The different prevalence of young women living with neither a partner nor children across countries mainly indicates different ways of organising family life over the life course or different timings in the process of family formation. This is an aspect more carefully analysed in the next section. To avoid the effect of such timing differences more effectively, we can observe how the group of women aged 30–34 behaves in different countries. These women mostly live in nuclear families (living with a partner and with children) in Western countries, although a significant proportion of women in this age group declare that they live both without a partner and without children. These constitute around 14 per cent of this age group in Germany (new and old Länder) and 16 per cent in Italy. However, what makes a substantial difference is whether these women, without apparent family responsibilities, have remained in the parental home or live in independent household – in Germany the vast bulk of the 14 per cent live in independent households (93 per cent), whereas in Italy a large majority of the 16 per cent lived in the parental home (76 per cent).

The main difference in this 30–34 age group lies in the proportion of lone mothers (without a partner but with children). Countries with the highest proportion of lone mothers in this age group are Sweden (12 per cent of women aged 33), France (12 per cent), Austria (11 per cent) and Germany (9 per cent), whereas in countries such as Spain, Italy and Belgium lone mothers do not account for more than 5 per cent of this group. However, the most differentiating feature is the proportion of lone mothers across all age groups in different countries. In many cases, lone mothers are a minority among young women and represent a much higher proportion among older women; France and Sweden are clear examples. This mainly reflects lone motherhood produced by partnership breakdown, and this is less frequent for young adult women. In countries such as Spain, which has a very low incidence of divorce, the proportion of lone mothers is only relatively important in the older age group. In other countries, however, lone motherhood embraces similar proportions of women regardless of their age, as in the United States and Canada. This reflects the situation where lone motherhood results not from breakdown of a long-term partnership but from rejection of shared parenthood (see Chapter 4.4 for the US policy response).

To sum up, the prevalence of different family forms (women's household position) varied substantially across age groups in the early 1990s in Western countries. In the 20–24 age group, the proportion of women who are living with a partner and women without both children and partner (mostly found in southern Europe) varied extensively. In the 30–34 age group, the main difference across countries is the prevalence of lone mothers. We look next at women's most common ways of establishing intimate relationships.

Diversity in intimate relationships: consensual unions, marital unions and living apart together

For a long time, the monolithic image of housewife marriage has been associated with the formation of a civil and/or religious union, because this was the socially legitimated site for sexual relationships and reproduction. This presumption no longer holds in many Western countries, as more women and men have premarital relationships, form consensual unions or maintain their autonomy while having an intimate relationship with a partner who lives in another household. The extent to which women adhere to these emerging types of intimate relationship across countries is now examined.

Figure 2.3 shows the percentage distribution of women according to the type of union and the percentage of women not living with a partner.[5] The sample has been divided into two large groups – young adult women (aged 25–34) and young middle-aged women (aged 35–44) – in nine Western countries. Two main facts stand out. On the one hand, a large country variation in the proportion of consensual (non-marital) unions is evident, with France at 19 per cent of women aged 25–34, as opposed to Italy and Spain with less than 5 per cent. On the other hand, it is very clear that the younger age group has a higher rate of consensual unions, which may indicate the progressive diffusion of alternatives among the younger generation. However, this statement should be taken cautiously, because consensual unions might simply be a prelude to marriage rather than a long-term arrangement, in which case it would be primarily concentrated in young adult women in any case. This seems to be the case in countries such as Italy, Austria and the UK.

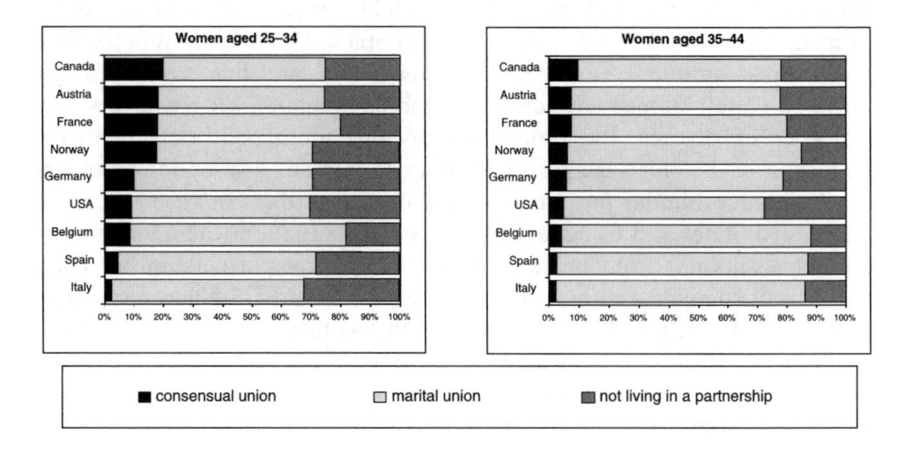

Figure 2.3 Types of union for women by age group: selected Western countries, early 1990s

Source: FFS standard record files; for survey years see note 1.

It is worth noting that there has been a general decline in the prevalence of marriage, which in most countries has been compensated for by the increase in consensual unions. However, this has not been the case in countries such as Italy or Spain, where consensual unions do not have a strong tradition and, consequently, there has been a sharp decline in the proportion of partnerships as a whole.

In the Nordic countries, however, consensual unions are popular for long-term relationships, although most partners with children have eventually married (Nikander 1998). Consensual unions are socially and legally regarded as equal to marriage, despite the majority of long-duration partnerships eventually being converted into marriages (Granström 1997). However, the interesting aspect is that marriages preceded by cohabitation seem to be far less stable than direct marriages in most countries (FFS country reports). This seems a puzzling finding, because one would expect a married couple with premarital experience to be better prepared for a stable relationship. The explanation must be a selection effect, probably related to women in consensual unions being more demanding on the relationship and, therefore, more exposed to the risk of breakdown.

It is also worth noting that in countries where consensual unions are uncommon among young middle-aged women, there is also a low proportion of women outside any type of partnership. Thus, in Italy and Spain, most young middle-aged women live in marital unions and less than 15 per cent do not live with a partner. In other countries, it is more common for this group of women to live outside any type of partnership: for example France (20 per cent), Canada (22 per cent), Germany (21 per cent) and the USA (28 per cent). Instead, in some of these countries, new forms of living arrangement become visible in this age group, such as so-called 'living apart together' (LAT, see Table 2.1). In France, 6 per cent of young adult women (aged 35–44) claimed to be in a LAT relationship, followed by Austria with 5 per cent. It might be hypothesised that these are countries with a greater degree of de-institutionalisation of the monolithic image of the housewife marriage mentioned above. However, I have some doubts about the meaning given to LAT relationships, because they might easily be confused with a boyfriend relationship instead of a deliberately chosen LAT relationship.

The incidence of LAT relationships is generally higher for the younger women (aged 25–34), which again gives the impression of a diffusion of emerging trends from the younger generation, although an intra-cohort analysis would be needed to confirm this. It might also be the case that LAT relationships among young women represent a way of testing the relationship rather than a stable and real alternative to a partnership. For instance, when young women were asked about their reasons for being in a LAT relationship, 77 per cent of German respondents said that it was because they wanted it that way, as opposed to Italians, only 46 per cent of whom claimed this. Furthermore, when they were asked later about future prospects, only 16 per cent of the Germans said that they intended to marry, as opposed to 51 per cent of the Italians. It also emerged in the FFS data that young middle-aged women (aged 35–44) living in LAT relationships were less willing than the younger women to convert their relationships into marriage.

There is another way to grasp the incidence of consensual unions, and this is to ask whether women have ever lived with someone whom they did not later marry. This is presented in Table 2.2, which shows higher percentages than Figure 2.3 for both age groups. The highest percentage of young adult women (aged 25–34) who have ever lived in a consensual union is reached in Austria, closely followed by Sweden and Germany. Southern European states such as Italy and Spain have the lowest rates. However, consensual unions will increase in southern European countries, as a slightly

Table 2.1 Percentage distribution of women living apart together (LATs), by age group (selected Western countries, early 1990s)

Country (year of survey)	*25–34*	*35–44*
Austria (1995–6)	10.3	5.3
Italy (1995–6)	9.9	1.8
Spain (1994–5)	9.8	2.8
France (1994)	9.6	5.7
Germany (1992)	9.6	4.0
Belgium (1991–2)	7.1	4.9

Source: FFS (standard record files).

Note: The question asked was 'Are you currently having an intimate relationship with someone who lives in a separated household?' Only these countries included questions about LATS.

Table 2.2 Percentage distribution of women who have ever cohabited with someone with whom they did not marry, by age groups (selected Western countries, early 1990s)

Country (year of survey)	*25–34*	*35–44*
Austria (1995–6)	58.3	46.4
Sweden (1992–3)	53.0	32.8
Germany (1992)	41.4	32.4
France (1994)	30.4	12.9
Finland (1989–90)	30.3	14.1
Canada (1995)	29.9	21.0
Norway (1988–9)	29.3	12.1
USA (1995)	27.4	22.5
Belgium (1991–2)	9.9	6.6
Spain (1994–5)	7.4	5.5
Italy (1995–6)	4.2	3.6

Source: FFS (standard record files).

Note: The question asked was 'Have you ever lived in the same household with someone with whom you had an intimate relationship but did not marry?'

higher proportion of the youngest women have been in consensual unions than have young adult women.

To conclude, alternatives to marital union are emerging, such as LAT relationships, consensual unions and living without a partner. However, the prevalence of these alternative living arrangements varies significantly across countries. These differences might be explained by the existence of policy disincentives or the dominance of traditional cultural values, which might progressively vanish.

New contexts for reproduction

The current process of de-institutionalisation of the traditional housewife family has given rise to a further separation between sexual and affective relationships, and reproduction. Marriage has lost its unique legitimacy for maintaining intimate and sexual relationships and for fostering childbirth. The most common partnership status of women at the birth of their first child varies across countries (see Figure 2.4). In countries like Sweden, it is more common to have the first child in a consensual union than in a marital union. The long tradition of consensual unions in Sweden, nowadays social and legally equal to marriage, means that women do not feel the moral obligation to foster childbirth within a marital union. However, it is much less common that young Swedish women have their first child outside any partnership (6 per cent), compared with North American women (20 per cent in the USA and 16 per cent in Canada), Germany (20 per cent) and the UK (39 per cent in 1999, quoted in Ermisch 2000). Some of the questions that

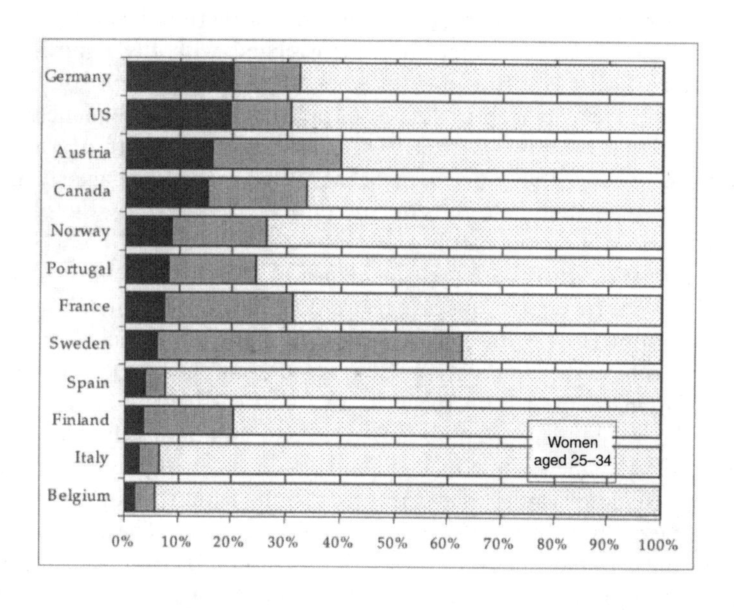

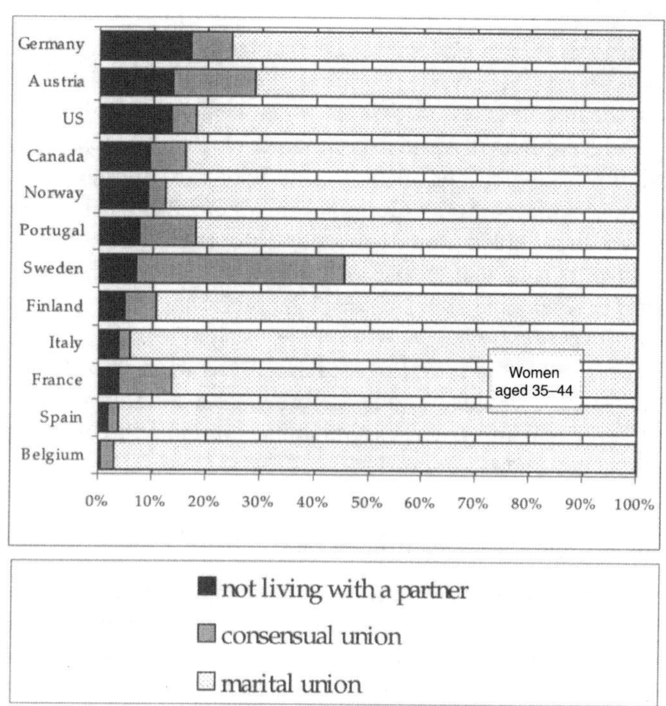

Figure 2.4 Women's partnership status at birth of first child: selected Western countries, early 1990s

Source: FFS standard record files; for survey years see note 1.

arise are how long these women stay in lone motherhood, whether this is a voluntary choice and whether this is correlated with the feminisation of poverty (see Roll 1992; Bradshaw *et al.* 1996). Certainly, lone motherhood has different social perceptions, as well as economic consequences, across countries (Duncan and Edwards 1999). If we compare both age groups in Figure 2.4, we see that only 9 per cent of young middle-aged Canadian women had their first child outside any type of partnership, whereas 16 per cent of young adult women did so.

The countries with the lowest incidence of a first child born to women aged 25–34 not living with a partner are Belgium, Italy, Finland and Spain. In these countries – with the exception of Finland – the most popular pattern is to have the child within marriage, despite the fact that in countries such as Spain children born to unmarried couples have the same rights as children born in a marital union. Portugal, as a southern European country, exhibits different behaviour to Italy and Spain. As many as 16 per cent of young Portuguese women had their first child within a consensual union and another 8 per cent without living with a partner. These figures break the presumed homogeneity of family life in southern Europe and point to the existence of a different gender culture in Portugal (see González and Solsona 2000).

When analysing the prevalence of certain living arrangements we need to take into account the extent to which they are constrained or enabled in a given social context. For instance, in Germany and Britain consensual unions are discriminated against compared with marital unions, because parents do not have the right of joint custody of the children (see Chapter 5 for Britain). Additionally, in Germany a system of marital tax splitting (incomes are first added and then split into two and taxed separately) primarily favours married couples with only one income rather than two-earner families (Federkeil 1997; see also Chapter 4.1).

In brief, the context of reproduction varies significantly across countries, although these differences are largely related to the popularity of different living arrangements as illustrated in the previous section. In the next section, a different analytical approach is adopted in examining the behaviour of one female birth cohort across countries.

The frequency and tempo of women's early life events

This section examines the timing and frequency of early life events for women born between 1956 and 1960. Four events occurring in early adulthood are examined using life-table procedures: leaving home, first partnership formation, and first and second births.

From a life-course perspective, family formation patterns are regarded as age-related events that require longitudinal observations. Hence a particular female birth cohort was selected, those born in 1956–60, for all the sample countries to capture differences in their life experiences. These women lived through the same historical period but in different national institutional contexts. The life history of this cohort can be reconstructed retrospectively up to the women's 35th birthdays in the majority of countries and is, therefore, the youngest cohort that could have been chosen.

Leaving the parental home

In general, most countries have seen a delay in the age at which young adults leave the parental home, largely as a consequence of longer periods in education and increased age at entry into the job market (Corijn and Klijzing 2001). In the specific cohort analysed here, there are sharp differences in the point at which they left their parental home for the first time (see Figure 2.5, which represents an age-specific life table, to be interpreted in terms of the cumulative experience of women's (1956–60 cohort) leaving home by age). Seven countries have been included, representing different timings and intensities of home leaving. The life events analysed in the next sections will also draw on this sample of countries, because the timing at home leaving might also determine the pattern of subsequent life events.

As Figure 2.5 shows, women left home at a comparatively late age in southern European states compared with Swedish women, which is the extreme case for leaving the parental home at an early age. Sweden is closely followed by the USA (despite the USA giving information on the age of last leaving the parental home, so that women might have left even earlier, returned to the parental home and left again). By their 25th birthday, 32 per cent of women born between 1956 and 1960 had not left the parental home in Italy, 24 per cent in Portugal and 23 per cent in Spain, but only 8 per cent in France, whereas virtually everybody had left home in Sweden. Furthermore, by their 28th birthday around 20 per cent of Portuguese and Italian women still lived in the parental home. These enormous differences will also affect the sequence and intensity of other life events, such as childbirth.

There are various explanations for these timing differences across countries. First, there are cultural differences, for instance in the fact that there is not a major social stigma in southern European countries if young adults remain at the parental home for a long period while unmarried. Adult children may even rejoin the parental home after divorce or separation, as in Spain (Solsona 1998), without this being perceived as inadequate or suspicious behaviour. In northern and central European countries, however, it is expected that at a certain age young adults will lead independent lives in their own households.

Second, in northern and central European countries young adults can, to a greater extent, rely on state support (for example, social housing or unemployment benefits), which is virtually non-existent in southern European states (Jurado 2001). Instead, in southern Europe the family bears the main responsibility for dependent children while they study, during unemployment,

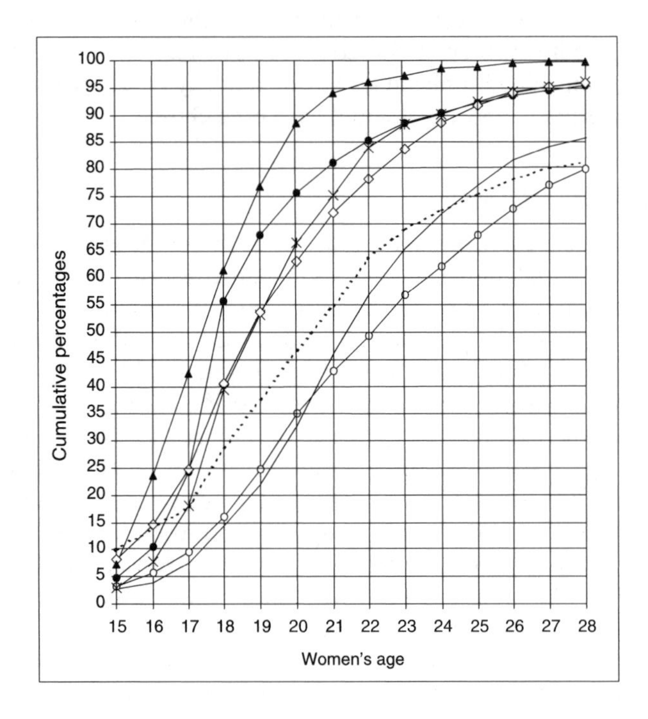

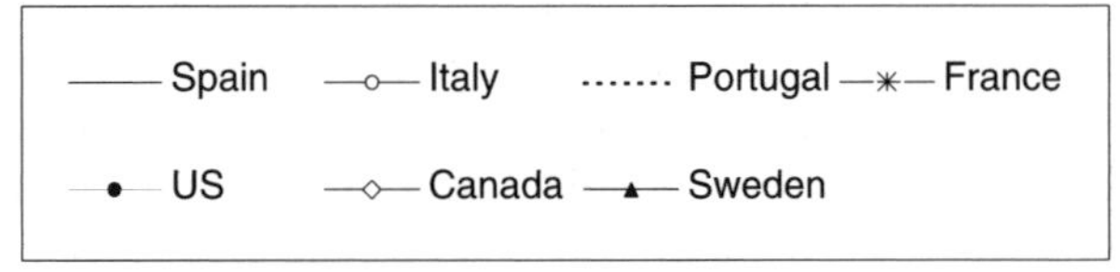

Figure 2.5 Cumulative percentage of women (1956–60 cohort) who had ever left the parental home, by age: selected Western countries

Source: FFS standard record files.

Note: Women were aged 34–9 in Spain, 34–40 in Italy, 36–41 in Portugal, 33–8 in France, 34–9 in US, 35–9 in Canada and 32–4 in Sweden at the time of the interview. The question asked in the USA was 'When did you last leave the parental home?' rather than 'What was your age at your first home leaving?'. The Swedish cohort consists of women born in 1959 only.

or while searching for a job. As argued by Bettio and Villa, young people in southern Europe acquire 'independence within rather than from the family' (1998: 146). For Italy, as an example, De Sandre *et al.* (2000) argue that this parental support has the positive effect of enabling women to surpass men in achieving high levels of education. This also means that children only leave the parental home thanks to a parental transfer of resources, which also implies overloading the mother with family responsibilities for a longer period. Interestingly enough, women's higher educational attainment is a crucial variable shaping the process of family formation, as we will see later in this chapter. A longer period of parental support has also been reported in countries such as Belgium, where children might remain at home until they acquire a job and their own income, despite better access to scholarships or unemployment benefits than in southern Europe (Lodewijckx 1999).

Timing differences in leaving home are even more marked when observed across educational categories in different countries (see Figure 2.6). In general, education normally has the effect of delaying certain transitions, such as forming an independent household or having a first child. Figure 2.6 shows that this delay is particularly manifest among highly educated women in southern European countries. Thus, in Italy, 29 per cent of women born between 1956 and 1960 with higher education had not left the parental home by their 30th birthday, while in France, virtually all women with the same educational attainments had left home by this age. Hence, not only do southern European women tend to leave the parental home at a rather late age, but also the timing is further postponed among women with secondary or higher education. Educational attainment has great potential for enabling women to organise their occupational and family life in the later stages of their lives, because they have accumulated human capital and job experience in the labour force, but in southern Europe this is achieved at the cost of delaying the process of leaving home – and at the expense of their parents.

Forming a partnership

Age at first partnership follows similar geographical patterns to leaving home (see Figure 2.7). However, there are some singularities. In some countries, women may have spent a considerable time between leaving their parental home and entering a new partnership (most common in northern and central Europe, Canada and the USA), while at the other extreme forming a partnership does not necessarily mean leaving the parental home at all but rather forming a family with two nuclei (Spain) or, in other southern Europe countries, entering a partnership (typically married) directly after leaving the parental home. Over 70 per cent of women in France and Sweden had formed their first partnership (either marital or consensual) by their 22th birthday, whereas only 46 per cent in Italy and 53 per cent in Spain had done so. This delay in the formation of a first union has an indirect effect on fertility, because – as was pointed out above – most childbirth is within marital unions in southern Europe. The delay is again more pronounced among more educated women, as Figure 2.8 shows.

Childbearing

The timing differences at first birth between countries is shown in Figure 2.9. It is worth noting that Portuguese women in the 1956–60 cohort had

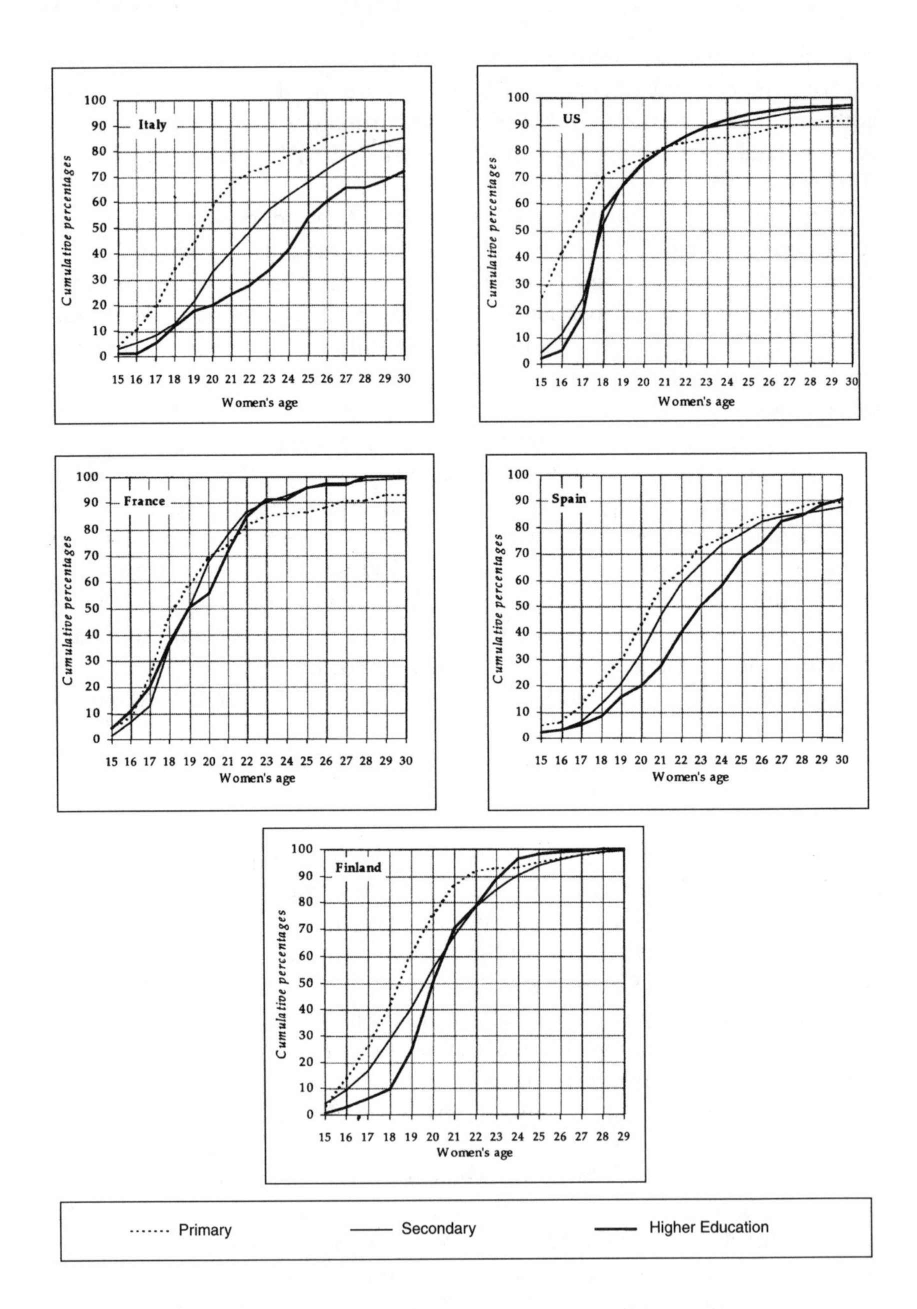

Figure 2.6 Cumulative percentage of women (1956–60 cohort) who had ever left the parental home, by age and educational level: selected Western countries

Source: FFS standard record files.

Note: Educational attainment was classified into three large categories as follows: a lower educational category (ISCED 0–2); secondary education (ISCED 5–6); and higher education (ISCED 3–4).

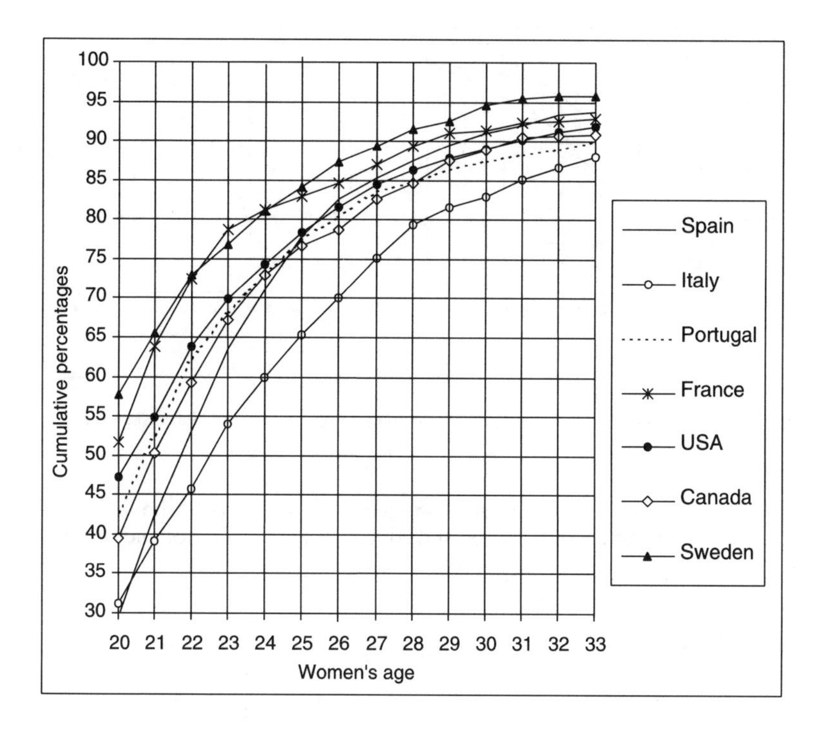

Figure 2.7 Cumulative percentage of women (1956–60 cohort) who had started their first partnership, by age: selected Western countries

Source: FFS standard record files.

Note: First partnerships include both marital and non-marital unions.

their first child at an early age, despite having left the parental home rather late, as shown in Figure 2.5. This means that these women, once they are in a partnership, do not wait long before having their first child. In contrast, Swedish women were the earliest to leave the parental home but waited longer to have their first child. By their 28th birthday, 82 per cent of women born between 1956 and 1960 had had their first live birth in Portugal, but only around 65 per cent in Italy and Sweden.

These cumulative percentages of women with a first child should be interpreted with caution, since some women have not yet reached their final fertility level (completed cohort fertility is calculated at the end of the childbearing years, around age 50). Figure 2.9 simply shows the timing of bearing the first child up to 33 years of age. It remains a puzzle how long the large percentage of women aged 33 who remain childless – at the extreme approximately 20 per cent Italy and Canada – will merely postpone motherhood, or reject or miss it altogether.

The pressure of the 'biological clock' may be felt particularly by women in higher education. Education seems to have a stronger effect on the timing

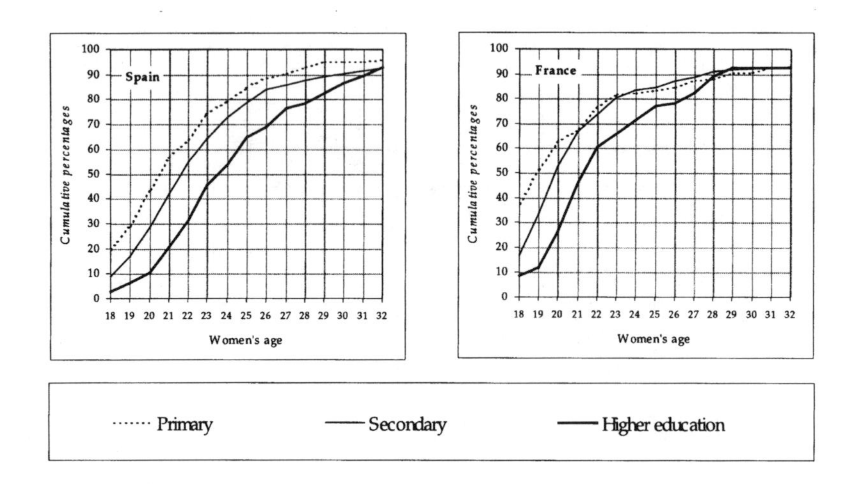

Figure 2.8 Cumulative percentage of women (1956–60 cohort) who had started their first partnership, by age and educational level: France and Spain

Source: FFS standard record files.

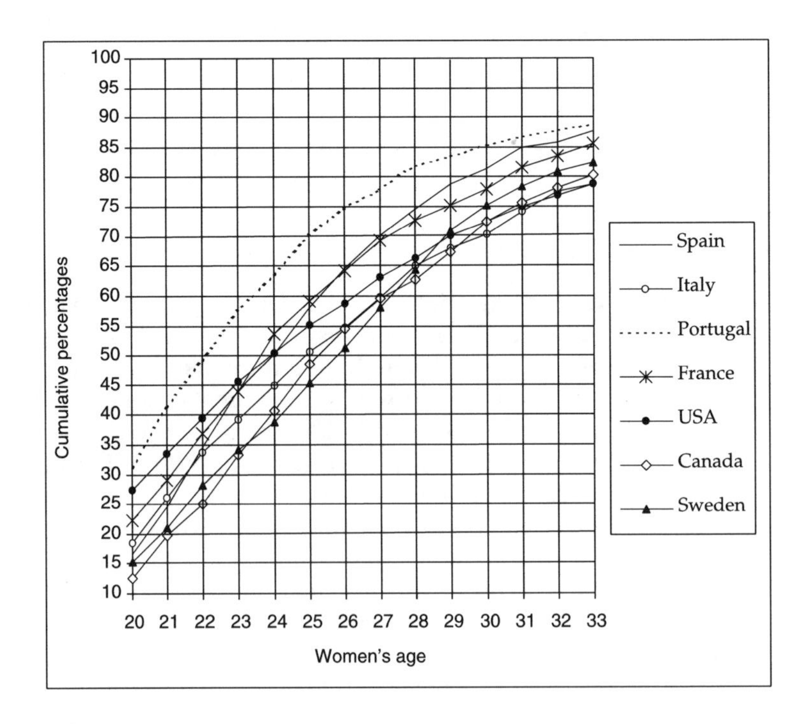

Figure 2.9 Cumulative percentage of women (1956–60 cohort) who had their first live birth, by age: selected Western countries, 1950–97

Source: FFS standard record files.

of the first child than the formation of a first union. Various examples are given in Figure 2.10. The peculiarity of this figure is that in no country did more highly educated women from the 1956–60 cohort catch up with the childbirth intensity (first birth) of their less well-educated contemporaries, although differences according to level of education lessen with age. Again, this varies between countries: for example, by the age of 35, 40 per cent of Italian women born between 1956 and 1960 with higher education had not had a first live birth, compared with just 23 per cent in France. This means that the higher proportion of childlessness is concentrated in educated women, who may experience stronger conflict between work and family roles in their early adult years. Indeed, a study of US women who postponed childbearing past age 30 in 1990 and 1995 showed that almost half of them remained childless by choice or necessity, despite being in a better position to combine work and family (Martin 2000). In countries with better public childcare services this difference might be less important, although many other factors must be determining women's fertility choices.

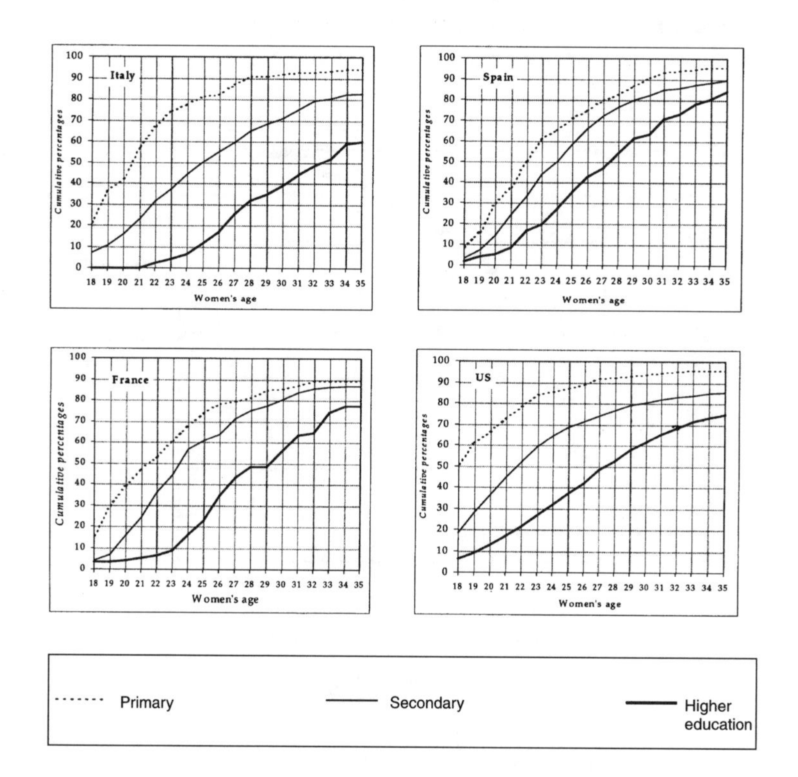

Figure 2.10 Cumulative percentage of women (1956–60 cohort) who had their first live birth, by age and educational level: France, Italy, Spain and the USA

Source: FFS standard record files.

However, Lesthaeghe and Willems (1999) argue that the European Union is close to levelling off in childbearing postponement, because the increase in female higher education and female employment during the reproductive age – two major factors in delay – will be very small in the near future. This might be the case as far as educational attainment is concerned, but it is less evident in the case of employment, in which there are still important differences between women and men, especially in the southern European countries (Forsberg *et al.* 2000).

Lastly, the interval between first and second live births has been analysed for France, Italy and Sweden (see Figure 2.11). Very nearly half of Italian women in the 1956–60 cohort gave birth to their second child 3.5 years after the birth of their first. The comparable figures for spacing births was 3.1 years in France and 2.7 per cent in Sweden. The shorter birth interval in Sweden has been related to both the postponement of the first child and the parental insurance system. When a mother has a second child up to 2.5 years after the first child, she is entitled to parental benefit at almost the level of her income before the first child was born (see Chapter 4.3).

To conclude, women born in the same period (1956–60) have organised their early family life in different ways across Western countries. These

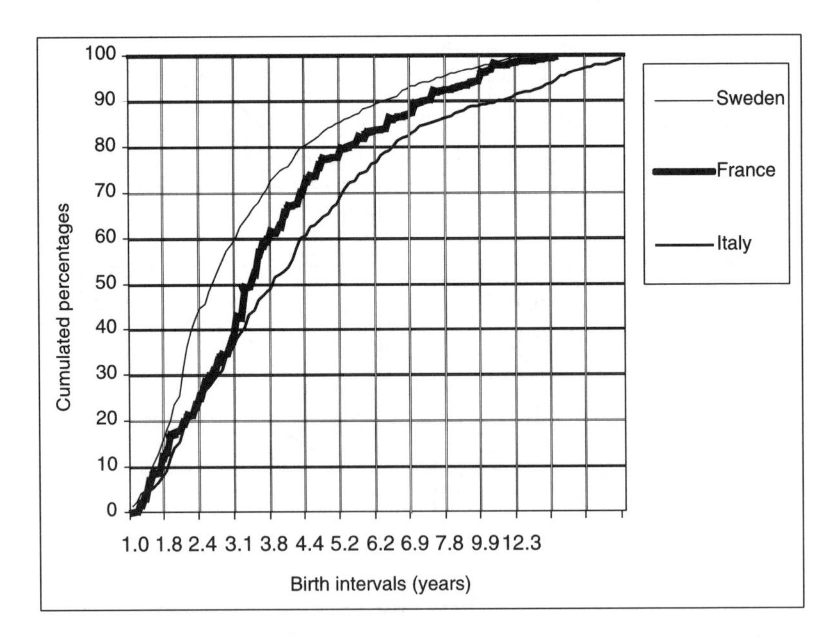

Figure 2.11 Time interval between first and second live birth (1956–60 cohort, women): France, Italy and Sweden

Source: FFS standard record files.

differences in timing and intensity might be partly attributed to diversity in values and gender expectations. This seems to be linked to the existence of different strategic reasoning across various categories of women (thus, highly educated women tend to delay family responsibilities for longer than their less well-educated counterparts) and the existence of different material constraints (for example, the relative availability of public support to enable young people to leave the parental home).

Conclusion and discussion

This chapter has provided a general description of Western families, taking as a reference point the female population and applying two different analytical perspectives. The first perspective focused on cross-sectional analysis of various living arrangements across Western countries in the late 1990s. The main differences between countries lie in the differing popularity of lone motherhood and consensual unions. However, the problem with cross-sectional observation is that we do not really know whether individuals in specific family situations will remain so for a long time or whether these will be only a short stage in their lives. The social and personal meaning of consensual unions, for instance, might change considerably according to their duration. This issue should be addressed further in demographic analyses.

The second part of the chapter focused on longitudinal analysis. Here I examined the demographic behaviour of the 1956–60 female birth cohort in their early phases of family formation. The main conclusion is that women born in the same period in different countries have had very different experiences concerning the quantum and tempo of various family events. The 1956–60 female birth cohort in southern European countries left the parental home rather later than in other Western countries, and they mostly entered new partnerships directly. In countries like France and Sweden, women spent more time between leaving home and building a new partnership, and they did not necessarily form a marital union. However, the most interesting differences appeared when we compared the behaviour of women according to educational attainment. More highly educated women tend to postpone most processes of family formation, but they catch up somewhat with women in other educational categories later in life. However, in most countries high educational attainment has a particularly strong effect on childbearing. By the time women reach 30, they are far from reaching the fertility (first child) of less well-educated women.

For authors such as Latten and Graaf (1997), more highly educated women are trend setters for the way family life is going to be organised in the near future. However, this observation opens up other questions, such as why highly qualified women cannot combine pursuing a career in the labour market and having children. Their lower fertility might simply be a strategy to reconcile paid work and family life, but this strategy might also cause unintended childlessness. The nature of the welfare state regime may be an important factor here, as women-friendly states such as Sweden can enable this reconciliation (see Chapter 4.3).

I began this article by empathising with the role of women as instigators of alternative living arrangements to the housewife marriage. I must end by posing the question of why, even in countries where women enjoy similar levels of economic integration and equality, so many differences in family life and family formation patterns persist. This is only one indication of the importance that culture and social policies must play in the configuration of current family life. These issues are followed up in succeeding chapters of the book.

Acknowledgement

Thanks to the Advisory Group of the FFS programme of comparative research for its permission, granted under identification number 76, to use the FFS data on which this research is based.

Notes

1 For further details of the survey procedures, see the technical annex of the FFS standard country reports. Sample size, age range and survey year of the countries included in the chapter are as follows: Austria (4,500 women aged 20–54 in 1995/96); Belgium (3,200 women aged 21–40 in 1991/92); Canada (4,200 women aged 15–54 in 1995); Finland (4,200 women aged 22–51 in 1989/90); France (2,900 women aged 20–49 in 1994); Germany (6,000 women aged 20–49 in 1995/96); Italy (4,500 women aged 18–42 in 1993); Norway (4,000 women aged 20–43 in 1988/89); Portugal (6,000 women aged 1,554 in 1997); Spain (4,000 women aged 18–49 in 1994/95); Sweden (3,900 women aged 20–49 in 1992/93); and the United States (10,500 women aged 15–44 in 1995). The data used in this chapter correspond to figures obtained directly from the standard country reports and indicators estimated from the standard record files.

2 There is an extensive literature on the influence of assumed family models on the construction of social policies. See, for instance, Naldini (2001) for Italy and Spain, Daly (1996) for Britain and Germany, Lewis (1992) for Britain, and Sainsbury (1994) for other European countries.

3 The total fertility rate (TFR) measures the sum of the age-specific fertility rates over the whole range of reproductive ages for a particular period. The TFR is interpreted as the number of children a woman would have during her lifetime if she were to experience the fertility rates of the period at each age. In contrast, complete fertility (CF) indicates the final family size of a specific true cohort. The TFR and CF may lead to different interpretations of the recent declines in birth rates, because the TFR exaggerates short-term fluctuations and changes in the age pattern of fertility. Thus, the increase in the mean age of childbearing that has occurred in most European countries partly explains the current low TFR rates.

4 Caution should be used in the comparison between age groups in Figure 2.2, as there are some differences in the groups by countries. The Belgian sample covered only the age range 21–40, whereas most countries cover the age range 20–44.
5 Canada, Finland and Sweden did not include the question about the respondent's current situation within the partnership and are therefore excluded here.

References

Becker, G. (1993; enlarged edition, originally published in 1981) *A Treatise on the Family*, Cambridge, Mass. and London: Harvard University Press.

Bettio, F. and Villa, P. (1998) 'A Mediterranean perspective on the break-down of the relationships between participation and fertility', *Cambridge Journal of Economics* 2(22): 137–71.

Blossfield, H.P. (ed.) (1995) *The New Role of Women: Family Formation in Modern Societies*, Boulder: Westview Press.

Boh, K., Bak, M., Clason, C. *et al.* (eds) (1989) *Changing Patterns of European Family Life: A Comparative Analysis of 14 European Countries*, London: Routledge.

Bradshaw, J., Kennedy, S., Kilkey M. *et al.* (1996) *The Employment of Lone Parents: A Comparison of Policy in 20 Countries*, London and New York: Family Policy Studies Centre and Joseph Rowntree Foundation.

Corijn, M. and Klijzing, E. (eds) (2001) 'Transitions to adulthood in Europe', *European Studies of Population*, Volume 10. Dordrecht: Kluwer Academic.

Crouch, C. (1999) *Social Change in Western Europe*, Oxford: Oxford University Press.

Daly, M. (1996) *The Gender Division of Welfare: The British and German Welfare States Compared*, Florence: European University Institute.

De Sandre, P. *et al.* (eds) (2000) *Fertility and Family Surveys in Countries of the ECE Region*, Standard Country Report 10o: Italy. New York and Geneva: UN Economic Commission for Europe and UN Population Fund.

Duncan, S. (1995) 'Theorising European gender systems', *Journal of European Social Policy* 5(4): 263–84.

Duncan, S. and Edwards, R. (1999) *Lone Mothers, Paid Work and Gendered Moral Rationalities*, London: Macmillan.

Ermisch, J.F. (2000) 'Employment opportunities and pre-marital births in Britain', ISER Working Paper 26, Institute for Social and Economic Research, University of Essex.

Eurostat (2000) *Statistiques sociales Européennes: Démographie. Thème 3: Population et conditions sociales*, Luxembourg: Official Publications of the European Communities.

Federkeil, G. (1997) 'The Federal Republic of Germany: polarization of family structure', in F.X. Kaufmann, A. Kuijsten, H.J. Schulze and K.P. Strohmeier (eds) *Family Life and Family Policies in Europe: Structures and Trends in the 1980s*, Vol. I. Oxford: Clarendon Press, pp. 77–113.

Forsberg, G., Gönas, L. and Perrons, D. (2000) 'Paid work: participation, inclusion and liberation', in S. Duncan and B. Pfau-Effinger (eds) *Gender, Work and Culture in the European Union*, London and New York: Routledge.

González, M.J. and Solsona, M. (2000) 'Households and families: changing living arrangements and gender relations', in S. Duncan and B. Pfau-Effinger (eds) *Gender, Work and Culture in the European Union*, London and New York: Routledge.

Granström, F. (1997) *Fertility and Family Surveys in Countries of the ECE Region*, Standard Country Report 10b: Sweden. New York and Geneva: UN Economic Commission for Europe and UN Population Fund.

Hufton, O. and Kravaritou, Y. (eds) (1998) *Gender and the Use of Time*, The Hague: Kluwer Law International.

Jurado, T. (2001) *Youth in Transition. Employment, Housing, Social Policies and the Family in France and Spain*, Aldershot: Ashgate.

Kaufmann, F.X., Kuijsten, A., Schulze, H.J. and Strohmeier, K.P. (eds) (1997) *Family Life and Family Policies in Europe: Structures and Trends in the 1980s*, Vol. I. Oxford: Clarendon Press.

Kuijsten, A. (1996) 'Changing family patterns in Europe: A case of divergence?' *European Journal of Population* 12, 115–43.

Latten, J. and de Graaf, A. (1997) *Fertility and Family Surveys in Countries of the ECE Region*, Standard Country Report 10b: The Netherlands. New York and Geneva: UN Economic Commission for Europe and UN Population Fund.

Lesthaeghe, R. and Willems, P. (1999) 'Is low fertility a temporary phenomenon in the European Union?' *Population and Development Review* 25(2): 221–8.

Lewis, J. (1992) *Women in Britain since 1945: Women, Family Work and the State in the Post-War Years*, Oxford: Basil Blackwell.

Lodewijckx, T. (1999) *Fertility and Family Surveys in Countries of the ECE Region*, Standard Country Report 10k: Finland. New York and Geneva: UN Economic Commission for Europe and UN Population Fund.

Martin, S.P. (2000) 'Diverging fertility among U.S. women who delay childbearing past age 30', *Demography* 37(4): 523–33.

McDonald, P. (2000) 'Gender equity in theories of fertility transition', *Population and Development Review* 26(3): 427–39.

Naldini, M. (2001) *The Family in the Mediterranean Welfare States*, London: Frank Cass.

Nikander, T. (1998) *Fertility and Family Surveys in Countries of the ECE Region*, Standard Country Report 10g: Finland. New York and Geneva: UN Economic Commission for Europe and UN Population Fund.

Oppenheimer, V.K. (1995) 'The role of women's economic independence in marriage formation: a skeptic's response to Annemette Srensen's remarks', in H.P. Blossfield (ed.) *The New Role of Women: Family Formation in Modern Societies*, Boulder: Westview Press.

Oppenheim-Mason, K. and Jensen, A.M. (eds) (1995) *Gender and Family Change in Industrialised Countries*, Oxford: Clarendon Press.

Popenoe, D. (1993) 'American family decline, 1960–1990: a review and appraisal', *Journal of Marriage and the Family* 55: 527–55.

Rendall, M.S. (1999) 'Entry or exit? A transition-probability approach to explaining the high prevalence of single motherhood among black women', *Demography* 36(3): 369–76.

Rivers, K.L. (2001) 'Has welfare reform reduced nonmarital births?' *Population Today* 9 (February/March).

Roll, J. (1992) *Lone Parent Families in the EC*, Brussels: European Commission.

Sainsbury, D. (ed.) (1994) *Gendering Welfare States*, London: Sage.
Solsona, M. (1998) 'Viure sol, viure amb família', in Enquesta Metropolitana de Barcelona 1995, 49–67. Barcelona: Institut d'Estudis Metropolitans.

Part II

Perspectives on family policy

3 Political intervention and family policy in Britain

3.1 Individualisation, assumptions about the existence of an adult worker model and the shift towards contractualism

Jane Lewis

Sociologists have used the concept of individualisation to refer to the way in which people's lives have come to be less constrained by tradition and customs and more subject to individual choice. This in turn can only be understood against the background of changes in the labour market and in social provision by the modern welfare state in particular. Elizabeth Beck-Gernsheim (1999: 54) has described the effects of individualisation on the family in terms of a 'community of need' becoming 'an elective relationship'. The family used to be held together by obligations based on solidarity and need, but also by the powerful prescriptions flowing from widespread acceptance of the male breadwinner model, with its idea of men bearing primary responsibility for earning and women for caring. Women's increased participation in the labour market in particular has eroded this model at the level of behaviour and even more at the level of prescription. As Beck and Beck-Gernsheim (1995) have argued, it has become difficult to mesh the labour market biographies of two adults with the demands of family life.

Politicians and policy makers have increasingly acknowledged one of the main manifestations of increasing individualisation – economic independence. In large part, their apparent acceptance of this dimension of family change at the end of the twentieth century was prompted by concerns about international competitiveness and the importance of adult participation in the labour market as a means of achieving it. This was as evident at the European as at the UK level (CEC 1993, 1995). This acceptance also stemmed from the emphasis on responsibilities as opposed to rights, which has marked the work of American commentators since the 1980s, and from a European social democratic focus on labour market insertion as a means of combating social exclusion; both these perspectives have informed 'third way' politics in the UK. The focus on work has involved a profound shift away from a set of assumptions based on the notion of a family with a male breadwinner towards a family model in which both men and women are assumed to be in the labour market, although to what degree remains unspecified. While in practice the male breadwinner model only ever became a social reality for middle-class women – and for a relatively short period of time – it exercised considerable prescriptive power in terms of the division of labour between men and women. The new set of assumptions is supported by aggregate statistics reporting women's labour market participation, which now rivals that of men but which is nevertheless very different in respect of the shorter hours that women work and in their wage rates. In turn, this means that there are substantial inequalities in earned income, which are particularly marked for mothers and fathers of younger children. Indeed, there are good grounds for arguing that the shift in assumptions about women's participation in the labour market on the part of policy makers has actually outpaced changes in the social reality.

This has serious implications, given that social policy making of all kinds is moving increasingly towards a contractual model. The government is seeking to promote contracts between its agents and individual citizens in a whole variety of fields, as well as with groups of citizens and between citizens themselves. Thus there is reference to contracts between the state and recipients of welfare benefits, to contracts between schools and parents, and between partners in intimate relationships in the form of premarital or cohabitation agreements. Behind these developments is an assumption that all individuals have an equal capacity to contract. This may be true in the legal sense, but inequalities in power and in access to resources makes this approach problematic. This section deals particularly with the social policy dimensions of this shift in the UK, while James (Chapter 3.2) and Maclean (Chapter 3.3) look at the implications for family law.

The adult worker model and the social reality

In the UK, Tony Blair's introduction to the document on welfare reform has been widely quoted as a summary reference to the Labour government's new approach to social provision: 'Work for those who can, security for those who cannot' (Cmnd 3805, 1998: iii) and is contrasted with the Beveridgean promise of security for all. How to draw the boundary between those who can and those who cannot work remains a major issue. The UK welfare reform document goes on to state that the welfare state based around the male breadwinner is increasingly 'out of date' (*ibid.*: 13). The problem is that a universalised adult worker model no more fits the social reality than did the male breadwinner model of the past. It is the new 'ought to be' but much less the new 'is'.

Part of the new political ideal is to promote social inclusion, but part of the ideal is also that wages will enable more self-provision in the social arena (especially in respect of pensions). There are signs that ideas about the new welfare contract are moving from social contributions to individually defined contributions, premised on the idea that all adults are in the workforce. But this is an especially unreal assumption for women, given the unequal gendered division of unpaid care work and the fact that a disproportionate number of women are employed in low-paid, part-time, often care-related jobs. These shifts are most apparent in the UK among Western European countries, although the Netherlands has also moved with considerable speed away from one of the strictest male breadwinner regimes. The Scandinavian countries moved consciously to a more individualised adult worker model a generation ago, and in many other Western European countries the old employment contract based on the needs of a man in regular lifetime employment is also under question (Supiot 1999).

An adult breadwinner model may have more to offer women than policies based on male breadwinner assumptions. However, given the social reality of women's – and especially mothers' – lesser involvement in paid work and greater responsibility for unpaid work, it has the potential to raise new threats to their welfare unless issues to do with the unequal gendered division of work and hence of lifetime earnings are addressed.

During the last quarter of the twentieth century, research has revealed the extent to which the male breadwinner system no longer described behaviour for a significant proportion of families in Britain (Crompton 1999). In 1975, according to the General Household Survey, 81 per cent of British men aged 16–64 were economically active and 62 per cent of women. By 1996, this figure was 70 per cent for both men and women (ONS 1998: tables 5.8 and 5.9). But the precise nature of the erosion of the male breadwinner model, in Britain as elsewhere, is complicated. There has been no simple move from a male breadwinner to a dual-career model. Rather, in most Western countries some kind of dual-breadwinner model has become the norm. Often, given women's lower earnings and shorter working hours, this amounts to a more or less one and a half earner model.

This one and a half breadwinner model seems to describe the case in Britain. While the rate of married women's participation in the labour market increased hugely in the postwar period (from 47 per cent of women aged 16–59 in 1961 to 72 per cent in 1996), as Catherine Hakim (1996) has pointed out, almost as many women were employed full-time in 1951 as in 1981 (30.3 per cent aged 20–64, as opposed to 31.6 per cent). Almost half of women workers are employed part-time. Only 8 per cent of men worked part-time in 1998, and most of these were either elderly or students, whereas 44 per cent of women did so (Thair and Risdon 1999). Furthermore, almost a quarter of women with children under 10 work fifteen hours or less per week (*ibid.*), and 23.7 per cent of all female employees work less than twenty hours a week (Rubery *et al.* 1998). Similarly, while the proportion of men's hourly wages earned by women who were working full-time rose from 63 per cent in 1970 to 80 per cent in 1995, the hourly wage rate of part-time women workers compared with male workers narrowed by only six percentage points over the same period and actually worsened relative to full-time women workers (Walby 1997: tables 2.4 and 2.6). By 1996/97, women's contribution to a couple's joint lifetime earnings ranged from 41 per cent for a low-skilled woman without children to 49 per cent for a high-skilled woman without children, but it dropped to 24 and 47 per cent, respectively, with the addition of two children. This finding reflects the large earnings gap between equally skilled men and women due to motherhood, and which hits low-skilled women particularly hard (Women's Unit 1999).

The gendered division of labour is still manifestly unequal in Britain, as in most Western countries (see Chapter 4 for the case-type countries of Germany, Spain, Sweden and the USA). Women assume more of the (unpaid) work of care, for children and for dependent adults. While economic activity rates among British mothers have risen rapidly, especially for those with children under 5 (from 40 per cent in 1986 to 54 per cent in 1996), the vast majority of those women work part-time and continue to take major responsibility for childcare. In respect of adult care, representative sample surveys have revealed that the largest category of carers for adults are spouses and that as many as half of these are husbands (Arber and Ginn 1991). Nevertheless, women are the largest group of unpaid carers, and there is substantial evidence to suggest that they do much more by way of intimate personal care tasks. Indeed, when there is a female carer on hand there is less likelihood of formal public care being provided (Lewis 1998). This in turn makes policies based on an assumption that an adult worker model exists problematic. Thus, for example, when the British government swung from treating lone mothers as mothers to treating them as workers in the late 1990s, they did so regardless of the fact that a majority of married mothers actually work part-time.

Policy and contractualism

An adult worker model as a basis for policy making is not necessarily a bad thing for women, given the wider policy assumptions about the extent to which people will have to take more responsibility for providing for themselves, for example in respect of pensions. It all depends on the terms. In all likelihood, it is an improvement on the male breadwinner model, which served to reinforce female economic dependence while failing to recognise and compensate women's role as carers adequately. But problems arise when governments legislate on the basis of an 'ought to be' rather than an 'is', especially when, in the case of women's behaviour in respect of paid and unpaid work, the social reality is so complicated.

In respect of welfare reform, the Labour government's emphasis on 'welfare to work', a minimum wage, labour market activation programmes (such as the New Deals) and making work pay via new tax credit systems has taken forward the idea that all adults, women included, will be employed. The New Deal for Lone Parents made lone mothers part of the welfare-to-work strategy but was not at first made compulsory. However, with the introduction of a single gateway in 2001 combining the Employment

Service and those parts of the Benefits Agency that pay benefits to people of working age, lone mothers' benefits became conditional on an interview. While there is still no requirement that lone mothers become workers, the interview is work-focused. However, only just over half the lone parents attending an initial New Deal interview by December 1999 came from the target group of women with school-age children, who are seen as the most likely to enter the labour market (Millar 2000). As Barlow, Duncan and James point out in Chapter 5, this is likely to reflect the fact that women themselves continue to put caring responsibilities first. As Evans (2001) has remarked, the incentive structures of the British system prioritise the move into work and reinforce the view that welfare to work is a single-point transition. But this is unrealistic, given the nature of many of the jobs on offer and of the care responsibilities that women in particular bear.

The Working Families Tax Credit (WFTC), the centrepiece of Labour's policies to make work pay, seeks to encourage labour market participation, especially by lone mothers, and includes a childcare tax credit. However, its effect on women with partners may be equivocal, because it is administered on the basis of joint earnings and may thus reduce the incentive for partnered women to take low-paid jobs (Rake 2001; McLaughlin *et al.* 2001). In fact, as Lister (2000) has pointed out, policy may still be confused about the extent to which women are in the end conceptualised as being fully individualised. Both increased means testing and the move towards tax/benefit integration work in the opposite direction to individualisation and the promotion of an adult worker model. Thus, the New Deal for the Partners of the Unemployed (mainly women) treats them both as having an independent relationship to the labour market and as dependants. Their access to the programme is dependent on their being the partner of an unemployed man. Thus, while ideas about individualisation are clearly expressed, it is still assumed that married women can depend on their husbands as and when necessary.

Policies to address the issue of unpaid work are less coherent and less well funded than those addressing the issue of increasing labour market participation in the UK. This remains the case, even though the very existence of something like the National Childcare Strategy marks a significant departure for a country that has, since 1945, denied a role for the state in reconciling family and workplace responsibilities (Hantrais and Letablier 1996). The childcare tax credit, introduced as part of the WFTC, meets 70 per cent of the cost of care for one child to a maximum of £100, or £150 for two. It is aimed mainly at lone mothers; partnered parents are eligible only if both are in work. It also assumes that employment precedes childcare, whereas the process of arranging work and childcare tends to be chicken and egg for the women involved. Other European countries have much more developed cash benefits and services for the care of children (*ibid.*).

The danger is that new assumptions regarding an adult worker model will underpin further moves towards an individual contractualism that overestimates women's economic independence and capacity for self-provision and insists on an unfair reciprocity that ignores the unpaid care work that must be done and that many women (and some men) wish to do (see Chapters 5, 6, 12 and 13).

References

Arber, S. and Ginn, J. (1991) *Gender and Later Life*, London: Sage.

Beck, U. and Beck-Gernsheim, E. (1995) *The Normal Chaos of Love*, Cambridge: Polity Press.

Beck-Gernsheim, E. (1999) 'On the way to a post-familial family. From a community of need to elective affinities', *Theory, Culture and Society* 15 (3–4): 53–70.

CEC (1993) *Growth, Competitiveness and Employment. The Challenges and Ways forward into the 21st Century*, Luxembourg: Commission of the European Communities.

—— (1995) *Equal Opportunities for Women and Men*, follow-up to the White Paper on Growth, Competitiveness and Employment. Brussels: Commission of the European Communities, DG-V.

Cmnd 3805 (1998) *New Ambitions for our Country. A New Contract for Welfare*, London: Stationery Office.

Crompton, R. (ed.) (1999) *Restructuring Gender Relationships and Employment. The Decline of the Male Breadwinner*, Oxford: Oxford University Press.

Evans, M. (2001) 'Welfare to work and the organisation of opportunity. Lessons from abroad', CASE Report 15. London: London School of Economics.

Hakim, C. (1996) *Key Issues in Women's Work*, London: Athlone Press.

Hantrais, L. and Letablier, M.-T. (1996) *Families and Family Policies in Europe*, London: Longman.

Lewis, J. (ed.) (1998) *Gender, Social Care and Welfare State Restructuring in Europe*, Aldershot: Ashgate.

Lister, R. (2000) 'Overview of UK welfare reform', paper presented to US/UK Welfare Reform Seminar, University of Bath, May 2–5.

McLaughlin, E., Tewsdale, J. and McCay, N. (2001) 'The rise and fall of the UK's first tax credit: The Working Families Tax Credit, 1998–2000', *Social Policy and Administration* 35(2): 163–80.

Millar, J. (2000) *Keeping Track of Welfare Reform. The New Deal Programmes*, York: Joseph Rowntree Foundation.

ONS (1998) *Living in Britain: Results from the 1996 General Household Survey*, London: Stationery Office.

Rake, K. (2001) 'Gender and New Labour's social policies', *Journal of Social Policy* 30(2): 209–32.

Rubery, J., Smith, M. and Fagan, C. (1998) National working-time regimes and equal opportunities, *Feminist Economics* 4(1): 71–101.

Supiot, A. (1999) *Au-dela de l'Emploi*, Paris: Flammarion.

Thair, T. and Risdon, A. (1999) 'Women in the labour market. Results from the Spring 1998 LFS', *Labour Market Trends* (March): 103–27.

Walby, S. (1997) *Gender Transformations*, London: Routledge.

Women's Unit (1999) *Women's Individual Income 1996/7*, London: Cabinet Office.

3 Political intervention and family policy in Britain

3.2 The Family Law Act, 1996

Adrian James

> Pending full implementation of the Act, core features of the divorce process survive unchanged since the passage of the first Matrimonial Causes Act of 1857.
>
> Advisory Board on Family Law 2000: 5

The story of the law relating to divorce in England and Wales has been well documented (see, for example, Allan 1991; Burgoyne *et al.* 1988; Goldthorpe 1987; James and Wilson 1986; Phillips 1988; Stone 1990), and there have been many important changes since the Matrimonial Causes Act of 1857. However, as the above quotation makes clear, some of the main features of the divorce process have remained unchanged for nearly a century and a half, a situation that the Family Law Act 1996 (hereafter referred to as the Act) was intended to address. However, the fact that the Advisory Board on Family Law (ABFL) felt compelled to make this observation is, perhaps, indicative of a degree of frustration about the difficulties of implementing the Act.

The ABFL was established by the Lord Chancellor to provide him with independent advice on the implementation of the Act, which he recognised would be a difficult and lengthy process, not least because two of the key components of the Act – the provision of information to those wishing to divorce prior to the formal commencement of proceedings and the provision of publicly funded mediation – were to be subjected to extensive independent evaluation prior to being implemented. However, it also became clear, not least because of strong opposition from self-appointed defenders of 'family values' during the passage of the Bill, that making fundamental changes to those core features of divorce that had remained unchanged for so long would be a politically sensitive process. The aim of this section is to identify the principal assumptions underpinning the government's policy and to suggest some reasons why these assumptions may yet prove to be the downfall of the Act.

Part I of the Act spells out the principles that underpin its main provisions, which clearly embody and reflect the government's thinking, *viz.*:

- The institution of marriage should be supported.
- Couples who are contemplating divorce should be encouraged to take all practicable steps, including marriage counselling, to save their marriage.
- Marriages that have irretrievably broken down should be ended with minimum distress to the parents and children, in a manner designed to promote as good a continuing relationship between the parties and any children affected as is possible, without incurring unreasonable costs in ending the marriage.
- Any risk of violence to the parties or children of a marriage should, in so far as is reasonably practicable, be removed or diminished.

In framing this legislation, therefore, the government sought to address a wide range of concerns. Foremost among these was addressing the problem of the high divorce rate by bolstering the institution of marriage, which was seen by the government as the only proper foundation for the family (a view subsequently made explicit in the Supporting Families Green Paper; see Chapter 3.3). In addition, however, there was also growing pressure to introduce a number of reforms: these were intended to make the divorce process less damaging; to protect the welfare of children in such situations; to lessen the amount of conflict so often associated with divorce; to improve the protection of women and children against domestic violence; and, permeating all of these concerns, to lessen the cost of divorce to the taxpayer. The government therefore faced the unenviable task of framing legislation that would reconcile these disparate objectives without also being seen to be making divorce easier.

This wide-ranging agenda emerged from certain significant developments from the mid-70s onwards, a period in which the divorce rate climbed steadily. Important among these was the progressive reform of the divorce law during this period, making it increasingly an administrative as opposed to a judicial process, in conjunction with the development of the mediation movement (James 1990). This sought to encourage parents to agree on how to resolve disputes arising from divorce, to promote mediation as the preferred method of dealing with such issues, and to persuade successive governments of the effectiveness of such an approach, as well as its social and economic benefits. The unfolding of these arguments can be charted through the work of the Law Commission (1988, 1990), which led to the publication of a consultation paper (Lord Chancellor's Department 1993). This was followed eighteen months later by the government's proposals (Lord Chancellor's Department 1995), which led directly to the framing of the Bill that was introduced in November of that year and eventually reached the statute book on 4 July 1996.

Part IV of the Act, which brought together provisions for dealing with domestic violence and regulating the occupation of the family home into a single set of civil remedies, was introduced (with Part I) without demur in October 1997. However, the remainder of the Act contained major innovations that were more contentious, having been the focus of heated debate during the passage of the Bill through Parliament. In particular, Part II contained the most hotly contested innovation – the final and complete removal of the concept of fault from divorce by making irretrievable breakdown, to be demonstrated by the passage of a defined period of time after the filing of a statement of the breakdown of a marriage, the sole ground for divorce. The government consequently decided to pilot the key provisions contained in Parts II and III and to evaluate their impact before finally implementing the remainder of the Act.

Two main mechanisms incorporated into the Act were designed to achieve the ambitious objectives that supported this fundamental reform of the divorce process – information meetings and publicly funded mediation. The Act made information meetings a necessary precursor to the formal commencement of divorce proceedings. They reflected the view that 'the system should require divorcing couples to consider carefully the consequences and implications of divorce … [which] should not be so easy that the parties have little incentive to make a success of their marriage' (LCD 1995: para. 3.1, p.17). It was therefore envisaged that everyone contemplating divorce should be required to receive information, presented both verbally and in writing, about the availability of services such as marriage guidance, as well as family mediation, legal advice, the likely cost of these services and their eligibility for state funding.

This provision was seen as a means of encouraging people to consider whether divorce was the best course of action, of ensuring that everybody had access to the same kinds of information about divorce and related matters, and to raise awareness of support services. Although it was clearly regarded as important to promote information about marriage guidance, the intention was also clearly 'to encourage couples to consider family mediation rather than arm's length negotiation through lawyers or litigation' (*ibid.*: para. 7.7, pp.57–8). The process of piloting information meetings, in the course of which a range of different models and methods were to be considered, commenced in 1997.

Publicly funded mediation was provided for in Part III of the Act. This was implemented in March 1997 in order to allow the proposed arrangements to be piloted by the Legal Aid Board (now the Legal Services Commission). As a result of its consultations, the government had concluded that 'Mediation should not be compulsory, but … there should be a definite encouragement to couples to use family mediation' (*ibid.*: para. 5.21, pp.42–3). The reasoning behind this conclusion was that couples might not seek mediation without such 'encouragement'; that marriages that were capable of being saved were more likely to be identified through mediation than through the legal process; that spouses should be encouraged to take responsibility for the breakdown of their marriage and to minimise any bitterness and hostility associated with this; and that couples should be encouraged to look to their post-divorce responsibilities as parents. The Act therefore required applicants seeking legally aided legal representation in divorce proceedings (with certain exceptions, such as in cases where the existence of domestic violence was seen to make mediation inappropriate) to attend a meeting with a mediator in order to assess their suitability for mediation.

It was the responsibility of the Legal Aid Board to pilot a rolling programme for the introduction of these provisions, phase I of which began in March 1997. The pilot not only sought to identify the most appropriate form of contracting with providers but was also intended to ensure the availability of a range of different suppliers of mediation, including the not-for-profit sector and lawyer providers, with coverage in all areas of England and Wales by the end of the pilot period. The entire process was to be evaluated independently, with particular attention being given to assessing the cost-effectiveness of mediation and its impact on the legal costs associated with divorce, since this was effectively the first time that public money had been made available to support mediation in divorce.

The government's expectation was that the combined effect of these provisions would mean that more couples would be diverted from seeking divorce into reconciliation; that more of those who wished to continue with divorce would do so through mediation rather than legal representation and litigation; that mediation would prove to be cheaper and more cost-effective than other options; and that the combined effects of these changes would represent a saving on the public purse.

However, it is clear that the government's assumptions about the way the public would respond were oversimplified and that people appear reluctant to accept this new approach to divorce. The reasons for this are complex and, until both reports have been published, it would be premature to seek to explain why the pilots have not had the effect hoped for by the government. However, the ABFL believes that part of the explanation for this is that 'the way in which, for good practical reasons, the Act has been implemented has led to a lack of nexus between the mediation provisions in Part III and the more fundamental changes in Part II' – in other words, that the pilot information meetings were not coordinated with the mediation pilots.

However, the evidence published to date suggests that the reasons are more complex than this and that part of the explanation lies in the fact that there are deep-seated aspects of professional culture and social attitudes that have so far proved resistant to fundamental change. Thus, for example, there is evidence of considerable resistance from within the legal profession to both publicly funded mediation and information meetings (Davis 1999: 633; McCarthy 2000: 551). As McCarthy reports, 'The interim results showed that only 7 per cent of those attending an information meeting went on to attend mediation' (2000: 553), although a much higher proportion indicated that they would be willing to consider mediation later on in the process.

The evidence also suggests that the majority of people assume they need, and prefer to give precedence to obtaining, legal advice rather than mediation. Indeed, 39 per cent of those who attended meetings were more likely to want to seek advice from a solicitor than if they had not attended a meeting (Lord Chancellor's Department 1999). Recent research on the work of solicitors in divorce (Eekelaar *et al.* 2000) has revealed the complexity of such work, but it also provides strong evidence of why the role of the solicitor is so highly valued by so many. As Davis (1999: 634) argues:

> Lawyers provide partisan support, coupled with an authoritative account of the norms of legal settlement – both of which are valued ... The provision of public funding for mediation has not, to date, altered this picture ... if mediation is conceived as an alternative to lawyer negotiation it is an alternative that appeals to only a minority.

It also seems clear that most of those attending the pilot information meetings found them useful: 'immediately following an information meeting, the majority of parents reported feeling better informed about various topics relating to children, including how divorce affects children, family mediation and family court welfare services' (Richards and Stark 2000: 485). However, information meetings do not appear to have been successful as part of a marriage-saving policy. Indeed, only 13 per cent of those attending took up the offer of attending a meeting with a marriage counsellor. Less than half of these did so with the hope of saving their marriage (Lord Chancellor's Department 1999), and it seems likely that interventions designed to achieve this need to be made available at an earlier point in the marriage (McCarthy *et al.* 2000).

It is evident that the Act represented an attempt to use the law to influence social behaviour, and it has been criticised as a form of social engineering (Eekelaar 1999), even though the information meetings pilot steered away from overt persuasion and the mediation pilot did not involve compulsion. In its present form, the Act offers 'no guarantee that couples will be influenced to change their behaviour if only one party receive[s] the information' (Walker 2000: 334), an observation that is also of relevance to the lower than expected take-up of mediation, which also depends on the engagement of both parties and which the Act, in its current form, has so far failed to deliver: 'in the absence of coercion, or of a major cultural change, mediation is a minority choice' (Davis 1999: 634). Arguably, this is because the Act failed to acknowledge the complex nature of the decisions made by individuals facing marital breakdown. It therefore seems likely that the use of some degree of compulsion may have to be part of any measures introduced if the changes desired by the government are to be achieved.

The failure of the Act in this respect has been recognised by the Advisory Board on Family Law (2000), which acknowledges that:

> simply amending the law is insufficient to bring about the change of culture implicit in such an approach ... The underlying philosophy of the Act is very different to that which people have grown accustomed to,

> and it is to be expected that it will take time and careful advocacy to lead to its general acceptance.
>
> para. 2.5, p.6

As a consequence of the government's disappointment over the outcome of the pilot studies, in January 2001 the Lord Chancellor announced that the remainder of the Act would not be implemented. The government has indicated that it remains committed to the principles behind the Act, which continues to command widespread support among interested professionals (see Thorpe and Clarke 2000). However, the apparent lack of public support for the proposals contained in the Act must now mean that the future shape of any changes is increasingly uncertain, especially in view of the traditional political sensitivity associated with divorce law reform. As the Lord Chancellor's Advisory Board commented shortly before the announcement of the non-implementation of the Act:

> there remains a strong sense of unfinished business and uncertainty over the future, and if this is to be dispelled, it will be necessary to develop and publish a strategy that matches public advocacy of these principles to their practical implementation in the law.
>
> *ibid.*: para. 2.6, p.6

In the light of the government's decision not to proceed with the implementation of the Act, that sense of uncertainty and unfinished business is now even more pronounced and the challenge set down by the ABFL remains. However, as part of formulating such a strategy, it is essential to take account of the growing body of research that details the lives of those facing divorce, the complexity of the decisions they face and the many factors that influence the choices they make (see for example Neale and Smart, Chapter 9, this volume). Policies and policy makers tend to abstract issues from the micro-contexts of behaviour and thus to ignore the many and often quite subtle variations in the definitions, emotions and motivations that come into play in such potentially fraught situations as marital breakdown and divorce. Any political strategy relating to law, no matter how well it matches principles to practical proposals for implementation, is doomed to fail if it does not take adequate account of research into such issues. This is one of the central themes of this book.

References

Advisory Board on Family Law (2000) Third Annual Report. London: Lord Chancellor's Department.

Allan, G. (1991) *Family Life*, Oxford: Basil Blackwell.

Burgoyne, J., Ormrod, R. and Richards, M. (1988) *Divorce Matters*, Harmondsworth: Penguin.

Davis, G. (1999) 'Monitoring publicly funded mediation', *Family Law* 29: 625–35.

Eekelaar, J. (1999) 'Family law: keeping us "on message"', *Child and Family Law Quarterly* 11: 387–96.

Eekelaar, J., Maclean, M. and Beinart, S. (2000) *Family Lawyers: The Divorce Work of Solicitors*, Oxford: Hart Publishing.

Goldthorpe, J. (1987) *Family Life in Western Society*, Cambridge: Cambridge University Press.

James, A. (1990) 'Conciliation and social change', in T. Fisher (ed.) *Family Conciliation Within the UK: Policy and Practice*, Bristol: Family Law.

James, A. and Wilson, K. (1986) *Couples, Conflict and Change*, London: Tavistock.

Law Commission (1988) *Facing the Future: A Discussion Paper on the Ground for Divorce*, Law Commission No. 170. London: HMSO.

—— (1990) *Family Law: Ground for Divorce*, Law Commission No. 192. London: HMSO.

Lord Chancellor's Department (1993) *Looking to the Future: Mediation and the Ground for Divorce: A Consultation Paper*, Cmnd 2424. London: HMSO.

—— (1995) *Looking to the Future: Mediation and the Ground for Divorce: The Government's Proposals*, Cmnd 2799. London: HMSO.

—— (1999) *Information Meetings and Associated Provisions within the Family Law Act 1996: Summary of Research in Progress, June 1999*, London: Lord Chancellor's Department

McCarthy, P. (2000) 'Providing information – the views of professionals', *Family Law* 30: 550–4.

McCarthy, P., Walker, J. and Hooper, D. (2000) 'Saving marriage – a role for divorce law?' *Family Law* 30: 412–16.

Phillips, R. (1988) *Putting Asunder: A History of Divorce in Western Society*, Cambridge: Cambridge University Press.

Richards, M. and Stark, C. (2000) 'Children, parenting and information meetings', *Family Law* 30, 484–8.

Stone, L. (1990) *The Road to Divorce: England 1530–1987*, Oxford: Oxford University Press.

Thorpe, L.J. and Clarke, E. (2000) *No Fault or Flaw: The Future of the Family Law Act 1996*, Bristol: Family Law.

Walker, J. (2000) 'Information meetings revisited', *Family Law* 30: 330–4.

3 Political intervention and family policy in Britain

3.3 The Green Paper *Supporting Families*, 1998

Mavis Maclean

In October 1998, the government published a Green Paper for discussion entitled *Supporting Families*, Britain's first formal governmental family policy statement. It covered a wide range of issues, encompassing the work and interests of a number of government departments. The chapters were divided into services and support for parents, financial support for families, the balance between home and work, and better support for serious family problems. So many different expectations awaited this publication that it could never have satisfied all comers. In retrospect, however, compared with the policy implications of a political landscape that had lacked integrated family policy statements of any kind, this Green Paper is worth re-examining and merits at least qualified enthusiasm.

The revival of political interest in the family stems from the early 1980s when, as the welfare state began to roll back, the family was required to fill the space. As the ideas of the Conservative government's Family Policy Group began to filter through to the national press, we heard of concerns about the break-up of the traditional family associated with a high rate of divorce and increasing numbers of one-parent families, and at the same time a determination in government that the family, not the state, should provide 'welfare'. Malcolm Wicks (1987), then director of the independent Family Policy Studies Centre, which collated information and offered valuable commentary, had to admit that the family 'always was the main source of welfare'. The then Conservative Prime Minister Margaret Thatcher, in a speech to a women's voluntary association, the WRVS, at its annual conference in 1981, said:

> it all really starts in the family, because not only is the family the most important means through which we show our care for others ... it's the place where each generation learns its responsibilities towards the rest of society. Statutory services can only play their part successfully if we don't expect them to do things for us that we could be doing for ourselves.

This was the period when Ferdinand Mount (1982) referred to the Stalinist powers of health visitors, the public health nurses who have a statutory right to enter the homes of young children to check their health and development; the 'nanny state' was anathematised, and the absence of an official family policy was in effect a very clear policy of privatisation of care.

Since 1997, we have had a New Labour government that takes pride in its family policy, and indeed it would be difficult now for any government to contemplate a policy approach that offers to do anything except support families. The difficulty lies in what is meant by a family, and what kind of support is to be offered to which kind of family groups. Under New Labour, we have moved on from the privatisation of the 1980s, but it is not yet clear how much change there has been or how much more can be expected. It is perhaps surprising that the impetus for change has come, with the energetic support of the Prime Minister, from the Home Office, with its responsibility for public order, the police and prison services, where Jack Straw as Home Secretary has taken a close interest in the matter. We might perhaps have expected the Department of Health, with its longstanding interest in child welfare, to be at the forefront, or even the Lord Chancellor's Department, which has a Family Policy Division and through family law reform has had a major impact on family life over the last twenty years. The introduction of no-fault divorce in 1970, the abolition of illegitimacy in 1987, the Children Act taken forward jointly with the Department of Health in 1989, and most recently the child support legislation of 1991, have altered the landscape for what Dame Brenda Hale described in a lecture for the Economic and Social Research Council (1997) as the key points in family life, 'hatching, matching and dispatching'. The Home Office interest in family support springs from its interest in juvenile delinquency and thus in approaching the family as an ally in the battle for social control. Social order and a cohesive society, it is hoped, may be achieved through stable family life and full adult participation in the labour market.

This administrative origin within the Home Office, among policies for social control rather than social welfare, is a little worrying, but let us be positive and look in detail at what the Green Paper puts forward. What kind of family is discussed? Is it the kind of family depicted in advertisements for healthy foods, particularly breakfast cereals, the model beloved of the Conservative administration of the 1980s, with a male breadwinner, domestic mother and two children? Or are other forms of family life included in the New Labour perspective? Does the Green Paper take account of serial partnership and cross-household parenting obligations? What of care for the elderly, and alternative forms of household among ethnic minority families?

On page 52 of *Supporting Families* we are told that 'children come first', that they need stability, that governments help and support but do not replace parents, and that all families are included. Parenting lies at the heart of the policy. This is good news in that it encompasses a wider spectrum of family experience than the earlier breakfast cereal model. One-parent families and families with members in different households are not excluded, and parental relationships are not always expected to coincide with marriage. In this the policy chimes with the underlying assumptions of the Children Act 1989, which introduced the concept of parental responsibility, irrespective of the legal relationship between the parents. But an element of social control is also present. Parents are referred to as the source of stability as well as nurture.

The practical proposals – including the setting up of the National Family and Parenting Institute to give authoritative advice to parents in the context of academic arguments often reported in the popular press, such as whether or not divorce has detrimental effects on children – have already had an impact and will continue to develop. But the funding of a parent telephone helpline again indicates the adoption of an underlying rational actor model, which is no longer regarded as viable by experts in the area (see, for example, Barlow and Duncan 2000; see also Chapter 5). But at least health visitors are no longer described as Stalinist, and the partnership between volunteers and new parents in the Sure Start scheme has every chance of working well where there is a good infrastructure. The financial support may be the key part of the package, in particular the Working Families Tax Credit and the New Deal for Lone Parents. The achievement of redistribution towards children in poor households is becoming a more openly acknowledged aspect of policy and may yet become a major election issue. The Labour Party opened its election campaign on 13 March 2001 with a letter to party members from the Chancellor, Gordon Brown, itemising a children's tax credit worth £500 per year for most families, combined with maternity pay of £75 for twenty-six weeks and two weeks paid leave for new fathers.

The first term of office of the New Labour government has been a fascinating time for policy analysts, as we watched a government of whom much was expected delivering a considerable part of its family policy by stealth and finding ways of packaging its policies in ways that are considered by the spin doctors to be acceptable to the voters in potentially marginal constituencies. This administration has taken a long-term approach to staying in power. I would argue that the Green Paper indicates a serious move towards being inclusive of a variety of family situations and begins to appreciate that individuals do not enter a family-type box and stay there. Every household is in a state of change and development. Today's lone parent is tomorrow's second wife. Every child in poverty will grow up and may become a low earner. The language employed is often that of social control, but the underlying values have moved a long way towards being positive about diversity in family life.

It is also fascinating to see the developing convergence of policy through the different sources of government activity, including penal policy, economic policy and family law reform. The often-voiced aim of government to develop a more cohesive, less fragmented approach to policy, in what is termed 'joined-up government', does indeed begin to acquire credibility as it becomes clear that child support is another way of looking at child poverty and pension splitting is part of female labour market participation and the male breadwinner model.

In the family law sections of the Green Paper, those with which I am most familiar, there are a number of encouraging paragraphs. The section 4.44–49 on making financial arrangements after divorce recognises the problems associated with the length of time currently taken to make these kinds of arrangement and argues for greater clarity and certainty for those approaching divorce by developing a number of guiding principles. Furthermore, the principles chosen reflect the excellent research carried out in this field over the last decade. The first principle is 'to promote the welfare of any child of the family under the age of 18 by meeting the housing needs of the children and the primary carer, and of the secondary carer, both to facilitate contact and to recognise the continuing importance of the secondary carer's role'. This represents a very careful assessment of whose interests come first, what these needs are, and how these mesh with the needs of both parents whether or not they have been married to each other or anyone else. The second principle is 'to take into account the existence and content of any written agreement about financial arrangements reached before or during marriage', again a measured approach to the topic of prenuptial agreements, showing an awareness of and attempt to deal with the acrimonious debate among lawyers that had arisen when the topic was first raised by the government. This principle is developed in detail, declaring that, having dealt with the needs of the children and the housing needs of the couple, the court would divide any surplus so as to achieve a fair result, recognising that fairness will generally require the value of the assets to be divided equally between the parties.

The final principle deals with the vexed issue of the clean break by declaring in favour of terminating financial relationships between the parties at the earliest practicable date. Defining this date remains problematic, but the previous principles give a clear indication that the needs of the children would be a primary factor, followed by the housing needs of both parents. The proposal reflects the strange British custom of investing all our resources in bricks and mortar and might look odd to a continental European accustomed to a flexible private rented sector or a substantial public rental sector. But this is not the place to consider the emerging issue of harmonisation of family policy in Europe.

The Green Paper goes on to discuss the provision of advice to couples entering or leaving marriage in a very proactive way, again revealing rational actor assumptions that are untested and unlikely to stand up to empirical investigation. But given a choice between the tough privatisation of the previous Conservative administration and a rather zealous 'do-gooding' that includes a concerted attack on child poverty presented as incentives to work, on balance the present strategy of 'tough love' is not so bad.

References

Barlow, A. and Duncan, S. (2000) 'New Labour's communitarianism and the rationality mistake', *Journal of Social Welfare and Family Law* 22(2): 129–43.
Hale, B. (1997) 'Private lives and public duties', Economic and Social Research Council annual lecture. Swindon: ESRC.
Mount, F. (1982) *The Subversive Family*, London: Jonathan Cape.
Wicks, M. (1987) *A Future for All*, Harmondsworth: Pelican Books.

3 Political intervention and family policy in Britain

3.4 Re-analysing the Black family

Tracey Reynolds

Introduction

The Black family in Britain continues to be under intense public scrutiny.[1] For example, during the media coverage of the Lawrence Inquiry in 1998, the Black family, in particular common-sense perceptions of it by the White majority, was once again in the media spotlight. However, the media coverage of the Lawrence family differed from the traditional negative representation of the Black family. The fact that the murdered teenager Stephen Lawrence came from a 'normal' (i.e. married, two-parent) family, and that somehow this made the Lawrence family different from the majority of problematical Black families in Britain, was continually emphasised.

Generally, the Black family in Britain has traditionally been recognised as a singularly female-headed household, with Black men occupying a marginal or absent role in the family as a result of Black women's dominant status. This therefore positions the Black family outside the normative understanding of the ideal family structure: married, two-parent, heterosexual households. Social research and policy investigating Black families in post-industrial societies such as Britain and the USA has focused attention on statistical evidence showing that today in Britain 51 per cent of Black families are female-headed. Such debates have acted to reify female-headed households as the sole family structure that Black people remain in during their lifetime (see Berthoud 2001). This tendency in research and policy debates to present Black, female-headed households as the unitary Black family model disguises the fluid and adaptive nature of Black family relationships and living arrangements and also the fact that, similar to families in other racial and ethnic groups, the Black family has diverse family and household patterns. This chapter aims to redress this imbalance in the literature by exploring the adapting and multiple Black family forms, household structures and family relationships.

The Black family in context: current concepts, themes and ideas

In the USA, policy makers examining the primary cause of poverty and deprivation across Black communities have explicitly attributed this to the high number of female-headed households. W.J. Wilson's (1997) study of Black family life points to the way that poverty has encouraged the displacement of Black men from the family. Unable to fulfil the traditional role of primary economic provider, Black men are therefore forced to live outside the family household. Ironically, female-headed Black households fall further into poverty because Black women's lower earning potential as a result of gender and racial inequalities in society leads to reduced family income and the greater potential for family poverty (Taylor *et al.* 1997). Policy makers in the USA have also linked high rates of welfare expenditure to the high incidence of female-headed households in the Black community. 'Welfare queen' and 'baby mamma' are explicitly racialised terms that have been used by policy makers and the media in the USA to position poor and Black female-headed households as 'undeserving' recipients of social welfare (Hill Collins 1998). The general consensus by right-wing and conservative commentators such as Charles Murray (1998) is that welfare benefits like Aid to Families and Dependent Children (AFDC), Medicaid, food stamps and public housing have directly caused the breakdown of the family and encouraged Black women to set up female-headed households.

By the mid-1990s, welfare spending in the USA had reached a new height with over 5 million families in receipt of AFDC. This resulted in increased calls, led primarily by the New Right conservatives, to reform welfare so that the primary responsibility for economic provision for poor families was returned to the family and increasingly removed from state hands. In 1996, the Personal Responsibility and Work Opportunity Reconciliation Act ended AFDC and introduced Transitional Aid to Needy Families (TANF). Alan Deacon (see Chapter 4.4) charts the shift in US welfare strategy during this period and the way that this marked a firm commitment by state and federal governments in the USA to create a new culture in which welfare receipt was viewed by those eligible for benefits as a temporary and transitory measure (i.e. while seeking employment or work-related training) and not as long-term permanent assistance. As a consequence, the new programme aimed to reduce the perceived benefits afforded to lone mothers under AFDC and shift the onus back on to the family, and in particular men, for economic responsibility for the family. Stringent new guidelines ensured that people previously eligible for benefits under AFDC were now denied benefits under TANF, and greater control of benefits made it easier to withhold or withdraw benefits to lone mothers. Deacon recognises that conservative policy makers' concern over the breakdown of the family, and in particular the Black family, formed the basis of these welfare reforms. Such an identification of the Black family as being on the point of collapse reifies its status as the 'undeserved'. So successful have right-wing policy makers been in the construction of Black people as the 'undeserving' recipients of welfare that they have been able to control the level of welfare provision given to poor Black people in the USA and reinforce a pathological viewpoint of Black family life (Gilens 1999). Indeed, this perceived exploitation of the welfare system by Black people has proved to be a 'vote catcher' for the last three Republican presidents (Ronald Reagan, George Bush and George W. Bush). This is despite extensive research showing that there is no direct link between the level of welfare provision to Black single mothers and the number of female-headed Black households in the USA (Moffit 1992).

The racial stereotyping of Black families, and particularly of female-headed Black households who are dependent on the state for welfare provision, also holds true for policy makers in Britain. However, in contrast to the USA, this racial stereotyping of Black lone-mother households is far subtler and occurs at an implicit level. Ann Phoenix (1996) identifies that there is an underlying moral and racialised context to policy makers' viewpoints concerning the 'deserving' and 'undeserving' recipients of social welfare, and that Black lone-mother households fall into the latter category. Policy attempts to reduce welfare expenditure on family income have been primarily thought of with the 'undeserving' households in mind. With regards to the 'undeserving' lone mother, a racialised Black identity is immediately assumed, so there is no need to refer to it explicitly in policy.

Two policies introduced during the 1990s and involving government intervention in family life to reduce welfare expenditure certainly support this view. In 1991, the Child Support Agency (CSA) was set up to monitor and legally enforce absent fathers' financial contributions towards their families while reducing the state's contribution to the family. Although the CSA acts as a universalistic system of obtaining financial provision from absent fathers, the disproportionate numbers of Black and other ethnic minority fathers who have been investigated by the agency suggest that there is a racial context to this policy (Hylton 1996).

A second policy initiative introduced during the latter half of the 1990s similarly enforced an implicit understanding of the 'undeserving' Black family. The New Deal for Lone Parents (NDLP) was set up in 1998 to offer advice and information to low-income single parents on training, financial incentives and affordable childcare provision so that they could (re)enter the labour market. While Black mothers have traditionally shown high rates of economic activity through full-time paid work, in recent years there has been an increase in unemployment among Black mothers under the age of 25 (Berthoud 2001; Reynolds 2001). On the one hand, various researchers have suggested that this increased rate of unemployment among young Black mothers represents a wider trend in 'Black youth' unemployment in Britain, whereby 30 per cent of Black women between the ages of 16 and 24 are currently unemployed (CRE 1997; Berthoud 1999). On the other hand, there is an (as yet underdeveloped) viewpoint that young Black mothers' reluctance to engage in full-time employment on the same scale as older Black mothers represents their support of a 'gendered moral rationality' that identifies moral costs to the children and family as a consequence of mothers working full-time (see Duncan and Edwards 1999).

Regardless of the differing rationales underpinning decreasing employment activity by young Black single mothers, policy makers in Britain have used the common perception of the welfare-dependent Black lone mother to their advantage. Despite Black people's minority status in Britain, Black lone mothers assume a highly visible role in the publicity material advertising the NDLP. Indeed, it could be argued that the image of the Black lone mother has acted as an important marketing strategy in publicising the initiative nationwide. By doing so, the notion of the Black single mother and her welfare-dependent household as the primary recipients of benefits is immediately reconfirmed in the public's imagination.[2]

Re-analysing the Black family: female-headed households and phases of family life

Today in Britain, an understanding of the family is no longer restricted to conventional assumptions that simply distinguish between single, nuclear and extended family households (see elsewhere in this book and Silva and Smart 1999). The Black family has been at the forefront of this debate concerning changing and varied understandings of the family primarily because conventional assumptions have never been flexible enough to deal with the many different and 'shifting' existing Black family structures and household patterns. Dorien Powell (1986), writing about the Black family, clearly recognised the dynamic and shifting nature of family relations and provides one of the few studies that offer a flexible and pluralistic understanding of the Black family and household structure. Powell developed a four-part typology of Black family relations to identify the fact that female-headed households are not a static, almost universal, given. Rather, they are one of many family forms, and most Black mothers move through several within their lifetime. The family forms were (1) single (complete absence of male partner); (2) 'common law' (joint residence without legal sanction); (3) married (joint residence and legal sanction); and (4) visiting relationships (those households where the male partner does not reside permanently in the household). The term 'visiting relationship' has its roots in the Caribbean and was first introduced to identify those fathers who lived outside the family household as a result of their inability to provide financially for the family but who were generally considered to be a part of the family by other family members and would regularly visit the family household. In the Caribbean, 'visiting' relationships dominate among the poor and lower social class groups, and the household it produces – female-headed – is considered by writers on the Caribbean as being representative of the adaptive capacities of low-income Black families to survive poverty and economic disadvantage (see Barrow 1996). Writers discussing the Black family in Britain, and in particular the prevalence of 'visiting' relationships among low-income working-class Black households, have applied and adopted these ideas of the correlation between the 'visiting' family patterns and poverty and economic insecurity to a British context (Dench 1996). The historical and cultural links between the Caribbean and Britain as a result of the postwar settlement of Caribbean people in Britain and, more recently, (re)migration and (re)settlement of Black people from Britain to the Caribbean (see Goulbourne and Chamberlain 2001) also make Caribbean family models highly relevant to this discussion.

Nonetheless, the view that female-headed households in Britain simply continue, and evolve from, a Caribbean tradition overlooks the fact that female-headed households are not the universal and singular family structure for Black families across the Caribbean region. Each Caribbean island is culturally distinct, and each island has its own customs, traditions and practices. Some islands, such as Jamaica, have a high prevalence of female-headed households, but even in this country the vast majority of female-headed households exist among the poor and lower social class groups in society, and by and large this reflects a cultural response to their adverse social conditions and circumstances (Pulsiphier 1994). In other Caribbean islands, married two-parent households comprise the largest family structure. For instance, 40 per cent of women in Barbados and 38 per cent of women in Antigua are married and live in 'traditional' nuclear households, compared with 31 per cent in Jamaica (Barrow 1996).

The concentrated focus on female-headed households has been at the cost of ignoring the other Black family forms and household structures that exist. Previous research has revealed and confirmed the sheer multiplicity and diversity of Black family households in Britain. In my own research (Reynolds 1999), a qualitative study of twenty Black mothers living in London, ten of the mothers were married. The remaining ten had family relationships and household structures that ranged from 'single' to 'visiting' to 'common law' relationships. A second study (see Edwards *et al.* 2000) involved me in interviewing a further twenty Black mothers. Again, half of the mothers in this study were in married/'common law' relationships, and half of them lived in a 'visiting' relationship.

Clearly emerging out of each of these two studies was the dynamic and fluid nature of family households, as the mothers moved through different relationships over a period of time. For instance, four out of the ten married mothers in the 1999 study were previously in 'visiting' relationships with their husband prior to marriage. Two of these mothers commented that they primarily saw this period as a 'getting to know you' phase before moving on to a 'common law' relationship and finally a married relationship:

ANITA: After we had the first child, we were spending all of our time together but I was used to my independence. At that stage in our lives I don't think either of us was ready to settle down and live together like man and wife and so we sat down together and decided that he would stay with us some of the time to see how things developed with us.

Obviously things worked out fine for us because we got married in the end.

Anita, aged 43, married; interview from 1999 study

TANYA: I am used to being on my own and doing my own thing and I couldn't ever imagine me being welded to a man's side ... About two years with him living here part-time I thought this isn't so bad and marriage just seemed to be a natural progression.

Tanya, aged 40; interview from 1999 study

The above quotations show that these mothers were not permanently fixed, in some pathological way, into a 'visiting' relationship. Instead, a 'visiting' relationship was considered a way to adjust to a change in their relationship status. Other married and partnered Black mothers that I interviewed moved from 'visiting' to 'common law' to marriage relationships as a consequence of external factors. For example, Maria, interviewed as part of the Edwards *et al.* 2000 study, openly admitted that her transition from 'visiting' to marriage was a result of pressure from her parents, who did not want her to be seen to be conforming to the negative public perceptions of female-headed Black households. Two other mothers from this study attributed their movement from 'visiting' relationship to marriage to changing levels of family income and in particular to the increased level of their partner's contribution to household income. These mothers' previous family arrangements can therefore be viewed as a rational response to their social and economic conditions. Dawn, for example, lived in a 'visiting' relationship with her partner while he was unemployed. It was only when he found a relatively secure job as a car mechanic and could contribute towards the family income that they decided to marry. Similarly, Diane married her partner when he obtained a permanent work contract that offered much greater job security.

These mothers' previous household arrangements (i.e. 'visiting' relationships) show that official statistics and data that record fathers as 'absent' from the household do not always accurately record what is actually occurring in Black family households. There are some, primarily low-income, Black mothers who live in 'visiting' relationships, and many others who have 'common law' relationships yet choose to declare themselves as single-parent households. One explanation for this could be that these mothers are rationally and strategically adapting their behaviour to meet the requirements of the benefit system. However, another reason clearly revealed to me by the mothers in both studies is that mothers who choose to live with their partners in 'visiting' and 'common law' relationships greatly valued the independent and autonomous status that they believe the term 'single' affords them. Thus, although official records tell us that over half of all Black families in Britain are female-headed households, in reality many of these live in two-parent households. Even in instances where the father lives outside the household on a permanent basis, he can still assume an active and participatory role in family life.

Conclusion

In Britain today the sheer variety of family forms makes it increasingly difficult for policy makers to define the family in conventional terms. The Black family offers one example, among many in Britain, of a social and cultural group that has many diverse family structures and household arrangements. Yet traditional definitions of the Black family in Britain and the USA present the female-headed household as a fixed and a unitary Black family structure. In reality, however, this household structure is one of the many stages of family life that Black women continue to move through during their lifetime. This choice of household arrangement is also indicative of these women's rational and strategic response to specific social and economic conditions that they face (for example, poverty).

This brief chapter purposely brings a cultural and racial dimension to the discussion of family practices and household structures in order to counteract the silence in family policy debates concerning the implications of racial and cultural difference for family arrangements in multicultural Britain. Its less than adequate attempts to address this matter primarily rests upon family policy's concentration on relationship form (i.e., marriage versus non-marriage) as opposed to relationship process (the support and commitment by family members as part of their daily lived experiences). It is only when relationship processes take a primary position in debates that family policy will be able to meet the challenge of understanding the multiple and varied family patterns that constitute family life in Britain today.

Notes

1 The term 'Black' in the British context refers specifically to people of African-Caribbean origin.
2 Black feminist writers have also played their part in reinforcing the idea that female-headed households are the primary family structure in Black family life (see Glenn *et al.* 1994).

References

Barrow, C. (1996) *Family in the Caribbean: Themes and Perspectives*, London: James Currey.

Berthoud, R. (1999) *Young Caribbeans and the Labour Market: A Comparison with Other Ethnic Groups*, London: Joseph Rowntree Foundation.

—— R. (2001) 'Family formation in multi-cultural Britain: three patterns of diversity', paper presented at one-day conference, Changing Family Patterns in Multi-cultural Britain. London: National Parenting and Family Institute.

Commission for Racial Equality (CRE) (1997) *Employment and Unemployment Factsheet*, London: CRE.

Dench, G. (1996) *The Place of Men in Changing Family Cultures*, London: Institute of Community Studies.

Duncan, S. and Edwards, R. (1999) *Lone Mothers, Paid Work and Gendered Moral Rationalities*, Basingstoke: Macmillan.

Edwards, R., Duncan, S., Alldred, P. and Reynolds, T. (2000) 'Partnered mothers and paid work', working paper, London: South Bank University.

Gilens, M. (1999) *Why Americans Hate Welfare: Race, Media and the Politics of Antipoverty*, Chicago: University of Chicago Press.

Glenn, E., Chang, G. and Forcey, L. (eds) (1994) *Mothering: Ideology, Experience and Agency*, London: Routledge.

Goulbourne, H. and Chamberlain, M. (eds) (2001) *The Caribbean Family in a Trans-Atlantic World*, London: Macmillan.

Hill Collins, P.H. (1998) *Fighting Words: Black Women and the Search for Justice*, Minneapolis: University of Minnesota Press.

Hylton, C. (1996) *Coping with Change: Family Transitions in Multi-cultural Communities*, London: Exploring Parenthood.

Moffit, R. (1992) 'Incentive effects of the US welfare system: a review', *Journal of Economic Literature*, 30 (March), 1–61.

Murray, C. (1998) untitled chapter in Rye, N. (ed.) *The Future of Welfare*, London: Social Market Foundation.

Phoenix, A. (1996) 'Social construction of lone-motherhood: a case of competing discourses', in E.B. Silva (ed.) *Good Enough Mothering?* London: Routledge.

Powell, D. (1986) 'Caribbean women and their response to familial experiences', in J. Massiah (ed.) *Women in the Caribbean*, Institute of Social and Economic Research, University of the West Indies.

Pulsiphier, L. (1994) 'Changing roles in the traditional West Indian houseyards', in J. Momsen (ed.) *Women and Change in the Caribbean*, London: James Currey.

Reynolds, T. (1999) 'African-Caribbean mothering: reconstructing a "new" identity, unpublished thesis, London: South Bank University.

—— (2001) 'Black mothering: paid work and identity', *Journal of Ethnic and Racial Studies*,

Silva, E.B. and Smart, C. (eds) (1999) *The New Family?* London: Routledge.

Taylor, R., Jackson, S. and Chatters, L. (eds) (1997) *Black Family Life in America*, California: Sage.

Wilson, W.J. (1997) *When Work Disappears: The Work of the New Urban Poor*, New York: Random House.

4 Political intervention and family policy in Europe and the USA

4.1 Cultural change and family policies in East and West Germany

Birgit Pfau-Effinger and Birgit Geissler

Introduction

Family obligations and the gendered division of labour within the family differ substantially, and European welfare states intervene in the family to different degrees, in various forms and with different aims (*cf.* Gauthier 1996; Millar and Warman 1996; Pfau-Effinger 1999). In particular, there are great differences in the social practice of motherhood, i.e. the degree and form of women's participation in paid work during the period of active motherhood. The impact of family policies on social practices is often seen as deterministic, with women acting according to the incentives and disincentives provided by welfare state policies. However, social practices cannot be explained as a simple reaction to welfare policies: individual behaviour also refers to cultural values and norms (see Hakim 1999). In this vein, Duncan and Edwards (1999) argue that mothers also act according to 'gendered moral rationalities', in which their priorities are differentially shaped by socially negotiated notions of what is 'the right thing to do'. An alternative position argues that women in general want to gain autonomy through employment, and therefore are oriented towards lifelong full-time employment. In this view, other choices such as part-time work or breaks in employment to undertake unpaid family work are caused by institutional restrictions, and therefore these choices are only second best. However, the assumption that there is a homogenous pattern of action and orientation for women with respect to family and paid work throughout Western Europe is not supported by empirical research (Pfau-Effinger 1998, 2000; Crompton and Harris 1998). Rather, we must examine the idea that women's social practices are heavily influenced by predominant ideals and values concerning the 'correct' division of labour and form of generational relations inside the family. It is necessary, therefore, to systematically include culture – the dimension of societal ideas, meanings and values – in any theoretical framework explaining the social practices of motherhood, and to theorise and analyse the ways in which culture, institutions, structure and social action are interrelated (Pfau-Effinger 2000).

Germany after reunification provides a good example for analysis of the relationship between family policies, cultural ideals of the family and the behaviour of individuals within the framework of the family. Until 1989, in West Germany on the one hand and the former GDR on the other, the institutional and cultural frameworks of the family, as well as family policies, developed in fundamentally distinct ways.

After reunification, the institutional framework of the family that had developed in West Germany was generalised to the whole of Germany. It was expected that the development of the family in both parts of Germany would thereby converge. Instead, the social practices of the majority of women, and therefore also the shape of the family, has remained substantially different in the two constituent parts. This is particularly true for the social practices of motherhood. Despite a now common framework of the form of the welfare state, the development of the family still seems to be characterised by two different developmental paths.

The aim of this chapter is to explain why, in the 1990s, within the same framework of family policies, two different forms of the family concerning the social practices of motherhood continue to exist in eastern and western Germany. The central argument is that in order to understand these differences, it is crucial to integrate the dimension of 'culture' into the theoretical framework of analysis. The discrepancy between the social practices of motherhood promoted by the West German type of family policies on the one hand, and the actual social practices of motherhood and childhood in East Germany on the other, can largely be explained by the 'longue durée' of cultural values and ideals of the family in East Germany.

West Germany: modernisation of the male breadwinner/female carer model

Cultural development in West Germany was rooted in the traditional male breadwinner/female childcare provider model and developed into a modernised version. In the 1950s and 1960s, a cultural model of the family primarily based on the notion of the housewife with male breadwinner family model was dominant. This conception reflected the cultural traditions of the urban bourgeoisie (Pfau-Effinger 1998). It conformed to the notion of a basic differentiation of society into public and private spheres. Women and men were considered to complement each other in their roles within the different spheres: men were regarded as breadwinners who earned the income for the family in the public sphere through gainful employment, whereas women were primarily regarded as being responsible for the work in the private household, including childcare. These separate competences were also based on a particular social construction of childhood, according to which children need special care in the family by their mother and to be supported extensively as dependent individuals.

Rapid modernisation in the decades after the Second World War meant that the dominant family model started to change as women increasingly questioned the traditional division of labour within the family. Important here were general processes of democratisation as well as a considerable expansion of the education system. Social actors, such as the newly founded feminist movement, also contributed to the development of a public discourse on gender inequality and justice. As a consequence, the housewife role – to the extent that it was not combined with the mother role – was increasingly seen as outdated and no longer able to compete with that of the employed woman. An important precondition was that women gained control over their fertility through the contraceptive pill, which led to a drop in birth rates (Willms-Herget 1985; Sommerkorn 1988).

Although women today are increasingly oriented towards professional qualification and continuous participation in the labour force, mothers still attach high priority to the task of caring for their children at home during the phase of active motherhood. Public childcare is viewed by most West German parents, mothers as well as fathers, as a complement to private childcare at home but not as an adequate substitute.[1] Within the now predominant male breadwinner/female part-time carer model, an employment break of several years for home-based childcare and part-time work during the phase of active motherhood is regarded as the most appropriate behaviour for women.

However, it should be borne in mind that because of the way the labour market has developed in Germany, women's orientation to gainful employment has only partly been realised in social practice. There are considerable numbers of 'involuntary housewives': the proportion of women who want to be employed is much higher than that of women who are actually employed (Holst 2000).

Change in family policies in West Germany in the postwar period lagged behind cultural change. After the Second World War, the welfare state was reconstructed as a conservative-corporatist welfare regime. Social provision was organised on the basis of the status of different social groups and the reproduction of existing hierarchies (Esping-Andersen 1990; Leibfried and Tennstedt 1985). Furthermore, family policies were directed at supporting the male breadwinner form of family, reflecting the broad acceptance of this model among the population in the 1950s and 1960s (Sommerkorn 1988).[2]

During a time of considerable change in the social practices and cultural constructions of motherhood and childhood, state policies were hobbling way behind women's emancipation efforts. Neither the possibility for mothers to stay at home to care for their children independently of a family breadwinner, nor the integration of mothers into the labour market, has been actively promoted (Pfau-Effinger and Geissler 1992). Since the 1970s, public provision of childcare facilities has been extended to a limited degree but has essentially remained insufficient in relation to demand (Kaufmann 1995). In 1996, an individual legal right for children between 3 and 6 to publicly financed childcare was introduced, even full-time if the parents need it, and largely influenced by European law. To date, however, public care facilities for young children under 3 remain scarce.

At the same time, the social rights of childcare providers are still inadequate and indirect in that they are derived from the income of the breadwinner. This causes great problems, especially for single mothers (Ostner 1995). In the last decade, however, some initial steps have been taken towards more autonomous income and social security for private childcare providers. In the mid-1980s, a parental leave system was introduced, which allowed parents to stay at home for a maximum of three years, eighteen months of which was to be paid on a means-tested basis. However, transfer income is below subsistence level, so in practice the law maintains the financial dependency of the caring parent, nearly always the mother, on the breadwinner, usually the father. Nevertheless, three years of child rearing are counted towards independent pension entitlements (Meyer 1997). In sum, though, these changes in family policy did not dissolve the cultural principle of financial dependency of the carer (in other words, women) within the family.

Development of the family in the former GDR

In the former East Germany, a dual-breadwinner/state carer model was stipulated for women by the totalitarian state at the cultural level. It substituted the male breadwinner model, which had been dominant in Germany, at least at the cultural level, although less in social practice, since the turn of the century (Rosenbaum 1982). The state and the Socialist Party had a monopoly in defining the main family model, and from the start efforts were made to devalue the housewife role culturally by defaming it publicly (Quack and Maier 1994). Alternative cultural models were marginalised (e.g. Trappe 1995). For those generations of women who were born and grew up in the former GDR, the combination of motherhood with full-time paid work, which gave them financial autonomy, was a central element of their identity (Nickel 1999).

Family policies in the former GDR aimed to implement the dual-breadwinner/state carer model of the family in social practices. Full integration of women into gainful employment was equated with gender equality, which was regarded as a major goal of socialist policies. Comprehensive control of children, their socialisation and education was also a central political objective of the state. Accordingly, increasing women's employment was supported as key by the government, whereas any decision by women in favour of the housewife role was not. The right to and duty of employment for women and men was fixed in the constitution of the GDR, and wage structures were such that families usually needed two full-time incomes to be able to afford an average standard of living (Nickel 1999). At the same time, the model promoted by family policies was also based on a rather strict division of labour in the household – the idea of the 'Mutti' (mum) being responsible for the care of the children beyond her working time – and also on a rather hierarchical social construction of gender relations (e.g. Quack and Maier 1994; Schenk 1995). The state infrastructure of childcare institutions was extended to support the mother in fulfilling her employment duties, and women were increasingly integrated into the system of professional education. Moreover, a maternal leave scheme was introduced, based on one year of maternal leave during which an income substitute was paid. Before reunification, the employment rate of women increased to a very high level, up to 91 per cent.

The development of gender culture and social practices in East Germany in the new framework of family policies

Since reunification, West German family policies, as well as the cultural ideas on which they are based, have come to represent the main institutional framework for the social practices of motherhood and childhood in eastern Germany. Policies offer women substantial incentives to choose a role as housewife and mother – full- or part-time – instead of full integration into paid work. However, research into attitudes towards the family, as well as into behaviour, shows a high degree of continuity in the cultural orientations and social practices of motherhood among East German women. Many more East German women want to be employed full-time (85 per cent) instead of being a housewife or working part-time, and on balance are more in favour of a much shorter family break than are West Germans.

The lasting differences between the cultural ideas and social practices of motherhood in East and West Germany can be explained, I would argue, by the 'longue durée' of the traditional gender cultural model of the GDR. The fact that practically no cultural alternatives to the dual-breadwinner/state carer existed for forty years may have contributed to the ability of this cultural model substantially to survive the transformation of the former GDR (Nowossadeck 1994; Beer and Müller 1994). It also seems as if there is little intergenerational change (Dölling 2000). Indeed, in East Germany civil society is developing very hesitantly, so that public discourses and reflections among the citizens are still not much in evidence. In comparison with West Germany, therefore, no real forum to discuss issues of gender relations has developed. Finally, it also seems as if the traditional family model in East Germany is used as a kind of cultural demarcation with the West, as a part of the East German identity and in which East Germany turns out to be more 'progressive' than the West.

Conclusions

The way the family is structured, and individuals act in their everyday life in the framework of the family, is not merely based on restrictions and incentives to behaviour by family policies. It is fundamentally rooted in the functioning of other central institutions of society such as the labour market, as well as, crucially, in the ways that the family, 'motherhood', 'fatherhood' and 'childhood' are culturally constructed in that society. These cultural constructions can vary within societies between social groups. Furthermore, these change. Thus the social practices of relevant social groups – as in the East German example discussed here – can in part differ from the aims of state family policies, whether these refer to more traditional, more innovative or, as in this case, to partial cultural ideals about the family. Therefore, if the impact of family policies on the everyday practices of individuals in the family is examined, it needs to be analysed in its societal context. The field of mutual interrelations between family policies, labour market development, cultural ideals about the family and the social practices of individuals has to be addressed. As this analysis has shown, this field is not necessarily coherent, but it can be characterised by various discrepancies, contradictions, asynchronies and conflicts.

Notes

1 Data produced by the ISSP (International Social Survey Programme) from 1994 shows that 72 per cent of West Germans believe that a pre-school child will suffer if its mother is employed.

2 The degree of redistribution of income by the state between social classes was limited, however. As a consequence, as implied above, a substantial section of the working class could not afford to practise housewife marriage.

References

Beer, U. and Müller, U. (1994) 'Sich-zurechtfinden in einer neuen realität: Barrieren und potentiale', in G. Engelbrech and P. Beckmann (eds) *Arbeitsmarkt für Frauen 2000 – Ein Schritt vor oder ein Schritt zurück?* Beiträge zur Arbeitsmarkt- und Berufsforschung 179, Nuremberg: Institut für Arbeitsmarkt- und Berufsforschung, 628–45.

Crompton, R. and Harris, F. (1998) 'Explaining women's employment patterns: "orientations to work" revisited', *British Journal of Sociology* 49(1): 118–36.

Dölling, I. (2000) 'Ganz neue inhalte werden im vordergrund stehen: die arbeit zuerst. Erfahrungen junger ostdeutscher frauen mit dem Vereinbarkeitsmodell (1990–1997)', in I. Lenz, H.M. Nickel and B. Riegraf (eds) *Arbeit.Zukunft. Geschlecht.*, Münster: Verlag Westfälisches Dampfboot.

Duncan, S. and Edwards, R. (1999) *Lone Mothers, Paid Work and Gendered Moral Rationalities*, London: Macmillan.

Esping-Anderson, G. (1990) *Three Worlds of Welfare Capitalism*, Cambridge: Polity Press.

Gauthier, A.H. (1996) *The State and the Family*, Oxford: Oxford University Press.

Geissler, B. and Oechsle, M. (1996) *Lebensplanung Junger Fraue. Die Widersprüchliche Modernisierung Weiblicher*, Lebensläufe: Deutscher Studien Verlag.

Hakim, C. (1999) 'Models of the family, women's role and social policy', *European Societies* 1(1): 33–58.

Holst, E. (2000) *Die 'Stille Reserve' des Arbeitsmarktes*. Opladen: Leske und Budrich.

Kaufmann, F.X. (1995) *Zukunft der Familie im Vereinten Deutschland. Schriftenreihe des Bundeskanzleramtes*, Bd 16. Munich: Beck.

Leibfried, S. and Tennstedt, F. (1985) 'Einleitung', in S. Leibfried and F. Tennstedt (eds) *Politik der Armut und Spaltung des Sozialstaats*, Frankfurt/M.

Meyer, T. (1997) 'Retrenchment, reproduction, modernization. Welfare politics and the decline of the German breadwinner model', paper presented to the Third ESA Conference, Essex University.

Millar, J. and Warman, A. (1996) *Family Obligations in Europe*, London: Family Policy Studies Centre/Joseph Rowntree Foundation.

Nickel, H.M. (1999) 'Ambivalenzen des Wandels: Ostdeutsche Frauen im Transformationsprozeß', in C. Honegger, S. Hradil and F. Traxler (eds) *Grenzenlose Gesellschaft?*, Opladen: Leske & Budrich, vol. 2: 127–37.

Nowossadeck, S. (1994) 'Paradigmenwechsel beim rollenverständnis ostdeutscher frauen? Eine auswertung empirischer untersuchungen', in P. Beckmann and G. Engelbrech (eds) *Arbeitsmarkt für Frauen 2000 – Ein Schritt vor oder ein Schritt zurück?* Beiträge zur Arbeitsmarkt- und Berufsforschung 179, Nuremberg: Institut für Arbeitsmarkt- und Berufsforschung, 615–27.

Ostner, I. (1995) 'Arm ohne ehemann? Sozialpolitische regulierung von lebenschancen für frauen im internationalen vergleich', *Aus Politik und Zeitgeschichte. Beilage zur Wochenzeitung Das Parlament*, B 36–7, 1, September.

Pfau-Effinger, B. (1998) 'Gender cultures and the gender arrangement – a theoretical framework for cross-national comparisons on gender', *Innovation. The European Journal of Social Sciences* 11.

—— (1999) 'Change of family policies in the socio-cultural context of European societies', *Comparative Social Research* 18.

—— (2000): *Kultur und Frauenerwerbstätigkeit in Europa. Theorie und Empirie des internationalen Vergleichs*, Opladen: Leske und Budrich.

Pfau-Effinger, B. and Geissler, B. (1992) 'Institutioneller und soziokultureller kontext der entscheidung verheirateter frauen für teilzeitarbeit – ein beitrag zur soziologie des erwerbsverhaltens', *Mitteilungen aus der Arbeitsmarkt- und Berufsforschung* 25(3): 358–70.

Quack, S. and Maier, F. (1994): 'From state socialism to market economy: women's employment in East Germany, *Environment and Planning A* 26(8): 117–32.

Rosenbaum, H. (1982) *Soziologie der Familie. Untersuchungen zum Zusammenhang von Familienverhältnissen, Sozialstruktur und sozialem Wandel in der deutschen Gesellschaft des 19*, Jahrhunderts, Frankfurt am Main: Suhrkamp.

Schenk, S. (1995) 'Neu- oder restrukturierung des geschlechterverhältnisses in Ostdeutschland?' *Berliner Journal für Soziologie* 5(4): 475–88.

—— (2000) 'Familienstrukturen, geschlechterverhältnisse und die flexibilisierung der beschäftigung in Ostdeutschland', in I. Lenz, H.M. Nickel and B. Riegraf (eds) *Arbeit.Zukunft.Geschlecht.*, Münster: Verlag Westfälisches Dampfboot.

Sommerkorn, I. (1988) 'Die erwerbstätige mutter in der Bundesrepublik: Einstellungs- und problemveränderungen', in I. Nave-Herz (ed.) *Wandel und Kontinuität der Familie in der Bundesrepublik Deutschland*, Enke: Stuttgart: 115–44.

Trappe, H. (1995). *Emanzipation oder Zwang? Frauen in der DDR zwischen Beruf, Familie und Sozialpolitik*, Berlin: Akademie Verlag.

Willms-Herget, A. (1985) *Frauenarbeit. Zur Integration der Frauen in den Arbeitsmarkt*, Frankfurt/M., New York.

4 Political intervention and family policy in Europe and the USA

4.2 Family policy and the maintenance of the traditional family in Spain

Lluís Flaquer

Introduction

In analysing the nature of Spanish family policy a paradox emerges. The maintenance of a strong traditional family in democratic Spain has been not so much the result of a political will to uphold it but rather due to the lack of debate on what should be the proper place of the family in the edifice of welfare. This debate has been avoided because, since Franco's death in 1975, family policy has come to be identified by most Spaniards as one of the most distinctive features of the former Fascist regime.

I define traditional families as households organised around the principle of the male breadwinner with a wife doing unpaid caring and domestic work. In addition, traditional families are understood as welfare providers in charge of care services and economic protection for their members, as well reproductive units geared to the rearing and socialisation of children.

In the last few decades, the modernisation of Spanish society has been impressive (see Almeda and Sarasa 1996). Spain has seen one of the highest rates of growth of real GDP *per capita* since 1960 in the OECD (Castles 1998). After the death of Franco, the political system was democratised in 1978, when the new constitution was drafted; and particularly since its entry into the European Community in 1986, Spain has become another Western European country rather than a sort of political outcast. Cultural changes, for example in media, communications, leisure and consumption, have also been marked. However, despite these important developments in the cultural, economic and political fields, Spain has retained a very traditional family system. It shows the largest household size in the European Union and is one of the EU countries in which there are fewer people living in one-person households and more people living in households consisting of couples with children. Divorce rates and the proportion of lone-parent households are also low compared with most other EU countries, and the formal employment rates of married women, and particularly of mothers, are among the lowest in the EU (see Chapter 2).

This 'family paradox' continues in the policy field. For while Spain is one of the European nations in which the force of kith and kin seems most apparent, the importance of the family in public policy is marginal. There is no comprehensive family policy, and the role of explicit measures is quite limited. With the exception of recent laments about a low fertility rate and its consequences for the viability of the pension system,[1] the place of the family in the political arena seems to have faded into oblivion over the last twenty years. According to Eurostat data, Spain devoted only 1 per cent of its expenditure to social protection of families and children in 1995, in contrast to the EU average of 8 per cent (see Table 4.1). However, these extreme data do not offer an overall picture of the situation. In order to assess correctly the way in which traditional families are maintained, the whole Spanish tax–benefit system must be taken into consideration.[2]

Tax, benefits and families

The current Spanish child support system is grossly inequitable and regressive, and this has a considerable effect on family incomes. In Spain, two different schemes officially relate to the economic protection of families:

Table 4.1 Social protection benefits by function: EU 1995, as a percentage of total benefits expenditure

	Family and children	*Unemployment*	*Sickness and health*	*Old age survivors*	*Disability*
Spain	1	16	29	45	8
Italy	4	2	21	66	7
Netherlands	5	11	29	37	16
Portugal	6	6	33	43	12
Germany	7	12	29	42	7
Belgium	9	15	22	45	7
France	9	8	29	44	6
Ireland	9	19	36	26	5
UK	9	6	26	39	12
Sweden	11	11	22	37	12
Denmark	12	15	18	38	11
Austria	13	7	24	47	8
Finland	13	14	21	33	15
EU average	8	8	27	45	8

Note: Data for Greece not available.

Source: Eurostat (ESSPROS).

child allowances and tax relief. Child allowances covered all workers contributing to social security until the end of 1990, when they became means-tested. Considering that since 1971 the monthly value of the allowance per child had been frozen at the increasingly minimal amount of 250 pesetas (about £1.00), it seemed necessary to undertake a reform. So in 1990 the Socialist government updated the benefit level to 3,000 pesetas per child and set up a non-contributory scheme, at the same time introducing a means test whereby only low-income families would be eligible for the benefit. As a result of this important reform, child benefits were transformed into a significant means of social assistance (Meil 1994).

During the 1990s, therefore, child support was carried out through a dual system of tax relief for high- and middle-income families and child benefits for low-income families. In accordance with the philosophy of the reform, the latter initially received more favourable treatment than the former. Tax credits were lump-sum deductions from tax payable, so their absolute amount was unaffected by the taxpayer's income. However, the level of child allowances was not updated in the 1990s, while the amount of tax relief was increased regularly, so that the value of both benefits has tended to converge. With the 1998 Income Tax Act passed by the People's Party conservative government, upper- and middle-class families were granted fiscal advantages over those on lower incomes. In the new Act, tax allowances take the form of deductions from income subject to tax, so that under progressive tax schedules their value grows as income increases. Thus, while the same social security benefits are paid to all children irrespective of their order of birth, tax allowances for dependent children are increased both with the amount of income and with the children's order of birth. Moreover, parents on low incomes are only entitled to benefits for children under 18 years of age, whereas parents liable to pay income tax can claim allowances for children under 25. All these new tax regulations have overturned the very spirit of the 1990 child benefit reform of favouring the poorest families by devoting more resources to them, and child support has become more regressive as well as less visible. The analysis of these legal provisions clearly shows that the fight against child poverty has not found its way, as yet, on to the political agenda in any strength.

Maintaining the traditional family: housing and unemployment benefits

There are also other transfers to families that are not nominally considered part of family policy but have family protection as their main purpose, in particular tax credits for the promotion of home ownership and unemployment benefits. An overview of family protection should also bear in mind these kinds of transfer because, as in the case of Spain, they can be very substantial and may even contradict the official statements of other public policies (Flaquer 2000). The analysis of these implicit alternative provisions of family policy may reveal how traditional family patterns are endorsed in a disguised way.

Spain has one of the highest rates of home ownership in the European Union, and growth in this sector in the last three decades has been intense (Castles 1998).[3] The significance of home ownership in Spain and other Mediterranean nations can be interpreted as a form of family self-protection in the face of an absence of universal child benefits and a relatively low coverage by social services. In addition, owner occupation in Spain is strongly supported by generous fiscal incentives; indeed, tax expenditure on home ownership is about 2.5 times higher than that for social housing (Flaquer 2000). Here again, the lion's share of housing expenditure is for high- and middle-income families. One of the unintended consequences of encouraging home ownership, instead of investing in social housing, is that young people stay in their parent's home while they save money to buy a property. This results in delayed formation of new families and hence keeps the birth rate down.

As we can see from Table 4.1, Spain spends twice as much on unemployment as the European average, even though the expenditure level had already been cut by reducing benefit entitlements in 1992/93 (Consejo Economico y Social 2000). This high spending level is partly due to the existence in Spain of dramatically high unemployment rates in comparison with other European countries.[4] However, this is only a partial, and too simple, conclusion: in order truly to understand the real effects of this kind of public expenditure, it is necessary to dissect the characteristics of the Spanish labour market.

Together with Italy, Spain shows one of the lowest female activity rates in the European Union and by far the lowest female employment rate.[5] These characteristics are partly related to a peculiar structure of the labour market. Since the early 1980s, it has been plagued by persistent internal imbalances and inequalities in terms of age and sex. Not only has unemployment become increasingly feminised, but women also account for the bulk of the worst forms of unemployment, including being first-time job seekers and being out of work for long periods. On the other hand, men are more likely to belong to a well-protected and permanent core of the labour market, which includes about two-thirds of employees – but only 37 per cent of the total workforce (Cousins 1999). Since the introduction of fixed-term contracts by the Socialist government in 1984, their number has grown to the extent that one-third of the workforce now has this kind of contract (Bentolila and Dolado 1994). Women and young people in particular, and virtually all new entrants to the labour market, are more likely to be in this kind of insecure and often less rewarding employment. Another form of segmentation of the labour market is provided by the existence of a huge informal sector, estimates of the importance of which range from 15 to 25 per cent of GDP (Moreno 1997). Although by the end of the 1990s the unemployment record had improved to a great extent, these labour market inequalities have hardly changed.

It should be kept in mind that this segmentation of the labour market goes hand in hand with an overprotection of heads of household, usually middle-aged men. One illustration of this special status is that contracts for people aged 30–45 specify higher redundancy payments than for other age categories. Privileging the core workforce in the face of growing unemployment means the strengthening of the insider–outsider divide. In effect, the high wages and job security enjoyed by (chiefly male) insiders are also what causes the exclusion of their sons, daughters and wives (Esping-Andersen 1999). Of all family status categories, heads of household are the least likely to be unemployed, including long-term unemployment, and the most likely to get unemployment benefits (Flaquer 2000). An important category of unemployed people is not entitled to benefits. As only workers with a previous contribution record can claim unemployment benefits, in a labour market segmented by age and sex, this means that family heads, mostly older men, can take up these advantages to the exclusion of many young people and women who are seeking their first jobs, who are often working in the informal economy or were contracted on a fixed-term basis.

Considering that no national social assistance safety net exists in Spain, adult family dependants can only rely on their respective family heads. If unemployment benefits may be taken as a provision for supporting families, the fact that they are mainly paid to older family heads implies an indirect upholding of traditional patterns of family organisation. The Spanish labour market favours the dependent family formation of women through marriage and in this way reinforces the institution of marriage (Jurado Guerrero 1999).

Equal opportunities and the lack of family policy

In turn, these effects of the Spanish tax and benefit structure have negative consequences for the development and operation of measures to reconcile work and family life. In fact, discrimination against women stems not only from the arrangements of the labour market but also from the lack of family-friendly provisions. One of the shortcomings of Spanish equal opportunities policies in the field of employment is that they treat women as workers rather than as mothers, thereby ignoring their family position (Frotiée 1994). This is partly because in Spain, after Franco's death, there was a break with previous family policy, which shifted from an outright defence of the traditional family to an equal opportunities approach. Paradoxically, this left women's position as carers unacknowledged.

During the democratic transition, the family issue was not tackled explicitly. While the family practically disappeared from the political agenda, no debate was launched as to what should be the division of tasks between the family and the welfare state. This was partly a consequence of the emphasis placed on the traditional family under the Franco regime. As family policy was a sort of emblem of Francoism, a backlash against it ensued with the change to democracy as it became associated with the fascism and dictatorship of the old regime. Thus, in post-authoritarian Spain the policy area of the family has been characterised by an avoidance of policy making (Valiente 1997). This meant leaving in place many old measures, which continued to languish unchanged without being utterly remodelled, unlike most other social policies, or even updated.

However, as a result of the Socialist government's action during the 1980s, health care was made universal, the pensions coverage was greatly increased and education was considerably expanded. But the social security system was not radically reformed, so there was a sense of continuity between the former fascist and the democratic welfare systems (Cousins 1999; Consejo Economico y Social 2000). In particular, the idea that in each household there is a main breadwinner deriving his (*sic*) income from paid work, which acts as an umbilical cord between welfare agencies and his dependants, was not questioned by policy reformers. Even if the male breadwinner family model was not explicitly defended as such, it was latent through a number of mechanisms that were mostly invisible to social actors. Rather than a sought-after effect, the maintenance of the traditional male breadwinner family model was the result of the set of complex circumstances discussed above.

On the other hand, these developments after the democratic transition were accompanied by the rise of equal opportunity policies for women. What was characteristic of this new trend was that fresh measures were construed as *opposed* to family policy, not as complementary to it. While family policy was thought of as regressive, equal opportunity policies for women were considered politically progressive. Another characteristic of this new outlook is that it was legal in character, rather than based on an emphasis on social services. A stress on the acknowledgement of gender rights and a fight for equal opportunities in the labour market took precedence over the provision of services for women, such as childcare facilities. The lack of a public system of day care facilities for children aged 0–3 is one of the obstacles to the reconciliation between work and family in Spain. This means that working mothers with young children have to rely on private sector facilities or on traditional solidarity networks, thereby reinforcing kinship obligations and values and hence the traditional family structure.

In other respects, the situation of the reconciliation between work and family is much better, but again the segmentation of the labour market affects the operation of existing measures. This is the case with maternity leave. Even if statutory provisions regarding maternity leave are around the European average, the improvements in Spanish legislation are counteracted by the precarious character of employment described above. Maternity leave comprises sixteen weeks paid leave for working mothers, plus two extra weeks for multiple births (Escobedo 1999). However, in 1998 only 41 per cent of women giving birth were entitled to paid maternity leave. Nevertheless, this represents a considerable improvement over the last few years, with a take-up of only 30 per cent in 1995.[6]

The 1999 Act for the reconciliation between family and work does not approach family policy in a comprehensive way but mainly consists of some improvement to already existing schemes and the incorporation of EU legislation. It does not provide for paid parental leave, although it gives guarantees against the dismissal of pregnant women and enhances the sharing of maternity leave between working fathers and mothers. Nevertheless, as no incentives are provided, less than 1 per cent of eligible fathers make use of these facilities.

Conclusion: change and persistence in the traditional family

In Spain, women's interests are poorly articulated and their mobilisation is quite limited. For one thing, the Spanish unions are male-dominated because women membership is very low, and they defend men's interests rather than women's. On the other hand, the position of the Spanish feminist movement towards family policy is ambiguous. Since 1975, family policy has been seen as a remnant of the fascist past, and state intervention itself was not sought because it was considered an intrusion into the family domain. This is probably one of the reasons why Spanish feminists often insist on the need for men to share household chores and care, rather than press for the provision for services by the state. It is widely believed that the quality of services provided by family members is superior to those supplied by the market or by the state (Bettio and Villa 1998). In addition, family services are also more valued because a sense of moral obligation is attached to their provision.

On the other hand, collaboration between members of different generations and the pooling of resources among kin provide some of the transfers and services that in other European countries are entrusted to the state. One of the main characteristics of the Spanish welfare system is that it is taken for granted that the family acts as a very important provider of social protection and therefore there is no need to develop comprehensive family policy measures. The combination of family caring responsibilities and paid work is perceived as a woman's private affair rather than as a public concern. Women thus compete for equal opportunities in the labour market without questioning the dominant patterns of family life (Escobedo 1999).

It is true that in the last two decades most women, especially those in the younger generation, have adopted egalitarian views, sometimes quite radical, on gender relations. But these views are at variance with the permanence of a quite traditional division of labour within the household. We can discern a dissociation between women's egalitarian aspirations in the labour market and the continuity of a strong sense of moral obligation in kinship relations. While in Spain a very intense debate on gender has taken place, deliberations on the significance of kinship obligations and values and the role of family policies in the welfare system have been virtually lacking.

The strong implicit assumption about the division of labour between the family and the state will only be challenged by political will or by the gradual evolution of female employment. Considering that in the last ten years women's participation in the labour market has been on the increase,[7] this will put more and more pressure on the family as a welfare provider in a scenario in which falling fertility contributes to a the ageing of the population. While no sudden breakthrough is in sight in the short term, in the long run this welfare system will be hardly viable. Taking into account that it creates a lot of inequities among women, key variables in its transformation are the position of the feminist movement and a better expression of female interests through mass organisation.

Notes

1. Spain had a total fertility rate of 1.15 in 1998, the lowest in the EU (Eurostat 2000). In a list of 187 nations, Spain had the fourth lowest fertility rate. According to UN estimates, Spain is projected to have the oldest population in the world in 2050, with a median age of 55 years (United Nations 2001).
2. Eurostat does not take tax expenditure into account in its social protection data.
3. As in Ireland, eight out of ten dwellings were owner-occupied in Spain in 1996, compared with an EU average of six out of ten (Eurostat 2000).
4. In 1995, the Spanish unemployment rate was 22 per cent, compared with the EU average of 11 per cent (Eurostat 2000).
5. The Spanish female activity rate was 36 per cent in 1996, compared with an EU average of 45 per cent; in the same year, the female employment rate was 32 per cent, against an EU average of 50 per cent (Eurostat, 2000).
6. Author's calculations.
7. The Spanish female participation rate, defined as female labour force of all ages divided by female population aged 15–64, has risen from 37.7 in 1987 to 47.1 in 1997 (OECD 1999).

References

Almeda, E. and Sarasa, S. (1996) 'Spain: growth to diversity', in V. George and P. Taylor-Gooby (eds) *European Welfare Policy: Squaring the Welfare Circle*, Houndmills: Macmillan.

Bentolila, S. and Dolado, J. (1994) 'Spanish labour markets', *Economic Policy*, 53–99.

Bettio, F. and Villa, P. (1998) 'A Mediterranean perspective on the breakdown of the relationship between participation and fertility', *Cambridge Journal of Economics* 22: 137–71.

Castles, F. G. (1998) *Comparative Public Policy: Patterns of Post-war Transformation*, Cheltenham, UK and Northampton, Mass.: Edward Elgar.

Consejo Economico y Social (2000) *La Proteccion Social de las Mujeres*, Madrid.

Cousins, C. (1999) *Society, Work and Welfare in Europe*, London: Macmillan.

Escobedo, A. (1999) 'Work–family arrangements in Spain: family adjustments to labour market imbalances', in L. den Dulk, A. van Doorne-Huiskes and J. Schippers (eds) *Work–Family Arrangements in Europe*, Amsterdam: Thela Thesis, 103–29.

Esping-Andersen, G. (1999) *Social Foundations of Postindustrial Economies*, Oxford: Oxford University Press.

Eurostat (2000) *Living Conditions in Europe. Statistical Pocketbook*, Luxembourg: Commission of the European Communities.

Flaquer, L. (2000) 'Is there a Southern European model of family policy?' in A. Pfenning and T. Bahle (eds) *Families and Family Policies in Europe*, Frankfurt-am-Main and New York: Peter Lang.

Frotiée, B. (1994) 'A French perspective on family and employment in Spain', in M.-T. Letablier and L. Hantrais (eds) *The Family–Employment Relationship*, cross-national research papers, fourth series. *Concepts and Contexts in International Comparisons of Family Policies in Europe*, Loughborough: European Research Centre, 30–40.

Jurado Guerrero, T. (1999) 'Why do Spanish young people stay longer at home than the French? The role of employment, housing and social policies', PhD thesis submitted to the European University Institute, Florence.

Meil, G. (1994) 'L'évolution de la politique familiale en Espagne: du salaire familial a la lutte contre la pauvreté', *Population* 49(45): 959–84.

Moreno, L. (1997) 'The Spanish development of southern welfare', Working Paper 97–04. Madrid: IESA-CSIC. Online: http://www.iesam.cisc.es

OECD (1999) *OECD in figures: statistics on the member countries*, Paris: OECD Observer.

United Nations (2001) *World Population Prospects. The 2000 Revision. Highlights*, New York: Population Division. Department of Economic and Social Affairs.

Valiente, C. (1997) 'The rejection of authoritarian policy legacies: family policy in Spain (1975–1995)', MIRE Florence Conference, *Comparing Social Welfare Systems in Southern Europe*, Vol. 3, 363–83. Paris: MIRE.

4 Political intervention and family policy in Europe and the USA

4.3 Working and caring for children: family policies and balancing work and family in Sweden

Ulla Björnberg

Introduction

Since the 1960s, the two-earner family has become normal in Sweden. By 1988, more than 85 per cent of mothers were in the labour market (Barn och Deras Familjer 1999). This early breakthrough of the two-earner family model in Sweden was supported by a number of social reforms, with a direct influence on individual choice concerning employment and family. This chapter section will first describe these reforms and then go on to outline the moral and political rationales underlying them.

The institutional context[1]

Parental insurance

In 1974, maternity insurance (dating from 1954) was replaced by parental insurance. According to the regulations, parental leave is available to both parents, regardless of whether they are married or simply cohabiting. The important point is that both forms of parenthood are acknowledged as equal (unlike in Britain, see Chapter 5). The insurance is accompanied by labour regulations guaranteeing the right to return to the workplace after the leave period. Currently (2001), the leave period is twelve months with 80 per cent income replacement and ninety days with a flat rate of 60 Swedish kronor (about £6.00) a day (the 'guaranteed days') – 450 days in all. In principle, all months are transferable between parents except for two (one reserved for the mother and one for the father). Normally, mothers take 90 per cent of the parental leave, but the rule that two of the twelve months are not transferable was introduced in order to encourage fathers to take at least one month parental leave (the 'daddy month'). The amount paid is subject to an income of roughly 276,700 Swedish kronor (about £19,600). To be eligible for parental insurance, parents must be insured for sickness benefit for at least 180 consecutive days before the first day of planned parental leave. And to be eligible for the 80 per cent coverage for the first 180 days, the insuree's income must be higher than the guaranteed 60 Swedish kronor rate for a minimum of 240 consecutive days prior to the birth of the child (Riksförsäkringsverket (National Insurance Board) 2000). Under the same legislation, parents are entitled to sixty days of 'temporary parental leave' per child (under 12) a year. This is for parental care if the child is sick, or the childminder is sick. Additionally, fathers are entitled to ten days leave after birth ('daddy days') to be with the mother and the newborn baby.

Unemployed parents who have had an income entitling them to sickness benefit are also entitled to parental allowance. The basic point is that there should be proof of the intention to work in paid labour. Unemployment benefits and parental allowance cannot be paid simultaneously. Labour market attachment for both parents is a necessary precondition for parental leave. Thus, if the mother is a housewife, the father cannot stay at home on parental leave.

Parental insurance is thereby tied to very strong incentives to be employed and to work full-time for at least six months before giving birth. This is also apparent in how the employment pattern of young women has developed: almost all have been employed prior to the birth of their first child, and most women are employed full-time; but when returning to the labour market after parental leave, many women start to work part-time (Sundström 1997). According to the parental leave package, a parent can demand part-time work until the child is 8, since part-time work can in principle be financed by parental insurance, that is within the 360 days that are covered at 80 per cent of normal income. There is also a rule that a parent can keep the eligibility level of income, upon which the insurance is based, for thirty-six months after the birth of the child. This rule has encouraged closer spacing between births (Hoem 1993). It also means that parents can keep their parental insurance at that level of coverage based on a salary for full-time work.

Following childbirth, parental allowance is paid to the parent who looks after the child. In principle, both parents cannot receive parental allowance at the same time, but the system is quite flexible, since parents can share days if, for instance, both work part-time. Days can even be taken on a quarter-day basis, dependent on agreement with the employer. Thus parents have the choice of splitting parental leave equally between them. However, unless the child is legally adopted, step-parents are not eligible for either parental allowance or leave.

Public and subsidised childcare

The right to parental leave, and benefits tied to that leave, presupposes that the child is cared for at home. Thus the leave can be regarded as a right of the young child to be cared for by a parent (or custodian – adopted children have the same rights) at home. This right has been connected to theoretical ideas on the importance of bonding in developmental psychology (Hwang 2000).

Apart from parental care during the first year of the child's life, the most prevalent form of childcare in Sweden is institutional childcare, which is financed by taxes and parents' fees. Parents pay a subsidised fee for each child – usually these fees are means-tested, based on household income. The number of siblings that are enrolled in childcare, and the number of hours that the child spends in childcare, are also taken into account. Fees remained fairly uniform throughout the country until 1993/94, when 85 per cent of the municipalities changed their systems and the levels of parental fees for childcare services. Since then fees and regulations for childcare services vary considerably between municipalities, which are the agents responsible for public childcare subject to the overall responsibility of the Ministry of Education, although a national ceiling on fees will be introduced in 2002. Emphasis is placed on the pedagogical goals of childcare rather than on simply taking care of children while the parents are at work.

Moralities and rationalities behind family policy for working parents

The growth of the welfare state was an important element in the development of the service-based economy, but a necessary precondition for this growth was a large tax base. Thus a pragmatic political goal in these reforms was to promote wage labour and so increase the number of taxpayers. However, the parental leave reforms were phrased as gender-neutral. In the political discourse of the time, it was stressed that equality between men and women was important to the reform. In turn, individual and mutual responsibility for family subsistence was seen as necessary for gender equality. Thus the father was appointed as a caring parent, not just a provider for dependent children.

In constructing the reform, a push dimension was therefore included in order to make fathers visible and morally responsible in taking parental leave, at least through the daddy days. This was later strengthened through the addition of the daddy month. In general, however, the options were set for a choice to be negotiated between the parents themselves. This left considerable room for manoeuvre in negotiations on the basis of highly gendered conditions, with the result that caring usually remained the mother's prime responsibility, even if fathers usually assisted to a greater or lesser extent.

Care of small children was also linked to employment and marked a dividing line between those mothers who were employed and those who were not. The benefits of giving birth as an employed mother contrast sharply with those available to mothers who are housewives (Åström 1992). This link to employment was emphasised and has been strengthened through the years. This is partly because income from paid work is considered the best way for families with children to support themselves, and to keep living standards of families with children as close as possible to those of households without children. Parental insurance is thereby regarded as support for financial self-help. Economic redistribution to families with children implies that the cost of children should be shared between society and the parents themselves as a norm, not just as a means-tested subsidy.

The ideological thinking behind this was based on a social democratic understanding of the relationship between family and state. Provision, socialisation and care of children are regarded as responsibilities to be shared between parents, society *and* employers. With the reform of parental leave, parents obtained rights and claims on society as well as on employers in particular, who in their turn took on obligations towards parents.

From the start, publicly provided childcare was seen as complementary to care provided by parents. The right of the small child to parental care during early childhood was a part of the ideology behind parental insurance, that of protecting the welfare of the child and encouraging bonding between parents and children. Public provision of childcare was included in a package of support for families not only to help them to earn an income but also for socialisation and pedagogical guidance. But childcare was also regarded as a way to provide a public guarantee of the welfare of the children. Indeed, public childcare has been widespread in Sweden since the end of 1900s, but until the 1960s, this was mostly intended to support lone mothers in poor circumstances: they could leave their children while they were working (Lindberg 1991). An extension of public childcare to all was discussed as early as the 1930s, led by the influential reformer Alva Myrdal and focusing on the *socialisation* of children, mainly in the urban environment. Myrdal considered urban life, particularly in poor and crowded areas, as unhealthy for children, who were playing in the streets with no pedagogical support and little adult supervision. She advocated extended provision of kindergartens to offer more qualified care of children and to give mothers the chance to work (Myrdal 1935). In turn, this fed into Alva and Gunnar Myrdal's influential writings on living conditions and welfare in Sweden and, investigated further by government reports, into the development of the Swedish welfare settlement from the 1940s onwards.

Moral and political dilemmas

The political discourse on family policy since 1990 has focused on the issue of public versus private arrangements for childcare and the ways in which society should support families. Childcare allowances for parents at home and subsidised shorter working hours for parents with children under 10 have been recurrent issues in this debate. The small but influential Christian Democratic Party, supported by the Conservative Party (*Moderaterna*), has taken a lead in advocating childcare allowances, while the dominant Social Democratic Party, the Left Party and the Green Party have, at the level of discourse, favoured shorter working hours. The argument for childcare allowances for parents at home has been represented as one of freedom of choice in childcare. It has been argued that, under the current system, those parents who want to care for small children at home after the parental leave period must do so at their own expense, and that very few families can afford to choose this alternative when subsidised childcare is linked only to public childcare. The Social Democrats, especially the women's section, have in contrast argued for subsidised shorter working hours for parents with young children. This position is represented as one of gender fairness, where under the current system women – when they become mothers – normally shorten their working hours at their own expense in order to give more time to their children and to the household.

Childcare allowances for children under 3 were introduced by the Conservative government in Sweden in 1994 but were abolished six months later by the incoming Social Democratic government. The allowance was taxed and was to be used for the costs of childcare, either provided by a parent at home, regardless of by whom, or for institutional childcare. Similar reforms were enacted in Finland in 1985 (Korpinen 2000) and in Norway in 1998 (Vigerust 2000). The experience of these reforms is that they are mainly used by women. More in-depth studies are needed to evaluate and understand the gender aspects of these reforms as well as the underlying motivation behind them. However, they do indicate a moral concern regarding care of children at home versus care elsewhere. This concern should not primarily be interpreted as meaning that institutional care *per se* is improper but rather that the conditions under which care and work can be combined are unsatisfactory. However, the commitments of employers to parental involvement and sharing between couples have not been a recurrent focus in the debates. I would also argue that care as a necessary part of life has been marginalised both in these debates and in the everyday lives of working parents themselves. Certainly, the effects of parental leave on gender equality have not been particularly marked. In 2000, women used around 90 per cent of the available leave days, a figure that has been reduced by only about 10 per cent since 1974 (Rfv 1998). Similarly, women took 60 per cent of temporary parental leave in 1999, a figure that has been fairly stable since 1989. The average number of days taken per child was seven in 1999 (Rfv website 2001).

Although parental leave covers a relatively short period of family life, it apparently has a strong impact on how the division of labour at home is put to practice in the longer run. Since mothers in most cases take long parental leave, a highly gendered pattern is set for sharing responsibilities for children and domestic work, which is subsequently not so easily changed. Women continue to adapt their work and leisure to the needs of the family, and men tend to take this adaptation for granted. Negotiations in the household result in women taking the main responsibility for children and household chores, even if men share the chores to some extent (Ahrne and Roman

1997; Andersson 1993; Bergsten and Bäck-Wiklund 1997; Björnberg and Kollind 2001).

Since the 1980s, the workforce has faced considerable changes in work organisation. Workers must adapt flexibly to changes in working hours, employment conditions and forms of work. Temporary employment has increased, and job insecurity is widespread among young women (Social Rapport 2001). These new conditions have brought stress and increased problems in balancing work and family, in particular among the majority of women working in caring jobs and services. However, the sharing of responsibilities at home has not kept pace with this development, so the burden falls all the more heavily on women. Arlie Hochschild (1997) has suggested that family responsibilities are becoming more marginalised under the pressures of working life. The boundaries between work and family are becoming blurred: through new technologies, such as mobile phones, e-mail at home, fax machines, etc., working life has invaded the home. Loyalty to the firm is demanded, either through the risk of dismissal for the temporarily employed or due to increasing measures from firms to increase loyalty to clients or to colleagues in network-based organisations and immediate chains of dependencies. Hochschild's conclusions seem to be valid for countries other than the USA, which was the focus of her studies, including Sweden.

Richard Sennet (1999) has analysed the trend towards flexibility in the labour market and its impact on social relationships and the social identity of employees under the new capitalism, also in a US context. He suggests that employees need to develop their personalities to be in line with new demands to behave smoothly, to be open to change at short notice, to be prepared to take risks and to remain independent of rules. According to Sennet, the new system breeds indifference and lack of trust, because people learn that they are replaceable. The flexible way of life presupposes autonomy and cooperation on a superficial level. He means that this kind of ethics stands in opposition to the kind of ethics that is needed in family relationships – loyalty, commitment, trust and long-term ties. The work ethic opposes the ethic of care, and parents will feel an urge to protect the family from negative influences, shortsightedness and temporary attachments (see also Chapter 6).

The points that these two analysts make are that the spheres of working life and of families operate under different kinds of ethics, and with different cultural understandings for individuals in them. The more paid work becomes integrated into home and family, the more it is likely that it will have a strong impact on the ways in which responsibilities and care are being carried out and negotiated. Gender equality at home, as a major discourse that women and men have to relate to in Sweden today, means different things to couples. It can, for instance, mean an equal amount of time spent on domestic work, or the equal splitting of chores, or equal access to economic resources, or mutual respect, or shared influence on major consumption decisions. For many women, the most important understanding of equality is mutuality in feelings of responsibility for children and domestic work, regardless of whether the final input in practical work is equal (Björnberg and Kollind 2001). In these negotiations, notions of guilt and debt are important and are used as currency in exchanges of inputs and in negotiations about commitments to children.

Women carry the main responsibility for taking care of the well-being of family members, especially children. The extent to which they feel that they fail to meet their criteria for taking responsibility for others, and for themselves, creates a moral dilemma that brings guilt. Taking responsibility for care is much more than simply doing practical caring. It includes invisible thoughts and considerations regarding the well-being and needs of the child, planning and thinking ahead, being available for the child, and being able to control as far as possible the conditions of the everyday life of the child (Elwin-Nowak 1999; see also Chapter 13). This is a heavy burden to carry and adds to feelings of stress, but it is not as visible as the practical caring work. To the extent to which women feel that there is a real sharing of responsibility and that the child's needs are satisfactorily met, her burden can be eased. This is probably the main reason why many women stress the sharing of responsibility as the most important dimension of gender equality in the home.

In an international context, Swedish family policy and childcare arrangements for working parents are relatively generous and are, more so than is usual, designed to stimulate gender equality at work and in the home. These policies have encouraged women to regard employment as an integrated part of their lives. In general terms, the Swedish experience of balancing work and care brings complex ambiguities and feelings of inadequacy in fulfilling responsibilities in caring. One reason is that the sharing of responsibilities between men and women at home remains askew. The more the conditions of work create a cultural distance between work and family, the more these moral dilemmas might be perceived as unsolvable. There is an evident risk of marginalisation of care in social relationships, and these problems demand that employers adopt a greater understanding of the needs of children and their working parents.

Note

1 This section builds on a more developed text on international family policy. See Björnberg (forthcoming).

References

Ahrne, G. and Roman, C. (1997) *Hemmet, Barnen och Makten. Förhandlingar om Arbete och Pengar i Familjen*, SOU 1997: 139. Stockholm: Fritzes.

Andersson, G. (1993) *Leva för Jobbet och Jobba För Livet. Om Chefsfamiljers Vardag och Samlevnadsformer*, Stockholm: Brutus Östlings Förlag.

Åström, G. (1992) 'En naturlig ordning om organisation efter kön', in Y. Hirdman and G. Åström (eds) *Kontrakt iKris*, Stockholm: Carlsson Bokförlag.

Barn och Deras Familjer (1999) *Demografiska Rapporter* 3. Stockholm: Statistics Sweden.

Bergsten, B. and Bäck-Wiklund, M. (1997) *Det moderna Föräldraskapet. En Studie av Familj och Kön i Förändring*, Stockholm: Natur och Kultur.

Björnberg, U. (ed.) (forthcoming) 'Family change and family policy in Sweden', in M. Alestalo and P. Flora (eds) *Family Change and Family Policy in the Scandinavian Welfare States*, Oxford: Oxford University Press.

Björnberg, U. and Kollind, A.-K. (2001) 'Individualism, loyalty and equality', unpublished paper, Department of Sociology, Göteborg University.

Elwin-Nowak, Y. (1999) 'The meaning of guilt: a phenomenological description of employed mothers experiences of guilt', *Scandinavian Journal of Psychology* 40: 70–83.

Hwang, P. (2000) 'Pappors engagemang i hem och barn', in P. Hwang (ed.) *Faderskap i Tid och rum*, Stockholm: Natur och Kultur.

Hochschhild, A. (1997) *The Time Bind. When Work Becomes Home And Home Becomes Work*, New York: Metropolitan Books.

Hoem, J. (1993) 'Public policy as the fuel of fertility: effects of a policy reform on the pace of childbearing in Sweden in the 1980s', *Acta Sociologica* 36: 19–31.

Korpinen, J. (2000) 'Child home care allowance – framing the Finnish experience', in L. Kallioma-Puha (ed.) *Perspectives of Equality – Work, Women and Family in the Nordic Countries and EU*, Copenhagen: Nord 2000:5.

Lindberg, M. (1991) *90 års barnomsorg 1874–1964. En utvecklingsstudie*, Norrköping: Institutionem för förskollärarutbildning.

Myrdal, A. (1935) *Stadsbarn. En Bok om Deras Fostran i Storbarnkammare*, Stockholm: Kooperativa Förbundet.

Riksförsäkringsverket (National Insurance Board) (1998) Statistikinformation Is1998:009,1998–05–11.

—— (2000) *Försäkringskassan Informerar*, Stockholm: Föräldraförsäkring.

Sennet, R. (1999) *När Karaktären Krakelerar* (*The Corrosion of Character*). Stockholm: Atlas.

Social Rapport (2001) Stockholm: Socialstyrelseln.

Sundström, M. (1997) 'Managing work and children: part-time work and the family-cycle of Swedish women', in H. Blossfeld and C. Hakim (eds) *Between Equalisation and Marginalisation: Part-time Working Women in Europe and the United States of America*, Oxford: Oxford University Press.

Vigerust, E. (2000) 'The Norwegian Act relating to supplementary cash benefit for parents of small children', in L. Kallioma (ed.) *Perspectives of Equality, Work, Women and Family in the Nordic Countries and EU*, Copenhagen: Nordic Council of Ministers.

Online: http://www.rfv/se/stati/famba/tillf.htm (10 January 2001).

4 Political intervention and family policy in Europe and the USA

4.4 Paternalism, welfare reform and poor families in the United States

Alan Deacon

The welfare system in the United States was radically restructured in the 1990s. The centrepiece of that restructuring was the abolition of a 'right to welfare'. For more than sixty years, the dominant form of welfare provision had been the Aid to Families with Dependent Children (AFDC) programme. The details of the AFDC programme had varied over the years, but in essence it provided means-tested benefits to poor women and their children. Those benefits were inadequate and deeply stigmatising, but they were benefits that could be claimed as entitlement. It was left to each state to decide what level of benefits it paid, but all were required by law to pay something to people whose income and resources fell below the limits defined by the federal government. That obligation was lifted by the cumbersomely titled Personal Responsibility and Work Opportunity Reconciliation Act (PRWORA) of 1996, which abolished AFDC and replaced it with a new programme called Temporary Assistance to Needy Families (TANF).

The ending of entitlement was a means to an end. The Act set out two central objectives of welfare reform: to 'end the dependency of needy parents on government benefits by promoting job preparation, work and marriage'; and to 'prevent and reduce the incidence of out-of-wedlock pregnancies' and 'encourage the formation and maintenance of two-parent families' (Duerr Berrick 1998: 5).

The first objective was to be met primarily through the introduction of time limits. No one was to receive welfare for more than two years without participating in work activities, or for more than a total of five years in their lifetime. The second objective was to be met through a series of provisions that withheld benefits from women who did not meet specific conditions regarding their own behaviour or that of their children. For example, the states were prohibited from paying TANF to mothers under 18 who did not live with an adult or did not attend school. They could also withhold benefits from mothers who did not help to identify the fathers of their children, did not attend school or had drug convictions. States were also given the option of introducing a 'family cap', that is of refusing to pay additional benefits to mothers who had another child when already on welfare.

These provisions were reinforced by changes in the way in which welfare was funded. The most important effects of these changes were to offer a significant windfall to states that reduced their caseloads and to reward states that met targets for the proportion of TANF recipients engaged in work activities or managed to reduce out-of-wedlock births without increasing the number of abortions.[1]

There is now an extensive literature on the US welfare reforms. This literature examines why those reforms took the form they did and discusses their impact both upon those on welfare and upon those in low-paid jobs (Bryner 1998; Mead 2000; Teles and Prinz 2000; Weaver 2000). The purpose of this chapter is a more limited one. It is to discuss the ways in which the 1996 Act sought to intervene in the structure and practices of poor families. In particular, it will show that the provisions of the Act were shaped by an important and protracted debate among US conservatives about how welfare reform could most effectively change the reproductive behaviour of poor women. The central issue in that debate was whether poor women should be viewed as rational actors who would respond to financial incentives or penalties, or as the dysfunctional poor who would respond only to compulsion. The chapter examines this debate and discusses which perspective has proved to be the more important influence upon the implementation of the Act. Before doing so, however, it is necessary to sketch in some of the background, albeit briefly.

The background to PRWORA

The story of the passage of PRWORA is simple in outline, complex in detail. The Clinton administration entered office in January 1993 committed to 'end[ing] welfare as we know it'. Clinton's proposals were based upon the ideas of David Ellwood, whose *Poor Support* had been published in 1988. Ellwood's starting point was that 'humane welfare will never be realised; too many suspicions and conflicts are built into the system' (1988: 237). The more adequate the level of benefit, Ellwood argued, the greater the threat to work incentives, or the more likely that it would create 'a potential incentive for the formation and perpetuation of single parent families' (*ibid.*: 21). The only way to escape from this Catch-22 was to redefine welfare as transitional assistance. The goal would be to equip recipients with the capacities and skills to enter or re-enter the labour force, and then require them to do so. A further goal would be to 'make work pay' by providing those in low-paid jobs with 'supplemental support' through the tax and child support systems. Indeed, Ellwood's original proposals would have ensured that a single parent escaped from poverty if she worked half time. However, remaining on welfare could not be an option: 'the long-term support system is jobs' (*ibid.*: 181).

Ellwood had previously established his reputation as a leading defender of welfare against the attacks of conservatives such as Charles Murray (De Parle 1996). This meant that the publication of *Poor Support* had a powerful impact. As Weaver explains, it 'legitimised among mainstream welfare scholars the idea of putting time limits on cash welfare benefits, albeit with a job guarantee at the end' (1998: 370). The impetus for reform was reinforced by the seemingly remorseless rise in welfare caseloads. The number of families in receipt of AFDC peaked at just over 5 million in March 1994, a rise of 30 per cent since 1989. These families included over 14 million people, 10 million of whom were children (Bryner 1998: 5–6). One American in twenty was dependent upon welfare when Ellwood became co-chair of President Clinton's task force on welfare reform early in 1993.

In the event, however, the publication of Clinton's plan was held up for over a year by arguments over its cost and the relative priority of reforms to welfare and healthcare. This delay proved to be fatal, because the Republican victory in the elections of November 1994 meant that Clinton faced hostile majorities in both houses of Congress. Moreover, the Republicans themselves were now deeply divided along one of the oldest fault lines in political thought, that between libertarianism and paternalism.

Welfare reform and the family

By the mid-1990s, the Republicans' welfare strategy was being subjected to two conflicting intellectual influences. The first was the so-called 'new paternalism' advocated by Lawrence Mead, and the second was Charles Murray's dramatic call for welfare to be withheld completely from lone mothers. These two dominant policy intellectuals of the Right shared a common belief in the need to restore the married family but held totally different views as to how welfare could help to bring that about.

According to Mead, the 'entire tradition of explaining poverty or dependency in terms of incentives or disincentives is bankrupt' (1992: 136). It is bankrupt, he argues, because the long-term poor do not respond to changes in the framework of financial incentives and sanctions in the way that Ellwood presumes. The reason why they do not respond is that they are not competent, functioning individuals who act rationally to further their interests. On the contrary, they are the 'dutiful but defeated', who will not take advantage of opportunities for advancement unless forced to do so. The problem lies not in a lack of opportunities but in public policies that condone self-destructive behaviour. Strategies that offer a job guarantee or attempts to 'make work pay', claims Mead, are popular with liberals because they assume that all the poor 'respond to the same suasions as the middle class'. However, the reality is different. The people who respond to such offers and incentives are 'mainly those who are already functional, already within the economy. No incentive has shown a power to pull many people across the line from nonwork to work. For that stronger medicine is required' (*ibid.*: 162).

This stronger medicine should take the form of work requirements, backed by severe benefit sanctions for non-compliance and administered through intensive case management. It is this close supervision and direction of the lives of recipients that is the defining feature of paternalism in welfare. Moreover, this combination of 'help and hassle' can also be used to ensure that the poor fulfil the other obligations of citizenship. During the 1990s, many states utilised the so-called waiver provisions to introduce a significant measure of paternalism into the old AFDC programme.[2] By the mid-1990s, thirty-one states had made welfare conditional upon satisfactory attendance at school (learnfare); seventeen states required teenage mothers to live with a parent or guardian; and twenty-one states withheld welfare from mothers who failed to ensure that their children were immunised or met other healthcare requirements (Bryner 1998: 201–5).

Mead's fellow conservatives have had no difficulty with his focus upon the behaviour of the poor. What has caused them problems is his emphasis upon the role of government and upon the need for an enlarged and transformed welfare bureaucracy. In this respect, the new paternalism challenges longstanding conservative beliefs about the inherent wastefulness and inefficiency of big government. At the same time, it contravenes the central tenet of the libertarian Right, that individuals should be free from government interference, provided only that their actions do not occasion immediate harm to others. These differences have been highlighted in the debate between Mead and Charles Murray.

For his part, Murray has always argued that the growth of dependency could be readily explained in terms of the 'perverse incentives' generated by welfare. Back in 1984, he wrote that there was no 'need to invoke the spectres of cultural pathology or inferior upbringing'. It was simply a question of the poor making 'rational choices among alternatives', and of people responding rationally to the reality of the world around them' (1984: 162). These incentives could not be removed by tinkering with the rules governing entitlement, and the only solution was to abolish welfare. At the time, this proposal was almost universally regarded as beyond the pale, but by the summer of 1994 something very similar had become 'the welfare reform prescription of a large number of significant Republican leaders and potential presidential candidates' (Teles 1996: 151). This hardening of the Republican Party's stance was in turn a reflection of its preoccupation with the apparent collapse of the married family, and especially of the poor, Black, married family.

The previous October, Murray had published a now infamous essay in the *Wall Street Journal* in which he had claimed that 'illegitimacy is the single most important social problem of our time', because 'it drives everything else' (29 October 1993). The inference was that there was little point in incorporating work requirements into AFDC. As he later told a British audience, a welfare Bill that succeeded 'in moving large numbers of women off the welfare rolls' but did 'nothing about the illegitimacy ratio' would have achieved 'nothing' (1998: 61). The impact of what Teles has termed 'Murray's ideological stink bomb' (1996: 157) was dramatic, and by early

1994 prominent Republican think tanks were calling for the withdrawal of AFDC and food stamps from unwed mothers. Empower America, for example, claimed that the need was not for 'tougher work provisions and job training' but 'to go after a system that fosters illegitimacy and its attendant social pathologies'. Similar arguments were put forward by Robert Rector of the Heritage Foundation, 'who became as influential among Republicans in 1995 as Lawrence Mead was in 1988' (*ibid.*: 152, 159).

It should be emphasised at this point that Mead did not question the central importance of the family. Indeed, he had written in 1991 that the 'inequalities' that stemmed from the workplace were 'trivial' compared with those stemming from family structure. 'What matters for success is less whether your father was rich or poor than whether you knew your father at all' (1991: 10). Mead's response to Murray was thus a pragmatic one. It was that government knew 'something about how to enforce work, but almost nothing about how to confine childbearing to marriage' (1997a: 69). He had a similarly pragmatic response to other conservatives, who argued that enforcing work obligations could be detrimental to the children of lone mothers (Wilson 1997: 342). Here again the issue was what public policy could actually achieve. The government knew nothing about how to make women better mothers, but it did know how to make them take paid employment. To children, 'functioning parents' were 'worth 25 Head Start programmes', and only parents who work have the self-respect needed to command the respect of their children (Mead 1997b: 15).

The Republicans in Congress sought to balance these conflicting arguments in the three Bills that they passed in July 1996. President Clinton vetoed the first two but signed the third into law on the eve of the 1996 presidential election campaign. Clinton's decision to sign what became PRWORA attracted enormous criticism. It was famously condemned as 'The worst thing Bill Clinton has done' by a former aide, Peter Edelman. Another critic was David Ellwood, who had resigned from the administration the year before. Ellwood described the new Act as 'appalling', since it offered claimants not 'two years and you work' but two years 'followed by nothing – no welfare, no jobs, no support' (1996: 26).

PRWORA in practice

The arguments over the impact of PRWOPA have been as fierce as those that surrounded its passage. There is some agreement about what has happened, but much less agreement about why it has happened. However, one point is beyond all dispute. The implementation of PRWORA has coincided with a truly remarkable decline in the welfare caseload. The number of people in receipt of welfare fell from over 14 million in January 1994 to just under 7 million in June 1999 (Weaver 2000: 343). The extent to which this fall can be attributed to the Act or to the strength of the US economy is a matter of dispute. At the very least, however, it can be said that large numbers of never-married mothers moved from welfare to work and that the economy generated jobs for them all. As Robert Lerman has pointed out, the unemployment rate for this group actually fell between 1996 and 1998 (1999: 237).

It is also true that poverty rates have fallen, albeit much more slowly than the caseloads. The proportion of Americans living in poverty declined from 13.7 per cent in 1996 to 12.7 per cent in 1998. In October 1999, the Center on Budget and Policy Priorities reported that the proportion of children in poverty was the lowest for twenty years and that the poverty rate for African Americans was at an all-time low (CBPP 1999: 1). However, this is not the whole story, since those families that remained poor were living in deeper poverty than before. Indeed, on the third anniversary of the passage of the Act the Children's Defense Fund claimed that the number of children living in households with an income of less than half the poverty line had risen by nearly half a million to 2.7 million between 1996 and 1999 (CDF 1999: 1).

The net result of all this has been a growing bifurcation of the poor in America. Those who have remained on welfare have experienced a further decline in their incomes, whereas some of those who have moved from welfare to work have been able to escape from poverty. Here again, however, the extent to which such women are indeed better off in work is a matter of dispute (Jencks 1997; Grant 2000). However, what is most important for the present discussion is that those women no longer had a choice. As Ann Orloff has recently noted, PRWORA eliminated 'caregiving as a base for making claims within the US welfare state' (2000: 133). TANF provides for a single mother on the grounds that she is a potential worker, not as someone with recognised responsibilities for the care of children. Lone mothers may be entitled to assistance with childcare if and when they take paid employment, but they can no longer 'maintain a household' without either 'access to a male wage' or themselves 'working for pay' (*ibid.*: 142). She goes on to argue that the lack of opposition to this change from 'women's equality organisations' reflects the fact that the great majority of married mothers were already in paid work: 'AFDC rules seemed to make possible staying at home to care for children at public expense – exactly what isn't guaranteed to any other mother or father' (*ibid.*: 152). Similarly, Theda Skocpol has argued that 'Americans cannot be convinced that parental work apart from at least part-time waged employment is socially honourable' (2000: 161).

There is a similar degree of consensus about the need to reduce the number of births outside marriage. However, the crucial difference is that there is far less agreement about how this reduction can be achieved. Rebecca Maynard, for example, has recently noted that after 'more than a decade of research, observers have found no magic formula for the prevention of teenage pregnancies' (1997: 101). It is perhaps not surprising, then, that a multi-state analysis of the welfare systems created under the Act found that most states were confused as to how they were supposed to attain 'the Act's anti-reproductive and marriage goals'. Indeed, the five states that had achieved the largest 'decreases in illegitimacy did not know what they had done to accomplish this, and, in fact, it appeared that at least some of them had done little or nothing at all' (Gentry *et al.* 1999: 15).

There are three points that can be made in conclusion. The first is that welfare reform in the USA has been influenced far more strongly by the new paternalism of Lawrence Mead than by the abolitionism of Charles Murray. Neither the Republican Congress nor the Clinton presidency was prepared to withhold welfare completely from lone mothers and their children. However, both were prepared to demand that those mothers accept a much greater level of surveillance and direction over their personal lives.

The second point is that to date this authoritarian approach has been far more successful in promoting paid work than it has been in promoting marriage or in reducing the number of births to teenagers. Once again this would appear to support Mead's argument that public policy is able to influence decisions about employment far more readily than it can influence decisions about marriage or childbirth. However, this was not the most important point at issue between Mead and Murray. The key question was whether or not a policy of forcing lone mothers to take paid employment would in time change the partnering and parenting practices of those mothers. There is simply no evidence to support or refute this notion; nor can there be for some considerable time.

The final point is perhaps the most important in relation to the aims and focus of this book. This is that both Murray and Mead work within an essentially economistic notion of rationality and choice. Murray starts from the premise that lone mothers will respond to financial incentives and sanctions, Mead that they would do so if they were sufficiently competent. Neither considers the 'multiple rationalities' discussed in Chapter 5, and both are exposed to the critiques developed in Chapters 12 and 13. Their response to those critiques would be to claim that there is strong public support for their position. The fact that the overwhelming majority of mothers in the United States are in paid employment effectively constrains public discussion of alternatives, especially for women on welfare.

Notes

1 In broad terms, the federal government in Washington had matched a state's spending on AFDC dollar for dollar. If more families were admitted to welfare, then the federal grant rose accordingly. This meant that welfare was relatively cheap for individual states, and especially for those with the lowest incomes per head, which received proportionately greater funding from the federal government. The 1996 Act replaced this matched funding with a block grant, which was based upon the amount each state had received in 1993 or 1994. The level of this block grant will be renegotiated as part of the reauthorisation of TANF during the 2000–2002 Congress.

2 The original purpose of the waiver provision was to allow individual states to experiment with new ways of delivering welfare. Under legislation passed in 1962, a state could submit a proposal for a demonstration project to the Secretary of State, together with a request that he waive the federal regulations

governing entitlement to benefit where this was necessary for the experiment to proceed. The crucial point was that the decision on whether or not to grant the waiver was taken by the White House, not by Congress. The original legislation had envisaged that the demonstration projects that were facilitated by the waivers would seek ways of making AFDC more successful. After 1986, however, the Reagan and Bush administrations used waivers to undermine AFDC. The first set of waivers allowed states to impose more stringent work conditions than were required by the existing legislation. However, the Bush administration encouraged a shift in emphasis towards the regulation of sexual behaviour and the deterrence of illegitimacy. In particular, waivers were used to overturn a Supreme Court judgement that a state could not deny welfare to a woman who was otherwise eligible on the grounds of her illicit sexual conduct (Teles 1966: 140).

References

Bryner, G. (1998) *Politics and Public Morality*, London: W.W. Norton.

CBPP (1999) 'Low unemployment, rising wages fuel poverty decline.' Online: http://www.cbpp.org/9–30–99pov.htm

CDF (1999) 'Extreme poverty rises by more than 400,000 in one year.' Online: http://www.childrendefense.org/release990822.html

DeParle, J. (1996) 'Mugged by reality', *The New York Times Magazine*, 8 December.

Duerr Berrick, J. (1998) 'Targeting social welfare benefits in the United States: policy opportunities and pitfalls', paper presented to Conference of the International Social Security Association, Jerusalem, January 1998.

Edelman, P. (1997) 'The worst thing Bill Clinton has done', *The Atlantic Monthly*, March 1997.

Ellwood, D. (1988) *Poor Support*, New York: Basic Books.

—— (1996) 'Welfare reform as I knew it: when bad things happen to good policies', *The American Prospect* 26.

Gentry, P., Johnson, C. and Lawrence, C. (1999) 'Moving in many directions: state policies, pregnancy prevention and welfare reform', paper presented to 21st Research Conference of the Association for Public Policy Analysis and Management, Washington, 6 November 1999.

Grant, L. (2000) 'Crossing the Atlantic: US welfare reform and the degradation of poor women', in H. Dean, R. Woods and R. Sykes (eds) *Social Policy Review* 12, London: Social Policy Association.

Jencks, C. (1997) 'The hidden paradox of welfare reform', *The American Prospect* 32.

Lerman, R. (1999) 'Retreat or reform? New US strategies for dealing with poverty', in H. Dean and R. Woods (eds) *Social Policy Review* 11, London: Social Policy Association.

Maynard, R. (1997) 'Paternalism, teenage pregnancy prevention, and teenage parent services', in L. Mead (ed.) *The New Paternalism*, Washington: Brookings Institution.

Mead, L. (1991) 'The new politics of the new poverty', *Public Interest* 103: 3–20.

—— (1992) *The New Politics of Poverty*, New York: Basic Books.

—— (1997a) 'Welfare employment', in L. Mead (ed.) *The New Paternalism*, Washington: Brookings Institution.

—— (1997b) 'From welfare to work', in A. Deacon (ed.) *From Welfare to Work: Lessons from America*, Institute of Economic Affairs.

—— (2000) 'The twilight of liberal welfare reform', *The Public Interest* 139, 22–34

Murray, C. (1984) *Losing Ground*, New York: Basic Books.
—— (1998) untitled chapter in R. Nye (ed.) *The Future of Welfare*, London: Social Market Foundation.
Orloff, A. (2000) 'Ending the entitlement of poor mothers: Changing social policies, women's employment and caregiving in the contemporary United States', in N. Hirschman and U. Liebert (eds) *Women and Welfare: Theory and Practice in the U.S. and Europe*, New York: Rutgers University Press. [also in L. Mead (ed.) *The New Paternalism*, Washington: Brookings Institution]
Skocpol, T. (2000) *The Missing Middle*, New York: W.W. Norton.
Teles, S. (1996) *Whose Welfare? AFDC and Elite Politics*, University Press of Kansas.
Teles, S. and Prinz, T. (2000) 'The politics of rights retraction: welfare from entitlement to block grant', in M. Landy, M. Levin and M. Shapiro (eds) *The New Politics of Public Policy II: The Persistence of Change*, Washington: Georgetown University Press.
Weaver, K. (1998) 'Ending welfare as we know it', in M. Weir (ed.) *The Social Divide: Political Parties and the Future of Activist Government*, Washington: Brookings Institution.
—— (2000) *Ending Welfare As We Know It*, Washington: Brookings Institution.
Wilson, J.Q. (1997) 'Paternalism, democracy and bureaucracy', in L. Mead (ed.) *The New Paternalism*, Washington: Brookings Institution.

5 New Labour, the rationality mistake and family policy in Britain

Anne Barlow, Simon Duncan and Grace James

Introduction: New Labour and remoralising social behaviour

Following its landslide election victory in 1997, the 'New Labour' government in Britain has adopted the express aim of changing social behaviour as part of its project of 'modernisation'. A major objective of this drive is to use legislation to sustain and induce particular types of partnership and parenting and to discourage other, less favoured, forms. This is because, as Prime Minister Tony Blair put it in a 1996 speech, while 'family values' are the key to a 'decent society', there is a 'moral deficit' that leads to an 'indifference to the undermining of family life' (Blair 1996a). Drawing on a communitarian discourse (see Etzioni 2000), governments should use the law to inculcate appropriate family values and so 'rebuild social order and stability' (Blair 1996b). This remoralising of the family links to a concern to extend paid work as a moral duty for citizens (*cf.* Lister 1998), or as the Prime Minister wrote in the popular tabloid newspaper the *Daily Mail*, 'If you can work, you should work' (10.2.1999). 'Work' in this discourse simply means paid work – unpaid caring work is not included, and those using benefits to support parenting, for example, are implicitly seen as work-shy and even immoral. Thus in launching the Social Exclusion Unit in his first major speech outside Parliament since the 1997 election, Blair (1997) talked of a growing underclass of unemployed young men and young single mothers, and the need to bring this 'new workless class back into society and into useful work'. It was, he went on, 'an offence against decency that work should be allowed to disappear … to be replaced by an economy built on benefits, crime, petty thieving and drugs'. In this speech, lone mothers' labour in bringing up children is not counted as useful, and 'society' seems to be limited to the employed. Receipt of benefits is not only set alongside criminality but is also held to mean both economic inactivity and personal idleness. This reform discourse was subsequently codified in policy terms in two 1998 Green Papers: *Supporting Families* and *A New Contract for Welfare*.[1] Both set out frameworks for much of the succeeding legislation in the first New Labour government up to 2001 (see also Chapter 3.3).

We examine the validity of this enterprise in terms of its underlying assumptions about family behaviour and decision making, and how this might be influenced through legislation. We argue that in its reform programme the government implicitly assumes a universal model of 'rational economic man' and his close relative the 'rational legal subject'. In this view, people take individualistic cost–benefit decisions about how to maximise their own personal gain. Change the financial and legal structure of costs and benefits in the appropriate way and people will modify their social behaviour in the desired direction. Alternatively, people may make sub-optimal decisions where they lack information about this cost–benefit structure. In this case, simply providing better information, or educating people so that they can access it and act upon it more effectively, will have the desired social effects. In either event, more people will marry, fewer will cohabit and divorce, and more young men and lone parents will take up paid work.

But what if this is not a correct assumption? Certainly, the assumption of rational economic man, and the theories of neo-classical economics that underlie it, have been vigorously challenged both in general and in their application to complex social decision making (see Chapter 12). Similarly, recent empirical research suggests that people do not act like rational economic man in making decisions about their moral economy (see also Chapters 9 and 13). Rather, people seem to take such decisions with reference to moral and socially negotiated views about what behaviour is expected as right and proper, and that this negotiation, and the views that result, varies between particular social groups, neighbourhoods and welfare states. These decisions are not simply individual, therefore, but are negotiated in a collective way. Calculations about individual utility maximisation, and in particular perceived economic or legal costs and benefits, may be important once these understandings are established, but they are essentially secondary to such social and moral questions. Decisions are still made rationally, but with a different sort of rationality to that assumed by the conventional economic and legal model.

Our point, therefore, is that people may take decisions on parenting, partnering and work on quite different grounds to that assumed by the New Labour government. If people do not act according to the model of rational economic man and the rational legal subject, then legislation based on such assumptions might well be ineffectual. This is what we have labelled the 'rationality mistake'. The proposals in the two Green Papers may be one example. At worst, for instance if a response to this weak effect is to introduce compulsion (as has happened with the attempt to move lone parents into paid work), then such policies might force large numbers of people to do what they consider to be morally wrong. Quite apart from the ethical implications of such a policy, it would probably still be inefficient.

The fate of the Child Support Act, a measure introduced by the Conservatives in 1991 to increase the financial contribution of absent biological fathers to the maintenance of their children, gives a good example. It was imposed from above by a government with a clear ideological agenda to mould and change family practices, and it assumed that people would act as 'rational actors' and change their social behaviour in response (Smart and Neale 1998). This disjuncture with how people actually behave has been reflected in, and compounded by, administrative bungling. The result has not only been large-scale refusal by both men and women to cooperate with the Child Support Agency (CSA), and considerable resentment by many who do, but also a wholesale discrediting of the legislation for its inefficiency and authoritarianism (see Burgoyne and Millar 1994; Clarke *et al.* 1994; Collier 1994; Millar 1996; Davis *et al.* 1998).[2] Will New Labour – despite a different political vocabulary – fall into the same trap? That this is not an inevitable trap is shown by the fate of the Family Law Act 1996 (Part II). Intended to extend the waiting time for divorce, and to better support marriage, this Act has now been abandoned in the face of pilot testing showing its unpopularity among the core voters of 'middle England' (see Chapter 3.2).

The following section outlines the nature of the 'rationality mistake', using the New Deal for Lone Parents (NDLP) as a case study. The next section goes on to examine New Labour proposals for reforming family policy in this light. This is followed by a section that counterposes the implicit assumptions of New Labour proposals against recent research into how people actually make decisions about family life. Concluding that New Labour is in danger of compounding a 'rationality mistake with a 'morality mistake', the final section sketches out some alternative policy directions.

The rationality mistake and the New Deal for Lone Parents

The New Deal schemes are a major plank of New Labour's policy goal of reconstructing welfare around paid work for all those of working age, including those like lone mothers (the vast majority of lone parents[3]) previously left out of labour market policies.[4] Briefly, the NDLP gives the lone parent a 'personal adviser' in the local job centre who provides a 'tailor-made' package of help and advice on jobs, benefits, training and childcare. A 'better-off' cost–benefit calculation is made of potential income in paid work versus current income, and lone parents are supposed to develop an action plan with their adviser (see Millar 2000). Originally introduced in eight pilot areas in 1997, the NDLP was extended nationally – without waiting for the pilot results – in 1998 to all lone parents receiving income support (a means-tested benefit for those without paid work or alternative income, and which supports a majority of British lone parents) and with children of school age. Originally a voluntary scheme, the NDLP will be made compulsory in 2002 and extended to all lone parents on income support whatever the age of their children. Repeat interviews are now demanded, and non-participants will lose benefits. So while taking employment (or training for employment) is not in itself compulsory, the pressure is certainly on to do so. This reversal of the previous policy position in Britain, where lone motherhood was seen as a legitimate reason for withdrawal from the labour market, is partly justified by a basic premise – as cited in the *Supporting Families* Green Paper (para 2.16) – that 85 per cent of unemployed lone mothers say they would like paid work if practical problems could be overcome.

Despite the government's rush to put the NDLP in place, it is worthwhile revisiting the pilot schemes run when participation was still voluntary. The evaluation reports show that only a quarter of lone parents in these areas agreed to take part, even including some who were not on income support and were not officially invited. About a third of these found paid work, although around 80 per cent of these were judged to have been likely to take paid work in any case, leaving an estimated 3.3 per cent success rate in moving lone parents off income support compared with non-participating areas (Finch *et al.* 1999; Hales *et al.* 1999, 2000a). These uptake figures are not only low, they are far lower than the 85 per cent of lone mothers quoted in the Green Paper as wanting paid work.

What are the reasons for this extremely low uptake rate? The qualitative research carried out by the evaluation studies reported that not all non-participating respondents actively opted out, quoting a number of particular and temporary reasons why they could not attend interviews (Hales *et al.* 2000b; Millar 2000), although we might reasonably assume that some of these reasons may have seemed more conveniently legitimate than expressing more fundamental doubts. Certainly, some non-participating respondents thought that they had little chance of an adequate job, and it could be that their knowledge of likely wages (usually low because of low hours worked and/or low wage rates), and likely job insecurity, coupled with the extra cost of travel to work, school meals and day care, mean that they saw the interviews as just a waste of their scarce time. This explanation would fit into explanations of the rational economic man type for the behaviour of lone mothers. The problem would be that the government had underestimated the level of constraints and overestimated the quality, rewards and availability of jobs. Lone mothers' own cost–benefit analyses would therefore usually have a different outcome to that imagined by the government or the NDLP personal adviser – it would be most rational, in this neo-classical sense, for them to remain on benefits.

However, there is another, and more fundamental, possible problem with the government's assumptions. It may well be that lone mothers are employing a different sort of rationality to the neo-classical model implicitly assumed. According to recent research, most lone mothers in Britain see their moral and practical responsibility for their children as their primary duty and that for many (although not all) this responsibility to be a 'good mother' is seen as largely incompatible with significant paid work (Duncan and Edwards 1999; Standing 1999; Von Drenth *et al.* 1999). Those lone mothers who chose not to take up paid work, far from falling into a deviant sub-culture that abhors self-reliance and social responsibility, did so on the basis of what they believed to be the morally proper thing to do as a mother.

Given this strong moral underpinning, their decisions about their non-involvement in the labour market were perfectly rational. These views of 'good mothering' are aligned with dominant conventional views about family life, and in this way unemployed lone mothers are not 'socially excluded' or in some sense 'outside society'. In contrast, the minority of lone mothers who did prioritise paid work, or saw it as integral to being a good mother, held views that are alternative to – or even 'deviant' from – dominant conceptions but were equally moral and rational. Furthermore, these alternative views of 'good mothering' are deeply social, mediated through lone mothers' experiences of being members of particular social groups in particular areas.

However, it is *paid* work that New Labour erects as a moral duty, not the unpaid caring that most lone mothers place first. This, we contend, is a 'rationality mistake'. Lone mothers make rational decisions about taking up paid work on quite different grounds to that assumed in the NDLP. Interviews with job advisers may be at best an irrelevance and at worst a threat. Unfortunately, it seems that the massive non-response to the voluntary stage of NDLP did not bring about any re-examination of its behavioural or economic assumptions. Rather, the government is to force its own assumptions upon lone parents through compulsory repeat interviews, with loss of benefits (which will inevitably affect children's lives) as sanction. According to Social Security Secretary Alistair Darling, this 'harsh but justifiable measure' is necessary to confront lone parents' 'poverty of ambition and poverty of expectation' head on (*The Guardian*, 11.2.1999). However, as this recent research shows, lone parents in fact have considerable ambition and expectations for their children, and they undertake considerable work in trying to achieve this, albeit unpaid caring work, which leaves them formally 'unemployed'.

We can call this response to policy inadequacy a 'morality mistake', and it appears on two levels. The first stage is to assume that people are not behaving 'rationally' (in terms of rational economic man and the rational legal subject) because of lack of information or, more pejoratively, ignorance. Hence, for example, the need for lone parents to have day care and labour market situations explained to them. If policy is still ineffectual – as seems quite likely – then this 'morality mistake' can move to a second, more authoritarian, stage. People are not behaving 'rationally' because of their own moral or cultural deviancy – lone mothers are wilfully irresponsible or morally inadequate. Compulsion can be justified and rationalised as the unfortunate effect of their 'poverty of ambition and poverty of expectation' or, more pejoratively, as resulting from the 'dependency culture'. Currently, government spokespersons seem to mix the two. The idea that people take what they consider to be morally appropriate decisions in their situation, and that they have worked hard in reaching these decisions in particular situations, is not considered. Ironically, in view of the theoretical claims of communitarianism, such legislation also rides roughshod over the varying community norms about parenting and paid work in which people reach such decisions.

In forcing its own version of rationality upon lone parents, the government risks making large numbers do what they consider to be morally wrong. In this way, the 'rationality mistake' – the false assumption that people act like rational economic man – is compounded by a 'morality mistake' – the false attribution of particular normative views. As we shall see, this is not surprising as 'rationality' is not divorced from 'morality', despite the strictures of neo-classical economics and rational actor theory (which in themselves can be seen as a perverse form of morality). These mistakes are underlain by oversimple assumptions about how people make important decisions about their family lives, with an overemphasis on individualistic economic rationality and a neglect of more collective moral judgements. In the next section, we examine New Labour's family policy proposals in this light.

New Labour's family policy: supporting families, or 'rationality' and 'morality' mistakes?

In New Labour's 'third way' family practices, or rather, 'the family' as an ideal form, come to play a pivotal role (see Chapter 6). For, unlike the neoliberalism of the New Right, in this communitarian discourse individuals and markets are both seen as socially embedded (Driver and Martell 1998). Economic success, therefore, demands both social cohesion and proper social morality. In practice, this social embedding has been taken to mean families, although the New Deal for Communities initiative and some related programmes have emphasised the importance of 'community' for disadvantaged inner city and social housing areas.[5] But proper family values, the key to a 'decent society', are in doubt given all the changes in families where there is increasingly a 'parenting deficit' – or so communitarian discourse goes. Mothers are out at work. Fathers may be absent. Hence children are left without moral guidance or emotional support. This is exacerbated by a 'moral deficit' where, Blair (1996a) claims, there is 'indifference to the undermining of family life'. Moreover, it is increasingly difficult for government to manage family life, where partnering, and even parenting, increasingly takes place outside formal marriage. Some commentators even see New Labour's interest in parenting as approaching the status of a 'moral reform crusade' (Coward 1998); certainly, the House of Commons Parliamentary Group on Parenting sees a national strategy for parenting as laying the foundations for 'social responsibility and self-discipline', which would 'promote important social objectives' (*The Guardian*, 9.6.1998).

The Conservative government's 'back to basics' campaign during the 1990s became quite open in proclaiming a moral agenda in favour of the traditional family, and it contained a strong element of vilification of other family forms, most notably lone motherhood (see Smart and Neale 1998;

Duncan and Edwards 1999). In contrast, New Labour proclaims moral tolerance. Nevertheless, it still firmly states that marriage is the ideal state and that living with two biological and preferably married parents is the best for children. Indeed, one of the new government's first initiatives in this area was to promote a 'national marriage week' early in 1998.

This somewhat contradictory position reflects a paradox set up by New Labour's version of communitarianism. On the one hand, there is a supposed parenting deficit, but on the other hand all adults below pensionable age have the ascribed duty to take on paid work. Traditional marriage, with two-parent married families, would seem to offer the best way of squaring the circle, for this is the family form that best allows the combination of parenting with paid work. Lone motherhood, in contrast, epitomises the contradiction between paid work and parenting – there is less disposable time for one parent to achieve either at adequate levels. The intricacies and ambivalences of step-parenting, cohabitation and all the other 'new family forms' just complicate matters and in any case are seen as more likely to lead to family breakdown. In these terms, parenting by both biological parents who are also married is therefore the best and most efficient family form in linking social morality, social cohesion and economic efficiency.

The 1998 Green Paper *Supporting Families* makes proposals to operationalise this preference. It is also particularly significant as the first cross-government social policy wholly conceived and developed under Tony Blair's leadership, and as such it lies at the core of New Labour's values (Travis 1998; Wintour 1998). *Supporting Families* can therefore be taken as a good indicator of the government's perspective. We will not comment here on all the proposals in the Green Paper (see Barlow and Duncan 1999), except to note that it is permeated by a neo-classical 'carrot-and-stick' view of family decision making. Supposedly, sub-optimal behaviour is the result of a lack of information, or a lack of ability to use it properly. Change this ('change the culture', as the Green Paper puts it in para 1.20) and more optimal behaviour will result – in this case, desired parenting or labour market behaviour. However, particular groups, such as the more disadvantaged in problem council housing estates or the sons of lone mothers, need to be educated, and instructed, as to what the right information is and, at times, coerced into the right behaviour. At times, this seems to lead to a 'blame the victim' approach to social problems. The activities of employers, for example, in providing low-paid or insecure jobs are not questioned. Rather, *Supporting Families* simply encourages employers, in unspecific terms, to introduce 'family-friendly employment', based on voluntary cooperation. No coercion here for those with anti-social behaviour![6] The point for us here is not only that this policy emphasis can be seen as resulting from New Labour's prescriptive and moralistic version of communitarianism, one that emphasises individual responsibility at the expense of socio-economic reform (Driver and Martell 1998), but also that this emphasis becomes naturalised where the sovereignty of individual preferences and behaviour is an axiom of the neo-classical version of social behaviour. This is, after all, the very foundation of rational economic man and, from this starting point, it does indeed make little sense to see the origins and causes of social problems as lying in wider social conditions, still less in the actions of employers and firms.

The most novel part of the Green Paper, and the one that maps out a basic response to family change, is chapter 4 – indicatively entitled 'Strengthening Marriage'. On one level, it claims that intervention aims to help the parenting relationship – whether married or not – to succeed. In any case, government competence is limited where 'families do not want to be lectured about their behaviour or what kind of relationship they are in' (*ibid.*: para 4.2). Yet at another level, the Green Paper states that the government's preferred parenting structure is marriage. As the preamble makes clear:

> marriage does provide a strong foundation for stability for the care of children. It also sets out rights and responsibilities for all concerned. It remains the choice of the majority of people in Britain. For all these reasons, it makes sense for the Government to do what it can to strengthen marriage.
>
> *ibid.*: para 4.8

What is more, the vast bulk of the chapter is concerned with how marriage can be supported and encouraged. Other possible partnership and parenting forms are hardly mentioned – despite the fact that in 1996 21 per cent of children were born to cohabiting parents, with another 14 per cent born to lone mothers. Both figures are increasing, and cohabitation is predicted to double by 2020. Yet only about half a dozen of the forty-nine paragraphs could have much relevance to such parents, and only three consider cohabitants. Nothing at all is said about same-sex parenting. What can the Green Paper say to all these parents other than 'get married'?

The chapter goes on to propose a number of measures to strengthen marriage. These include better preparation for marriage, such as a clear statement of rights and responsibilities, pre-nuptial agreements about the distribution of money and property, an enhanced role for marriage registrars in providing premarital counselling, modernisation and personalisation of the civil marriage service, access to mediation and counselling to support marriages in difficulty, and better information before divorce 'to increase the chance of saving more marriages' (para 4.12). Clearer rules on property division on marital breakdown are proposed to reduce conflict between married couples.

In contrast, proposals affecting cohabiting families are limited to just two suggestions. First is the introduction of a non-religious and public child-naming ceremony, which may also be used to stage the public signing of a parental responsibility-sharing agreement where parents are unmarried. This is designed to encourage public assertion of both parents' commitment to a child, whether or not they are living together. Second, the Green Paper rather grudgingly suggests that 'it might therefore be worthwhile' to produce a guide for cohabitants setting out their legal rights in relation to income, property, tax, welfare benefits and responsibility towards their children, to be made available in Citizens' Advice Bureaux and libraries (para 4.15). This does little to address the complexity and inadequacies of the law relating to cohabitation. While enforceable prenuptial contracts for those intending to marry are proposed, the Green Paper is silent on the issue of legally enforceable cohabitation agreements. There is no apparent recognition of the ongoing work of the Law Commission on home sharing for partners (Harpum 1995). Nor is there support for counselling to save cohabitation relationships, in sharp contrast to the proposed effort to be invested in saving marriages. The Green Paper therefore fails to acknowledge, let alone address, the need for better family law-based regulation of cohabitation relationships. And for lone parents the discussion is hardly about parenting at all (save for the negative assumption that their sons will lack male role models). The Green Paper sees the issue as simply getting lone parents into paid work, and in chapter 2 it basically repeats the NDLP proposals. In terms of policy discourses, lone mothers and cohabitees are seen more as a social threat. Only if cohabitees or lone parents marry will they be rewarded with the legal protection and government support that they and their children need.

The means of implementing this discourse, of strengthening marriage and reducing the threat of other family forms, is seen in terms of rational economic man and the rational legal subject. The government appears to believe that changing financial and legal parameters, as in the Green Paper, will thereby alter the calculations for people's decision making about partnering and parenting and will therefore in turn lead to the desired changes in behaviour. More lone parents will take up paid work, more couples will marry, fewer will cohabit, and fewer will divorce. The problem is that the basic assumption about how people make decisions about their moral economies – about how partnerships should be formed, sustained and dissolved; how parenting should be carried out; how this might be combined with paid work; and who does what sort of paid and unpaid work – might be incorrect. The whole enterprise might then become irrelevant – or even oppressive – because of this 'rationality mistake'. In the next section, we go on to counterpose these assumptions against recent empirical evidence about how people do make decisions about partnering and parenting.

Moral rationalities and family decision making

During the 1990s, family sociology turned more to what families actually do, rather than – as so often before – what they ought to do, or were assumed to do, and how deviant families and family members could then be seen in this light. As David Morgan (1996) put it, the focus is now on 'family practices' rather than on 'family problems'. The work of Janet Finch and her colleagues on family obligations has become something of a formative classic in this area (Finch 1989; Finch and Mason 1993) and has inspired a whole school of family research (see Silva and Smart 1999). The empirical focus is now on how notions of moral obligation and responsibility between kin might be changing in the context of rapid changes in family structures and other social changes like increasing female employment. Researchers have found that shared understandings about 'the proper thing to do' emerge over time and in specific contexts – there is no static concept of duty, or *a priori* moral rules in terms of abstract principles, and even less some rational economic calculation. Such understandings will also vary according to the different contexts of social groups, social places and social histories. This also means that these essentially moral decisions about care are often ambiguous and varying – there can be more than one 'right answer', depending on particular circumstances and histories. Similarly, socio-legal researchers established that people do not make rational cost–benefit responses to the law. Not only are many people generally unaware of legal frameworks about family life but also, when it comes to important decisions, the influence of social networks is the most important (Jacob 1992; Baker and Emrys 1993). Indeed, Bainham (1998) concludes that family law is inherently unenforceable unless it coincides with existing social norms, and at best it can set up a conceptual model of 'desirable' behaviour. At around the same time, theorists pointed out that 'ordinary people' do not have to be versed in the intricacies of moral philosophy in order to act morally or form moral judgements, and that moral and ethical reasoning are 'everyday social and textual practices' (e.g. Bauman 1993; Sevenhuijsen 1998). Moral decisions are not just the preserve of philosophers, religious leaders and politicians: they form the basis of everyday family life.

How people actually make these moral decisions, and how moral values are formed and how they inform action, now becomes crucial in understanding family behaviour. Certainly, this has important implications for the construction of social policy, at least in terms of its efficiency if not ethically. Put baldly, and with hindsight, this might seem obvious. It was just that much social research into families and decision making assumed that people were either passive respondents to external stimuli or rational economic men simply making decisions in terms of personal costs and benefits. In either case, they were fairly uniform. Exceptions were in some way deviant. The problem is that New Labour still seems to assume this.

So how do people in Britain see partnering, marriage and cohabitation, the focus of chapter 4 of the Green Paper on *Strengthening Marriage*. We draw here upon two complementary studies: a national (England and Wales) survey of attitudes and beliefs about cohabitation and marriage undertaken by the National Centre for Social Research in 2000 (Barlow *et al.* 2001); and a small in-depth pilot interview study of thirty mothers (eleven married, eleven cohabiting and eight lone mothers) carried out in 1998 in the contrasting social and labour market areas of Great Yarmouth in Norfolk and Merthyr Tydfil in South Wales (Barlow 1998).

Almost two-thirds of the interviewees saw marriage as an ideal family form, in that it symbolised stability and commitment. Interestingly, this included the majority of cohabitees as well as half the lone mothers. Similarly, in the national survey almost 60 per cent of respondents thought that marriage was 'still the best kind of relationship'. This ideal view therefore parallels the view of marriage taken in the 1998 Green Paper. However, and crucially, both interviewees and survey respondents took a different view of the moral reality of their own situations. Thus all the interviewed cohabitants had considered marriage, and all indicated that most people assumed they were married and that in any case no stigma was attached to cohabiting. But they had rejected marriage largely because they thought it made no difference to the success of their relationships and/or they had had previous bad experiences of marriage (they also – inaccurately – believed this rejection had no legal implications). Indeed, around half of these interviewees actively saw marriage as in some way threatening to their relationship, because it would change their partner's behaviour for the worse (lone mothers saw marriage more as a source of unhappiness and disappointment). A smaller group of cohabitants (four of the eleven cohabitees) did want to marry but saw cohabitation as a trial marriage. While these mothers saw the cost of a 'proper marriage' as a disincentive, they did not doubt the validity of cohabitation as a partnering and parenting form. In the national survey, only 28 per cent of respondents (married and unmarried) thought that marriage made couples better parents. Marriage was again more of an ideal rather than some superior family form in practice. At the same time, few of the married mothers in the interview study had actually got married because of its ideal characteristics, and around half had done so because of their wider social position in terms of religious beliefs or pressure from partners or parents.

Majority opinion, therefore, sees the ideal of marriage as just that, an ideal not always obtainable in practice. For many mothers in the interview sample, and particularly the cohabiting and lone mothers, cohabitation was seen as equal to, or even superior to, marriage. These views are not acknowledged in New Labour's 'social threat' view of unmarried families as replicated in the Green Paper.

The practical advantages of marriage given by the interviewees, whether married or not, are particularly illuminating. These do not refer to the superiority of marriage for partnering and parenting as supposed in the Green Paper. Rather, they referred to marriage as a social symbol. This symbolism was to be achieved in two major ways: through a change of name and through a full-blown 'white wedding' in church.

The desire by cohabitants to have the same surname as their children and partner was cited as a major reason for marriage, and this was a major reason for marrying given by four of the five mothers who had previously cohabited. It was the birth of children that commonly predicated this move. Conversely, most of the cohabiting mothers saw having a different surname to their partner and children as the greatest disadvantage of not marrying. (Two had formally changed their surname to that of their partner's, and another two families had adopted double-barrelled names). Female name changing is not a legal requirement, but it is rather a powerful tradition. Presumably, this is taken as a social signifier of a 'proper family', one that follows accepted gender norms about roles and responsibilities – this is the very reason why name changing is actually rejected by many professional married women and by those with 'alternative' feminist views.

It was also clear that the cohabiting mothers were not prepared to marry in a simple registry office ceremony. If they were to marry, it was on condition that they had a full-blown white church wedding.[7] It was the wedding as social display and symbol, not the institution or ideal of marriage as a partnership or parenting form, that was endowed with significance in the context of their lives. This is dramatically underscored by the fact that eight of these mothers had actually refused their partner's offer of marriage in a registry office! Those cohabitees in the 'trial marriage' group fully accepted that this might mean that they would never marry. These were the only unmarried respondents who indicated that financial incentives would have a decisive effect on their decision to marry, but only if this enabled them to have the highly desired white wedding in church.

This essentially social signifying role of marriage was buttressed by the 'common law marriage myth'. Nearly all interviewees, unprompted, firmly believed that the law treated cohabitees with children of the relationship in all respects as if they were married. Although the law has not recognised common law marriage since the Clandestine Marriages Act of 1753, both married and unmarried cohabiting couples volunteered this as an acknowledged legal status. Even in the (by necessity) prompted national survey, 56 per cent of respondents thought that common law marriage definitely or probably existed. Yet this is far from being an accurate reflection of the legal position: nearly all cohabiting mothers believed, incorrectly, that they would be entitled to a pension or other allowances on the strength of their partner's contributions; that they could make maintenance claims or claim a share of the joint house just as if they were divorced or widowed; and that unmarried fathers automatically gained the legal status of fatherhood if they jointly registered the birth. These proportions were lower in the national survey, perhaps reflecting the prompting of questions in the structured questionnaire, but still between 40 and 50 per cent of respondents wrongly thought that cohabitees possessed these legal rights of marriage. These beliefs are buttressed by the state having it both ways, for in assessing entitlement to means-tested benefits cohabitees are treated exactly like married couples! Similarly, the interviewed lone mothers commonly hated the CSA, linked to the misconception that accepting 'CSA money' would mean that they would be forced to allow fathers to contact their children. This had led two to refuse cooperation, despite a 40 per cent reduction in benefit levels. This ignorance of the law by lone mothers and cohabitees alike can have severe results (see Barlow and Duncan 1999, 2000) but in a wider sense is quite rational. This is because couples generally see their partnership, and its strength or weakness, in terms of a relationship, not in terms of an institution.

So marriage was often seen as an ideal state, but in terms of everyday moral adequacy few respondents saw marriage as a superior partnering or parenting form. It was the strength of a mother's relationship with her partner that was decisive, and this was unaffected by whether marriage had taken place or not. Similarly, marriage was seen as largely irrelevant to the welfare of children. Respondents, unlike government spokespersons, did not easily confuse partnering and parenting forms (married, cohabiting, etc.) with those processes (love, support, communication, etc.) that lead to the success or failure of these relationships. In this sense, the respondents took rather more sophisticated moral judgements than the government. People do not decide upon their moral economies according to the model of rational economic man and the rational legal subject. In this way, chapter 4 of the *Strengthening Marriage* Green Paper perpetuates the 'rationality' and 'morality' mistakes identified in the NDLP.

Some alternative policy directions

It is far easier to oppose than propose. What, a government spokesperson might retort, are the alternatives? An overall starting point is that uniform prescriptive policies are likely to be both inefficient and oppressive. There is also an overemphasis on social *forms* (such as paid employment, marriage) rather than social *relations* (working, caring, partnering, parenting). The alternative is to try to develop supportive and flexible legislative frameworks that do recognise the varying ways in which people take moral decisions. Ironically, communitarian thinking usually asserts that questions of values and morality are essentially local because they are embedded in, and relative to, particular 'communities' (Driver and Martell 1998). Unfortunately, New Labour's particular adaptation of communitarianism is in danger of prescribing moral values that ride roughshod over this plurality. Policies for partnering, parenting and paid work need to be locally and socially sensitive.

A first corrective to the 'rationality mistake' is that family policies need to respect local definitions of good parenting and partnering, including responsibility towards children. At the same time, parents and partners themselves, the recipients of policy, should be brought on board to allow them to express their needs and understandings and to find some degree of control over policies that affect their lives. As research on urban regeneration has also shown (Allen 1998), the opportunity to find some control over change is vital, otherwise policy intervention risks becoming just something that is done to you by more powerful outsiders.

Improved day care provision for lone mothers is a good example (see Duncan and Edwards 1999). Rather than being essentially seen, as in the

NDLP, as a means of parking children so that mothers can take paid work, policies should recognise that different groups of lone mothers have different ideas about what constitutes good day care and about how much day care is morally appropriate. Some prefer formal nursery provision for the whole day, while others are more likely to see relatives as the best carers, probably part-time, if they are willing to leave their children with anyone else at all. One national response might be to extend the day care 'disregard' to informal carers in calculating tax and benefits. On a local scale, it may be better in some areas to concentrate investment in day nurseries with professional staff but in others to develop initiatives to support care by relatives through training, back-up professional support and communal facilities. In other areas, there may already be quite extensive community and voluntary day care facilities, which some mothers prefer as being more in tune with their own circumstances and expectations, and these would need different forms of support again.

There are some problems with this strategy, which also raise more general, and quite crucial, issues about the distribution and definitions of work, caring and time. In the short term, this sort of bottom-up NDLP could risk the consolidation of social inequalities. Part-time informal day care might not be as socially or educationally advantageous as full-time professionally run nursery care, and in this way class and neighbourhood inequalities might be perpetuated or exacerbated. At the same time, however, if we take moral and cultural differences seriously, then we have to give different life models equal recognition. A possible way forward out of this dilemma is to emphasise that day care is for the benefit of children and in children's best interests, not simply a device for getting mothers into the labour market. As research also shows, British lone mothers do not simply want more day care; it is the type and quality of day care, including who would be looking after their children, that is crucial. Quality and purpose are just as important as quantity.

A bottom-up NDLP also risks perpetuating gender inequalities, for informal day care would be provided overwhelmingly by female relatives or friends and would thereby consolidate the distribution of caring work to the 'private realm' of women and families. (Even when it reaches the public sphere, formal care for young children is also a mainly female task.) This raises the question of the definitions of work and welfare. If we were to redefine 'work' as not just paid work but also work to care for children and the elderly, and at the same time redefine welfare to include the receipt of care, then we can see that 'welfare to work' is a misnomer: 'welfare' is not opposed to 'work', because most people receive and carry out both; welfare and work are mixed. Nor is care simply a barrier to paid work, or something that is simply necessary – both giving and receiving care are meaningful and valuable in their own right. If we take this on board, an implication is to remove the gendered and unequal valuations of full-time paid work, part-time paid work and unpaid work. These valuations do not just lead to income or resource inequalities, they also produce inequalities of time and status. Seen in this light, there is little advantage in lone mothers swapping day care for low-paid, part-time work at unsocial hours. Rather than erecting paid work – any paid work – as a moral duty it would be better to move towards moral and financial neutrality towards all forms of socially necessary work. An overall alternative, therefore, is that national 'welfare to work' should be redesigned as locally sensitive 'welfare and work'.

This redesignation provides a powerful challenge to the whole political philosophy underlying New Labour's welfare to work strategy, where it is paid work that provides the basis of both economic rationality and citizenship. As Selma Sevenhuijsen (see Chapter 6) points out, this latter view invokes a moral norm of self-sufficiency, and a related liberal view of human nature, which assumes that people are, or should be, detached individuals whose aim is autonomous and separate behaviour. We should all be Robinson Crusoes, or if we are not, welfare to work will help us to become one. In contrast, the morality arising out of giving and receiving care accounts, both philosophically and practically, for the relational and interdependent state of the human condition.

The argument with respect to cohabitation and marriage is similar. Rather than prescriptive policies focusing on form (marriage versus cohabitation), a more socially and communally aware communitarianism could develop policies to support partnering and parenting relations. The law should look at what a family does, rather than the form it takes, in ascribing legal rights and responsibilities. If the government so chose, it could endow cohabitation with rights and responsibilities similar to those held by married partners. This would provide legal security and state support for both partners and children within unmarried relationships. We can briefly note here how this is in contrast to some other European countries. In Scandinavia, for instance, cohabitation and marriage have long held equality before the law, and same-sex cohabitation, and more recently same-sex marriage, have been drawn into the same orbit. Lone mothers are just another type of worker citizen where all adults below pensionable age are treated as autonomous and supported in taking up paid work (see Chapter 4.3). A great advantage is that a large proportion of parents (up to 50 per cent) are not legally and politically marginalised. The Netherlands, Belgium, two autonomous regions in Spain (Catalonia and Aragon) and, most recently, France have also more closely approximated the legal rights of cohabiting couples to those of married couples (see Barlow and Probert 1999, 2000). In France, this change was achieved in two ways. First, the incorporation of a definition of cohabitation that encompasses both heterosexual and same-sex cohabitation into the French Civil Code has given cohabitees formal legal status combined with a safety-net package of rights. Second, by introducing PACS (*pacte civile de solidarité*: civil union or civil solidarity contracts, again available to all unmarried cohabitees whether heterosexual or same-sex), the French legislation now gives couples who have entered into a *pacte* the freedom to make their own binding legal arrangements. At the same time, it also guarantees legal rights similar to marriage for purposes including social security benefits, health insurance, inheritance and property division on the breakdown of a relationship. A duty, similar to that required in marriage, to offer each other mutual and material assistance is also imposed on these couples. The French state does not, therefore, view cohabitation as an exclusively selfish and uncommitted family form giving rise to individualistic behaviour – a commonly perceived, if unsubstantiated, view of cohabitation (Lewis 1999).

If these examples of inclusion are too radical in the face of English conservatism and the reactionary power of parts of the tabloid press, then some Commonwealth jurisdictions show partial moves in this direction. In Newfoundland, under the Matrimonial Property Act 1979, heterosexual cohabitees are permitted to opt into the matrimonial property legislation. In New South Wales, the De Facto Relationships Act 1984 enables heterosexual cohabitees who have been together for at least two years to apply for maintenance and property adjustment on the breakdown of a relationship. More recently, the Domestic Relationships Act 1994 in Australian Capital Territory extends the financial provision on breakdown of a relationship to all personal relationships (other than legal marriage) in which one provides personal or financial commitment and support of a domestic nature for the material benefit of the other. Even in Britain, the Scottish Executive is blazing the trail in its White Paper *Improving Scottish Family Law* (2000) by addressing the financial implications of cohabitation, suggesting that a legal claim should be available where a cohabitee has suffered economic disadvantage.

Certainly, the research findings show general public support in Britain for such an approach. In the 2000 national survey, 61.4 per cent of all respondents thought that cohabitants living together for ten years should definitely or probably have the same maintenance rights as married couples; 92.1 per cent thought they should have the same inheritance rights; and a massive 97 per cent thought that unmarried fathers should have the same rights as married fathers to make decisions about their child's medical treatment.

It is essential that New Labour redefines its communitarianism along these more pluralistic, voluntaristic and redistributive lines if lone mothers are to successfully balance their responsibility to their children with the opportunities of paid work, and if cohabitants are to become more successful partners and parents.

Notes

1 *Supporting Families: A Consultative Document*, London: the Stationery Office, 1998; *New Ambitions for Our Country: A New Contract for Welfare*, London, the Stationery Office, 1998.
2 While the incoming Labour government has attempted to simplify this legislation and streamline its operation, it remains committed to the legislation.
3 Although legislation normally refers to 'lone parents', the small minority of lone fathers are usually in substantial paid work and, in addition, are not positioned

as a social threat. This implicit distinction is a function of the gendered nature of parenting that is obscured in formal discourse.

4 Other New Deals target young people, the long-term unemployed, people on disability benefits; childless partners of the unemployed; and unemployed people over 50. The first two schemes account for the bulk of expenditure.
5 See Foley and Martin 2000 for summary, context and critique.
6 A basic framework of maximum working hours and extended maternity and parental leave has been enacted under the Employment Relations Act 1999, partly under the pressure of EU directives. However, the former are riven by exceptions, while the latter, especially where maternity leave over eighteen weeks and all paternity leave is unpaid, will effectively exclude low earners, who cannot afford to take them up. These low earners will include many lone parents and those living in inner cities that the government sees as most likely to display aberrant parenting behaviour.
7 All these respondents were in heterosexual partnerships and were apparently Christian, at least nominally.

References

Allen, T. (1998) 'Housing renewal: doesn't it make you sick', *Housing Studies*15(3): 443–61.

Bainham, A. (1998) 'Changing families and changing concepts – reforming the language of family law', *Child and Family Law Quarterly* 10(1): 1–15.

Baker, L. and Emrys, R. (1993) 'When every relationship is above average: perceptions and expectations of divorce at the time of marriage', *Law and Human Behaviour* 17(4): 439–50.

Barlow, A. (1998) 'Family structuring, legal regulation and gendered moral rationalities; some empirical findings', paper presented at Socio-legal Studies Association Annual Conference, Manchester Metropolitan University, 16 April (available from the author at Law Department, University of Wales, Aberystwyth).

Barlow, A. and Duncan, S. (1999) 'New Labour's communitarianism, supporting families, and the "rationality mistake" ', Working Paper 10, Centre for Research on Family, Kinship and Gender, University of Leeds.

—— (2000) 'Family law, moral rationalities and New Labour's communitarianism: Part II', *Journal of Social Welfare and Family Law* 22(2): 129–43.

Barlow, A. and Probert, R. (1999) 'Addressing the legal status of cohabitation in Britain and France: plus ça change?' *Web Journal of Current Legal Issues*: http://webjcli.ncl.ac.uk/1999/issue3/barlow3.html

—— (2000) 'Le pacs est arrivé: France embraces its new-style family', *International Family Law*, 182–4.

Barlow, A., Duncan S., James, G. and Park, A. (2001) 'Just a piece of paper. Marriage and cohabitation in Britain', chapter 2 in *British Social Attitudes: The 18th Report*, London: Sage.

Bauman, Z. (1993) *Postmodern Ethics*, Cambridge: Polity Press.

Blair, T. (1996a) speech to the CPU Conference, Cape Town, 14 October.

—— (1996b) in G. Radice (ed.) *What Needs to Change: New Visions for Britain*, London: HarperCollins.

—— (1997) 'The will to win', speech to launch the Social Exclusion Unit at the Aylesbury Estate, Southwark, 2 June.

Burgoyne, C. and Millar, J. (1994) 'Enforcing child support: the views of separated fathers', *Policy and Politics* 22(2): 95–104.

Clarke, K., Craig, C. and Glendinning, C. (1994) *Losing Support: Children and the Child Support Act*, London: Barnado's, Children's Society, NCH, NSPCC and SCF.

Collier, R. (1994) 'The campaign against the Child Support Act: errant fathers and family men', *Family Law*, 384–7.

Coward, R. (1998) 'Busybody's charter', *The Guardian,* 9 June.

Davis, G., Wikley, N. and Young, R., with J. Barron and J. Bedward (1998) *Child Support in Action*, Oxford: Hart Publishing.

Driver, S. and Martell, L. (1998) *New Labour: Politics after Thatcherism*, Cambridge, Polity Press.

Duncan, S. and Edwards, R. (1999) *Lone Mothers, Paid Work and Gendered Moral Rationalities*, Macmillan, London.

Etzioni, A. (2000) 'Internalisation, persuasion and history', *Law and Society Review* 34(1): 157–78.

Finch, H. and O'Connor, W., with J. Millar, J. Hales, A. Shaw and W. Roth (1999) 'The New Deal for Lone Parents: learning from the prototype areas', Research Report 92, Department of Social Security. London: DSS.

Finch, J. (1989) *Family Obligations and Social Change*, Cambridge: Polity Press.

Finch, J. and Mason, J. (1993) *Negotiating Family Responsibilities*, London: Routledge.

Foley, P. and Martin, S. (2000) 'A new deal for the community? Public participation in regeneration and local service delivery', *Policy and Politics* 28(4): 479–91.

Hales, J., Shaw, A. and Roth, W. (1999) 'Evaluation of the New Deal for Lone Parents: a preliminary assessment of the counterfactual', in House Report 42, Social Research Branch, Department of Social Security. London: DSS.

Hales, J., Lessof, C., Roth, W., Glover, M., Shaw, A., Barnes M., Elias P., Hasluck C., McKnight A. and Green, A. (2000a) Evaluation of the New Deal for Lone Parents: early lessons from the phase one prototype – synthesis report', Research Report 108, Department of Social Security. London: DSS.

Hales, J., Roth, W., Barnes M., Millar J., Lessof, C., Glover, M., Shaw, A., (2000b) *Evaluation of the New Deal for Lone Parents: early lessons from the phase one prototype – findings of surveys*, Research Report 109, Department of Social Security. London: DSS.

Harpum, C. (1995) 'Cohabitation consultation', *Family Law*, 25, 657.

Jacob, H. (1992) 'The elusive shadow of the law', *Law and Society Review* 267(3): 565–90.

Lewis, J. (1999) 'Marriage, cohabitation and the law: individualism and obligation', Research Series 1/99, Lord Chancellor's Department, London.

Lister, R. (1998) 'From equality to social inclusion: New Labour and the welfare state', *Critical Social Policy* 18(2): 215–25.

Millar, J. (1996) 'Family obligations and social policy: the case of child support', *Policy Studies* 17(3): 181–9

—— (2000) 'Lone parents and the New Deal', *Policy Studies* 21(4): 333–45.

Morgan, D. (1996) *Family Connections*, Cambridge: Polity Press.

Sevenhuijsen, S. (1998) *Citizenship and the Ethics of Care*, London: Routledge.

Silva, E. and Smart, C. (1999) 'The "new" practices and politics of family life' in Silva, E. and Smart, C. *The New Family Life*, London: Sage.

Smart, C. and Neale, B. (1998) *Family Fragments?* London: Polity Press.

Standing, K. (1999) 'Lone mothers and "parental" involvement', *Journal of Social Policy* 28(3): 479–95.

Travis, A. (1998) 'Straw plays Spock', *The Guardian*, 3 November.

Von Drenth, A., Knijn, T. and Lewis, J. (1999) 'Sources of income for lone mother families: policy changes in Britain and The Netherlands and the experiences of divorced women', *Journal of Social Policy* 28(4): 619–41.

Wintour, P. (1998) 'Nannying gives Labour pains', *The Observer*, 25 October.

6 A third way? Moralities, ethics and families

An approach through the ethic of care

Selma Sevenhuijsen

Introduction

It might be common knowledge by now that 'the' family is in many ways a powerful myth. It is not only a sociological myth, since there are many different kinds of family form and family practice, which shift over time and according to cultural context. It is also a political myth, since 'the family' is to a considerable extent constructed by state policies (family law, social policies) and by the idea systems of political institutions (political parties, advisory bodies, institutions of the welfare state). It matters how political theories conceptualise family, kinship and care and, at the heart of this complicated nexus, gender. As a contemporary illustration of the process by which a concept of 'the family' is implicated in political strategies, I will consider the contributions made by the British sociologist Anthony Giddens, especially in his book *The Third Way: The Renewal of Social Democracy* (1998).

Giddens presents his ideas as a middle road between neo-liberalism and 'old-style social democracy'. I focus primarily on the political philosophy underlying his approach, rather than current policy making. I therefore leave open the question of how far his ideas have influenced the policy of the Blair government in the UK, which has at times traded under the same banner of 'the third way'. Nevertheless, Giddens' merit is that he echoes New Labour thinking on the family in a manner that is systematic enough to allow a detailed critique. My main contention is that the feminist ethic of care can provide a useful vantage point from which to demonstrate both the weaknesses in Giddens' treatment of the family and the real possibilities for political renewal that lie in a potential 'third way' of thinking about democratic family practice that takes proper account of the ethics of care.

The normative framework of Giddens' third way

In the opening chapters of his book, Giddens lays down what in his view should be the crux of the normative framework of third way politics: a balanced relation between social justice, emancipation, equality and social cohesion. In a later section he substantiates these values further. He introduces five dilemmas for social democracy, *viz.* globalisation, individualism, the meaning of Left and Right, the value of political agency, and how to respond to ecological problems. He then states that 'the overall aim of third way politics should be to help citizens to pilot their way through the major revolutions of our time: *globalisation, transformations in personal life* and our *relationship to nature*' (Giddens 1998: 64).

Equality and freedom should be at the core of the third way's value system. Freedom to social democrats should mean autonomy of action, which in turn 'demands the involvement of the wider social community' (*ibid.*: 65). After the age of collectivism, third way politics should look for a new relationship between the individual and the community, a redefinition of rights and obligations. Old-style social democracy would be too much inclined to treat rights as unconditional claims. The prime motto for the new politics should therefore be *no rights without responsibilities*.

These notions are linked to two further core concepts, which are both relevant to his discussion of the family, that of *no authority without democracy* and *philosophical conservatism*. While the traditional Right looks to nation, government and traditional family life as a means of justifying authority and for ways to differentiate between right and wrong, and thus for moral judgement, social democrats should adhere to the idea that the only route to establishing authority is via democracy. The new individualism should not be seen as a threat to authority and solidarity but rather as a demand that authority be recast on an active and participatory base. The values of participatory democracy should in fact be applied to all spheres of social life. However, he qualifies these ideas by introducing the notion of philosophical conservatism. This norm should be adopted when dealing with the question of how to recreate social solidarity after the decline of tradition and custom, and how to deal with modernisation and economic growth in an era of environmental risk.

Modernisation should not be about 'more and more modernity' but should be conscious of the limits of modernising processes and about the need to 're-establish continuity'. Philosophical conservatism would suggest a pragmatic attitude of coping with change, a respect for past and history and, in the environmental arena, an adoption of the precautionary principle wherever feasible. 'The family' serves as the prime example of this notion of philosophical conservatism: sustaining continuity in family life, especially the well-being of children, should in Giddens' view be acknowledged as one of the most important goals of family policy. Woven through these ideas are notions of obligation and responsibility. Let me first discuss, then, the role of these notions in the general framework of the book before looking in more detail at the proposals for family policies.

The ethic of care versus contract and obligation

The notions of obligation and responsibility in third way discourse serve to bridge the gap between individual and society and to forge a new relationship between individual and community. In opposition to conservative ideology, Giddens does not want to see individualism as a threat to solidarity and the existence of social ties. As he states succinctly, we do not live in an age of moral decay but rather in one of moral transition, in which we have to live our lives in a more active way than was true for previous generations, and in which we have to find a new balance between individual and collective responsibilities (Giddens 1998: 37). At this point, it is important to note that he embraces human agency and self-fulfilment as positive normative goals, refusing to equate this with the notion of narrow-minded egoism that conservatives tend to ascribe to neo-liberalism.

However, the need for these metaphors of bridging (and thus the need for a 'third way') are created by the very discourse that Giddens uses in *The Third Way*. Despite his professed progressive intentions, a retrospective mood underlies his text, a mood in which the opposition between individual and society is accepted as given. He frequently uses metaphors of reparation for something that has been lost, such as when he states that third way politics should *re-establish* continuity, *recreate* social solidarity and *repair* the civil order. A feminist ethic of care denies such oppositions between individual and society in the first place. In three respects, the care ethic yields a different perspective on this topic than that provided by Giddens and related third way thinkers: first, with regard to the idea of human subjectivity; second, with regard to the ideas adopted about morality and politics; and, third, with regard to the underlying 'political sociology of care'.

As argued by a great number of authors, the ethic of care is inherently characterised by a *relational ontology*, both in the descriptive and in the normative respects. This is encapsulated in the idea that individuals can exist only because they are members of various networks of care and responsibility, for good or bad. The self can exist only through and with others, and *vice versa* (Gilligan 1987; Tronto 1993; Griffith 1995; Clement 1996; Hirschmann and DiStefano 1996; Sevenhuijsen 1998). In Giddens' approach, the need for obligations arises to counter the detachment that may arise in a society of atomistic, self-governed individuals: in this respect, his framework is permeated by the assumptions of contractual ethics. Conversely, the ethic of care takes the idea of self in relationship as the point of entry for thinking about obligations and responsibility. While the moral subject in the discourse of individual rights looks at moral dilemmas from the stance of the 'highest moral principles' and takes rights and responsibilities as a means of establishing relationships, the moral subject in the discourse of care already lives in a network of relation and (inter)dependence, in which he/she has to find balances between different forms of care: for the self, for others and for the relations between these.

As I have argued elsewhere, it is not 'duty' that guides her/him through recurrent moral dilemmas but rather situated questions of responsibility and agency, such as 'how can I best express my caring responsibility?' or 'how can I best deal with the relations between vulnerability, dependency and power?' (Sevenhuijsen 1998: 56, 1999). This comes quite close to the suggestion made by Janet Finch and others of taking the question of 'what is the proper thing to do' as a way of thinking about morality as a situated practice (Finch 1989; Finch and Mason 1993).

Nancy Hirschmann argues in her work on obligation that liberal theories on contract and consent cannot adequately deal with obligation, since they depart from a notion of equal and separate individuals. Liberal consent theories 'seek to understand how separate individuals can develop and sustain connections and still be separate; how they engage in relationships and still remain free' (Hirschmann 1992: 170). In contrast, a feminist approach would start from an understanding of obligations and responsibilities as daily human practices. Responsibility and obligation then become a basic standard against which other things are measured, such as the freedom to act as one wishes. The central question shifts to 'how can I achieve some freedom and yet remain connected?' Carol Gilligan, who has provided the groundwork for a feminist ethic of care, has outlined the difference it makes when we think along these lines:

> As a framework for moral decision, care is grounded in the assumption that self and other are interdependent, an assumption reflected in a view of action as responsive, and, therefore, as arising in relationship rather than the view of action as emanating from within the self, and therefore 'self-governed'.
>
> Gilligan 1987: 24

These observations also point to different modes of conceptualising the *relationship between morality and politics*. Political programmes that are based on constructions of individual holders of rights as the 'basic units' of society tend to see the law as the main guarantor of the existence of morality, and in many cases also to single out 'the family' as the primary locus for morality. As argued by Zygmunt Bauman (1993: 29): 'individual responsibility is then translated as the responsibility for following or breaching the socially endorsed, ethical legal rules'. According to Bauman, modernity thrives on the 'expropriation of the moral'. Modernity is fuelled by a deep-seated mistrust of the moral capacities of its subjects and thus aims to press its claims to moral truth by laying them down in legal imperatives, which are then supposed to educate those who are beyond the boundaries of 'proper morality'. Hence the continual urge to derive legal obligations from notions of rights.

The ethic of care implies a radically different account of the relationship between morality and politics and thus between obligation and responsibility. Because it starts from a relational ontology, it focuses primarily on the question of what politics could mean for the safeguarding of responsibility and relationship in human practice and interaction. Policy making needs a more sophisticated insight into the way in which individuals frame their responsibilities in actual social practices and how the moral dilemmas that go with the conflicting responsibilities of care for 'self, other and the relation between them' are handled. It would gain this insight from an attitude of initial trust in the moral capacities of individuals, and thus from an attitude of listening as a practice of democratic citizenship (Bickford 1996).

Social policies, and thus also family policies, should therefore be governed by responsiveness to the needs of those with whom they are concerned. It cannot be stressed enough that the 'caring attitude' is not confined to private interactions but should also count as a 'public virtue' that should enter the considerations of policy makers (Sevenhuijsen 2000a).

The relevance of these statements can be underlined further by pointing to the 'political sociology of care' that underlies the feminist ethic of care.[1] Care should best be seen as practice and disposition, as well as a social process. Berenice Fisher and Joan Tronto (1990) have proposed a definition of care as:

> A species of activity that includes everything that we do to maintain, continue and repair our 'world' so that we can live in it as well as possible. That world includes our bodies, ourselves and our environment, all of which we seek to interweave in a complex, life-sustaining web.

Joan Tronto (1993) has elaborated on how each of the four phases of care introduced by Fisher and Tronto (1990) corresponds to a specific value:

- *Caring about* consists of paying attention to the factors that determine survival and well-being and in establishing the need for care. The corresponding value is *attentiveness*.
- *Caring for* means taking the initiative for concrete activities, *responsibility* being the value that counts here.
- *Taking care of* is the concrete work of 'maintaining and repairing the world', carrying out the recurrent daily routines of caring work and developing a thorough understanding of these, and *competence* is the corresponding value.
- The fourth phase of care consists of *receiving care*. Here, open forms of interaction between care givers and care receivers are important as a check on the quality of care, *responsiveness* being the overriding value.

These four values – attentiveness, responsibility, competence and responsiveness – are thus the core of an ethic of care. To these can be added values like trust, honesty, respect and relational autonomy.[2]

Care can accordingly be conceptualised as a continuous social process and as a daily human activity. It should best be seen as a human practice that entails a set of moral orientations. These are aimed at the question of how needs should be interpreted and if and how they can be fulfilled. This is also why the care ethic cannot easily be seen as a version of duty ethics. The ethic of care does not presume that the caring actor has a universal moral obligation to care for the needs of others, an obligation that some writers derive from a 'feminine impulse to care on behalf of the other' (see, for example, Noddings 1984). According to Noddings, feminine care is inscribed in a Kantian ethic of obligation and duty: those acts should be considered as moral that are enacted from a universalisable feeling of duty.

In my view, it is more fruitful to stress that the care ethic implies being attentive to the other as inherently situated, and as different from the self. The implication of this point is that a pluralistic approach should guide policy formation as well as personal practice. The process of caring will typically bring together a variety of different actors (care givers and care receivers, private and public agencies, etc.), all with their own views on the caring process and with distinctive moral repertoires. Recognition of the moral agency of these actors calls for a new 'politics of needs interpretation' that takes full account of these local contexts of action and judgement.

The place of care in Giddens' conception of the third way

Against this background, it may become clear that in *The Third Way* Giddens discusses care in a rather paradoxical and defective manner. He mentions care in the chapter on family politics, stating that democratic family relations imply shared responsibility for childcare. Care is also mentioned in his chapter on the social investment state, where he says that the Left should accept the criticism of the Right that the welfare state is based too heavily on 'the motive force of protection and care' and thus 'does not give enough space to personal liberty'. Care and protection are nearly equated here. Together they are inscribed in a framework of control, where freedom, personal initiative and autonomy are constructed as their counterpart. By implication, care is conceptualised in terms of negative freedom, as an entity that stands in the way of self-fulfilment. This notion is far removed from the notion of the care ethic, that (good) care provides an indispensable contribution to human flourishing.

In his sociological observations and normative framework, Giddens also forgets to mention care where we might expect him to. The most remarkable passage in this respect is the one in which he writes about the meaning of involvement in the labour force as a means of attacking 'involuntary exclusion'. Work, he says, has multiple benefits: it generates income for the individual; it gives a sense of stability and direction in life; and it creates wealth for the wider society. But he also adds an important observation about the limits of the work ethic:

> Yet inclusion must stretch well beyond work, not only because there are many people at any one time not able to be in the labour force, but because a society too determined by the work ethic would be a

> thoroughly unattractive place to live. An inclusive society must provide for the basic needs of those who can't work and must recognise the wider diversity of goals life has to offer.
>
> Giddens 1998: 110

To see how painfully this remark misses its target, we need only reflect on the limitations of the work ethic as a guide to public policy in contemporary society. The quotation fails to address the importance of caring work in society and of the values of attentiveness and responsibility in creating humane relationships in daily social interactions. Also, a questionable distinction is made between those who can and those who cannot work. An outdated division between a category of 'self-sufficient workers' and 'dependent others', which is based on the independent male citizen-worker as the paradigm for citizenship, is thereby repeated (Fraser and Gordon 1994).

These contradictions can be overcome only by explicitly including the providing and receiving of care in ideas about 'the wider goals of life' and in our image of a society that 'seems attractive to live in' (i.e. in notions of the good life). In consequence, it should also be integrated into notions of collective agency and citizenship (Sevenhuijsen 1998).

In his paradoxical and defective discussion of care, Giddens misses the crucial sociological message of feminist theories on this topic: the notion that caring is a social activity in itself and that the moral orientation of care is crucial both for the provision of basic needs and for processes of social cohesion.[3] In this respect, it is striking that Giddens does not include care in his remarks on the 'transformations in personal life', which he nevertheless refers to as a major revolution of our times. In this context, he mainly talks about the individualism of the younger generation, although he does defend this against conservative worries about moral decay by pointing to their 'post-materialist' values and lifestyles. The problem with this approach is that it tends to reduce everything that happens in personal life to a matter of identity politics. In fact, these ideas are based on a separation between the psychological and the material elements of social life and human agency. The care ethic denies such a separation of material life and interpersonal relationships and points, by its insistence that care is work, to the interrelatedness of agency and morality and to the manifold gender subtexts in discursive patterns on the relation between paid work and care.

By omitting the social importance of care, Giddens also misses the *political* message of contemporary feminist theories of labour and care: that as many individuals as possible should have the opportunity to combine paid work and informal care in their life course. This is not just because there happen to be needy persons who cannot take care of themselves (and thus fall outside the category of 'responsible independent individuals') but because caring should be valued as an important human practice that contributes to the potential for moral agency. A democratic ethic of care starts from the assumption that everybody needs care daily (albeit care of different sorts and with different grades of intensity) and is (in principle at least) capable of giving care. We might conclude that a democratic and inclusive society ought to encourage its members to give both of these activities a meaningful place in their lives.

This point may be pursued by elaborating the moral and practical implications of the notion of care as a 'democratic practice'. As Joan Tronto has remarked, both caring as intimate involvement with others and caring in broader and more abstract long-term ways are essential to the roles of citizens in a democratic political system. Their development requires an involvement both in the intimate relations of daily life and in the more distant relations of public life (Tronto 1996).

The demand for equal access to different social spheres springs from the democratic moral impulse that individuals should have the ability to circulate in different roles and positions, where they can become acquainted with the needs and moral viewpoints of different social actors. Democratic life can flourish better when people have the ability to circulate between different positions of responsibility and can thus practice values like attentiveness, responsiveness and trust in their different walks of life.[4] The field of social policies and family politics is an important arena, where the policies supporting these notions should be developed. Again, we may wonder whether Giddens' proposals for a 'third way' are adequate in this respect.

Family practices, care and the search for new social policies

At several places in his book, Giddens argues for 'family-friendly' work environments. Again, however, his practical proposals are not sufficiently linked to his normative framework. The main problem in this respect in his version of the third way is that his normative image of citizenship is still principally grafted on to that of the wage-earning independent citizen. Access to paid work is constructed as the primary dimension of social inclusion. But this wage-earning citizen has to change in character, according to Giddens. In his ideal of the 'social investment state', citizens cannot rely on social rights and social security any longer to sustain their lives when the labour market fails. They must take their own responsibility and turn into 'responsible risk takers', the main subject position used by Giddens to construct his brave New Labour world of welfare policy and social citizenship. But there is a long way to go before access to paid work and the responsibilities for care are shared equally in gender terms. And Giddens' case at this point is not helped by the casual and self-contradictory way in which the concept of care enters his analysis.

Let us start with Giddens' proposals for a new family politics, in his own words a 'key test' for the new politics. In his section on 'the democratic family', he argues vehemently against conservative fears of the breakdown of the family and related arguments for a return to traditional family life and male authority. In his view, there is no way back: recapturing the traditional family would be a 'non-starter'. However, libertarian social democrats also get it wrong: their arguments for a 'proliferation of lifestyles', like one-parent families and homosexuals who raise children, are 'simply not convincing'. The (supposed) effects of divorce on children epitomise Giddens' concern for social cohesion: children in one-parent families would suffer not only economically but also from 'inadequate parenting and lack of social ties'.[5] A 'third way' in family politics would have to start from the normative notion of equality between the sexes. The idea of democratic family life suggests how individual choice and social solidarity might be combined. Formal equality, individual rights, mutual respect, autonomy and freedom from violence should serve as the normative framework for family relations, both between parents and between parents and children.

Care enters the story where Giddens states that the protection and care of children is the single most important thread that should guide family policy. Again, divorce and single parenthood serve as the negative counter-image here. Democratic family politics should enable shared responsibility for childcare, while the ability to 'sustain relationships through change, even radical change such as divorce', becomes paramount, even comparable in importance to flexibility and adaptability in the workplace (Giddens 1998: 94). This would imply introducing shared responsibility for childcare; the possibility of contractual commitments to children between parents but also between parents and non-parents (parenting contracts, separate from marriage); the enhancement of fathers' rights, for example to child minding and out-of-school care; and enhancing the responsibility (or even the obligation) of children to support ageing parents.

While care is certainly not absent in these proposals, it is striking that caring values are not mentioned in the normative framework for the new family politics. This should not come as a surprise, since as we have seen the basic approach in the book is informed by the idea of the individual rights holder as the basic unit of social life. In the end it is *contract* that has to secure relationship and responsibility in human life, instead of connectedness and 'lived' ties. The ease with which Giddens singles out care for children from wider networks of care, responsibility and dependency can also be questioned. It is as if the accomplishment of formal equality between the sexes leads to children being singled out as special 'objects of concern' for family politics. This concern is also rather one-sidedly perceived through a male gaze: reading between the lines, absence of the father is seen as one of the main concerns for family politics.

Starting from the notion of care as a democratic practice instead, the first social problem that should be addressed is the social inequality in the distribution of giving and receiving care, and of paid work and informal care structured along axes of gender, class and ethnicity. When we acknowledge the significance of care as a human practice, we should critically assess group privileges and systematic patterns of exclusion in these respects.

While the ethic of care would probably acknowledge the 'sustenance of relationship' as an important concern for family politics, it would not initiate its concerns at the point of the *failure* of relationship, i.e. divorce. It would prioritise social and political arrangements that enable adults of both sexes (and regardless of their sexual orientation) to participate in different forms of care: care for dependent children, care for partners and friends, care for dependent parents and, last but not least, care for the self.[6]

This would probably also contribute to a solution of the problem of absent fathers after divorce, since the presence of caring fathers *during* relationships between adults creates ties of care and trust that are based on daily practices of care, and that is likely to produce lasting commitment after the breakdown of the relationship. It would thus probably change the nature of 'divorce' as we know it. The primary arena for 'family politics' would then not be 'family law' (i.e. the regulation of kinship contracts) but rather the field of social policies: the policies that determine the regulation of working, the spending of time and the generating of income and maintenance, and related rights, duties and responsibilities.

It is at this point that we have to investigate the practical and moral suitability of the 'responsible risk taker' as the model for future social citizenship. in Giddens' view, social democrats should shift the relation between risk and security involved in the welfare state: 'people need protection when things go wrong, but also the material and moral capabilities to move through major periods of transition in their lives' (Giddens 1998: 100). Again, an approach from the ethic of care may clarify the shortcomings of these statements. Care should not be conceptualised as a safety net in times of misfortune and transition but rather as an ongoing social process that demands our attention daily and thus should figure prominently in any scenario for future social policy.

Many moral transitions in life have indeed to do with the demands and the failures of caring relations (Smart and Neale 1999). Giddens is in fact quite close to these insights when he draws attention to the limitation of the work ethic, and to the trend that more and more people are looking for 'opportunities for commitment outside of work'. Again, however, it is striking that he does not take the step of including care in these commitments: the working citizen remains in this respect the model for social citizenship.

In addition, the idea that people are more and more looking for 'opportunities for commitment outside of work' actually represents a male perspective, and in that sense it may not be a coincidence that caring is not adequately mentioned here. For women, after all, the situation is the other way around. At this moment in history, they are looking to extend their commitments from the home to the labour market and to social and political participation in a broader sense. For men, the situation is different. When engaging in care they do not need to claim access to a social domain that was formerly closed to them. Rather, they have to change their commitment to and identity in a sphere where they already live: the intimate life sphere, where they have to alter their way of dealing with responsibility and dependency. The point is that these intricate gendered relations of labour and care are part of the normative assumptions of modern welfare states and the creation of the 'modern individual'. Once we realise the extent to which not only work–family arrangements but also, for example, corporate cultures, urban planning and public transport arrangements are built on these gendered assumptions about labour and care, it may become evident that the development of new social infrastructures of care should receive high priority from policy makers.

What do these remarks imply, then, when evaluating the notion of the 'responsible risk taker' through the lens of care? In the care ethic, the notion of responsibility would certainly be crucial for social policy. But instead of deriving responsibilities from rights (a top-down model), the care ethic starts political reasoning from an understanding of interconnection and relationship, and thus from knowledge about daily practices of care and responsibility and the dilemmas contained therein.[7] Integrating the practice of 'care for the self' into notions of responsibility may contribute to current discussions on responsibility. By deconstructing the normative notion of the 'independent individual', the ethic of care undermines the entrenched patterns that have released men from daily caring responsibilities (for others and for themselves) and that have enabled them to count on women's availability to provide for their care needs. We may expect that in a situation where the practice of 'care for the self' is more 'normal' and where this is linked to the willingness to take responsibility for others and for relations of dependence, individuals will develop a wider range of moral sensibilities and thus also the capacity to take responsibility for their own actions and major life decisions. In this respect, the care ethic could be seen as a support for Giddens' new notion of human subjectivity.

However, the care ethic would be critical of giving the notion of 'risk' as much prominence as Giddens. It should be remembered that 'care' has, in his considerations on the social investment state, a negative undertone, as he associates it with control and opposes both these notions to personal liberty. From this perspective, it is evidently inconceivable that care might contribute to autonomy and liberty, or to the cultivation of human potential, goals that Giddens otherwise embraces as important for 'positive social welfare'. Again, the care ethic would stress that care is, on both an individual and a social scale, not something that protects individuals against risk but rather an ongoing social process that, when properly done, contributes to human flourishing.[8]

It should also be noted that it is often difficult to predict when either the need for or the availability of care will present itself in human life. It cannot be assumed that individuals will be able to predict their future needs for care before the event and to protect themselves against the failures of the caring arrangements around them. This would not only draw too heavy a bill on future social arrangements, it would also be an example of what Simon

Duncan and Anne Barlow have called the 'rationality mistake'. Important decisions about 'moral economies' are usually not taken in the form of simple 'cost–benefit' matrices but instead involve moral and negotiated views about what behaviour is expected as right and proper and what kind of lives people want to live (Duncan and Barlow 1999). This includes arrangements of care and responsibility. Now that social policies can no longer build on the full-time availability of women for daily care, we should be looking for innovative and flexible caring arrangements that can prevent 'caring gaps' coming into existence.

Gender-sensitive social policies: a third way?

Paradoxically, it is at this point that the notion of a 'third way' may contribute fruitfully to the design of new forms of social policy. The notion of care as a democratic practice accords with third way arguments for new public–private alliances and with the importance of a strong civil society, acting in cooperation with state agencies, in this case with the goal of establishing new 'social infrastructures of care'. But the care ethic also has something to add to third way thinking about human subjectivity and moral agency. Instead of talking about individuals as the basic units of social policy, we could take notions like 'selves in networks of care and responsibility' and 'working and caring citizens' as indices of moral subjectivity for social policy. Instead of deriving obligations from rights, we can start with knowledge about actually existing networks of care and responsibility. Instead of continuing to see care as a 'private affair' (and thus continuing entrenched patterns of domestication of care), we can reflect on how to align public and private responsibilities for care, and to include the values of care in the moral sensibilities that we bring to bear in our citizenship practices (Sevenhuijsen 1998; Tronto 1996).

This political attitude to care can be linked to a 'third way', since both these approaches cross the boundaries of traditional political thought systems. The notion of care as a democratic practice is at odds with old-style social democracy, where this has tended to insert issues of care into its normative parameters of solidarity and justice. This has left questions of care and compassion to conservatives and communitarians, who tend to link them to issues like 'family values' and to homogeneous notions of 'community'. But the care ethic is at odds with neo-liberalism and conservatism, because it argues for making care into a public virtue and wants to extend notions of equality and social rights to include practices of giving and receiving care. It is situated at the intersection between social democracy and neo-liberalism, while it gives weight to notions of responsibility and trust and in fact substantiates and grounds these further. It would share some of the current concerns about social exclusion and social cohesion but would again extend the parameters of the discussion by implying (the importance of) caring practices within these concerns.

When a norm of equality in access to the giving and receiving of care both in public and private contexts is combined with democratic notions of equality of voice (and thus with the values of attentiveness and responsiveness), it can be expected that the institutions of care have the capacity to generate loyalty and commitment on the part of those who participate in them and can thus work as vehicles for solidarity and social cohesion.

But on a more practical level, a potential alliance between the care ethic and a 'third way' in politics is also available. Both the design and the implementation of the new social policies have after all to be a collective endeavour of different social and political actors, and they thus call for new public–private alliances. Facilitating combinations of labour and care would mean the thorough reorganisation of the social arrangements of time and place for care and would, for example, imply the following:[9]

- the further introduction of flexible working hours and the right to part-time work without loss of job and social security;
- paid leave to care for children, sick relatives and friends;
- flexibility in retirement age and old age pensions;
- adapting corporate cultures to the presence of employees with caring responsibilities;
- adapting working and caring time, via the regulation of working hours and aligning public transport and shop opening times, to the needs of 'working and caring citizens';
- setting up arrangements to support lone mothers in caring for their children and earning a living;
- supporting men in further developing caring identities and caring practices;
- facilitating divorced parents in continuing to share childcare, both materially and emotionally;
- attuning schedules for professional home healthcare for the elderly to care by their relatives and friends;
- further adapting healthcare systems to users' needs and integrating considerations of daily care into medical practice;
- giving 'caring networks' a place in community work and in the school life of children; and
- building neighbourhoods in which persons of different generations can live together, and including caring facilities within them.

When considering both the philosophical and the practical implications of a political ethic of care, it may become clear that a notion of 'philosophical conservatism', as proposed by Giddens, is not adequate to approach future social policies regarding the family.

We are living in a period of change that could perhaps best be characterised as a transition from modernist forms of care policies, based on familial care and the heterosexual norm, to a politics that is better attuned to postmodern caring practices, situated in different social domains and in a diversity of lifestyles. A notion of philosophical conservatism does not suit this situation, since it frames these policies too much in a backward-looking way. Too often, attitudes of philosophical conservatism harbour traditional and male-biased assumptions, which are at odds with the needs for new normative frameworks in a post-feminist age.

When we want to assist people to 'pilot their way' through current moral transitions, we need creative and forward-looking policies that draw on the moral capabilities and existing responsibilities of citizens. Therefore, the new social policies should not be aimed at imposing a new normative construction of 'the family' but rather should be attuned to both existing and shifting family practices and caring practices, and the need for new ones. This will contribute to a further de-privatisation of care while acknowledging the intimate aspects of caring relations. The moral considerations of care can become part of the political quest for new divisions of responsibility between public and private life. And because moral attitudes are thus brought firmly into public life, this may also provide an alternative to conservative pleas for 'family values'. In that respect, the ethic of care provides us with an elaborated alternative to the acceptance of the traditional family as the norm for state policies.

Notes

1 This chapter both includes and elaborates on arguments developed in my other publications. See Sevenhuijsen 2000a, 2000b.
2 On care and trust, see Sevenhuijsen 1999 and Dillon 1992. On relational autonomy, see Mackenzie and Stoljar 2000.
3 For a similar critique, see Levitas 1998.
4 This forms a substantial addition to Giddens's normative framework for the 'democratic family'. He links democracy in the family rather one-sidedly with equality in rights and decision making.
5 In this and several other respects, Giddens's framework is permeated with Durkheimian notions about the functionality of the family and the role of fathers. Ruth Levitas' critique of New Labour ideology refers to a 'new Durkheimian hegemony' (*ibid.*: 178–89).
6 As argued by Weeks *et al.* (1999), the issue of care and responsibility for children raises, in an acute form, the legal status and social policy implications of the emergence of elective families and the public affirmation of lesbian and gay relationships. They argue for a concept of 'intimate citizenship'. Caring practices should form part of the status of citizenship, not only because citizenship arranges the rights and obligations that are connected to parenting and parent–child relationships but also because the status of citizenship should be built upon the recognition of the need for intimate desires, pleasures and 'being in the world'.
7 It is striking that Giddens uses the concepts of responsibility and obligation alternately, as if they mean the same.
8 The notion of 'human flourishing' as a guideline for public policy is elaborated on by the American philosopher Martha Nussbaum (2000). It is a broader concept than the concept of 'human potential' as used by Giddens. In his book,

this concept fits into a discourse of economic rationality and functionality, where inclusion in the capitalist economy is the primary motive for developing the capabilities of individuals.

9 Some of these measures are currently under consideration or are being implemented by the Dutch government, which is a coalition between social democrats and liberals and thus in a way an example of a 'third way' government.

References

Bauman, Z. (1993) *Postmodern Ethics*, Oxford: Basil Blackwell.

Bickford, S. (1996) *The Dissonance of Democracy: Listening, Conflict, and Citizenship*, Ithaca, NY: Cornell University Press.

Clement, G. (1996) *Care, Autonomy, and Justice: Feminism and the Ethic of Care*, Boulder, Colo.: Westview Press.

Dillon, R. (1992) 'Respect and care: toward moral integration', *Canadian Journal of Philosophy*, 105–32.

Duncan, S. and Barlow, A. (1999) 'New Labour's communitarianism: supporting families and the "rationality mistake"', Working Paper 10, Centre for Research on Family, Kinship and Divorce, University of Leeds.

Finch, J. (1989) *Family Obligations and Social Change*, Cambridge: Polity Press.

Finch, J. and Mason, J. (1993) *Negotiating Family Responsibilities*, London: Tavistock/Routledge.

Fisher, B. and Tronto, J. (1990) 'Towards a feminist theory of caring', in E.K. Abel and M.K. Nelson (eds) *Circles of Care: Work and Identity in Women's Lives*, New York: State University of New York Press.

Fraser, N. and Gordon, L. (1994) 'A genealogy of dependency: tracing a keyword of the U.S. welfare state', *Signs: A Journal of Women in Culture and Society* 19: 1–29.

Giddens, A. (1998) *The Third Way. The Renewal of Social Democracy*, Cambridge: Polity Press.

Gilligan, C. (1987) 'Moral orientation and moral development', in E. Feder Kitay and D.T. Meyers (eds) *Women and Moral Theory*, Totowa, NJ: Rowman & Littlefield.

Griffith, M. (1995) *Feminisms and the Self: The Web of Identity*, London: Routledge.

Hirschmann, N.J. (1992) *Rethinking Obligation. A Feminist Method for Political Theory*, Ithaca, NY: Cornell University Press.

Hirschmann, N.J. and DiStefano, C. (eds) (1996) *Revisioning the Political: Feminist Reconstructions of Traditional Concepts in Western Political Theory*, Boulder, Colo.: Westview Press.

Levitas, R. (1998) *The Inclusive Society? Social Exclusion and New Labour*, Houndmills: Macmillan.

Mackenzie, C. and Stoljar, N. (eds) (2000) *Relational Autonomy: Feminist Perspectives on Autonomy, Agency and the Social Self*, New York: Oxford University Press.

Noddings, N. (1984) *Caring: A Feminine Approach to Ethics and Moral Education*, Berkeley: University of California Press.

Nussbaum, M.C. (2000) *Women and Human Development: The Capabilities Approach*, Cambridge: Cambridge University Press.

Sevenhuijsen, S.L. (1998) *Citizenship and the Ethics of Care: Feminist Considerations on Justice, Morality and Politics*, London: Routledge.

—— (1999) 'Too good to be true? Feminist Considerations about Trust and Social Cohesion', *Focaal*, 207–22.
—— (2000a) *De plaats van zorg. Over de betekenis van de zorgethiek voor sociaal beleid*, Utrecht: Universiteit Utrecht.
—— (2000b) 'Caring in the third way: the relationship between obligation, responsibility and care in Third Way discourse', *Critical Social Policy: A Journal of Theory and Practice in Social Welfare* 20: 5–37.
Smart, C. and Neale, B. (1999) *Family Fragments?* Cambridge: Polity Press.
Tronto, J.C. (1993) *Moral Boundaries. A Political Argument for an Ethic of Care*, New York: Routledge.
—— (1996) 'Democratic caring, caring for democracy: justice, power and inclusiveness,' unpublished paper, New York.
Weeks, J., Donovan, C. and Heaphy, B.. (1999) 'Everyday experiments: narratives of non-heterosexual relationships', in E. Silva and C. Smart (eds) *The New Family?* London: Sage.

Part III

Family practices

7 Sociological perspectives on the family

David Morgan

Introduction

The object of this chapter is not so much to outline the numerous and various sociological perspectives on the family but to examine the process of theorising or sociologising itself. More specifically, the aim is to explore what is entailed in the bracketing of the two words 'sociology' and 'family'.

All such bracketings, such as 'sociology and religion' or 'sociology and art', are inherently problematical, and 'sociology and family' shares in these problems while presenting a few additional and particular ones. In part, the discussion is about the relative weighting to be given to the two words when they appear, perhaps in the title of a textbook, together as 'the sociology of the family'. If the stress is to be given to the latter term, the implication would seem to be that there is something special, distinct or unique about 'the family' and that the sociological task is to explore the social consequences of this group and possibly some of the social processes that take place within it and the social forces shaping or distorting the family. In any event, the sociologist is required, to a greater or lesser extent, to take 'the family' as given. The very use of the definite article, as Bernardes and others have argued, would suggest this to be the case (Bernardes 1997; Morgan 1996).

If, on the other hand, the stress is to be placed on the term 'sociology', the implication would seem to be that the family as a social institution and family processes are part of a wider set of social relations and processes and that the task of sociology, as a generalising science, is to explain or understand the family in terms of more general principles. Within this broad category we may perhaps distinguish the pluralists, who admit a variety of sociological (together, perhaps, with other non-sociological) accounts, and the imperialists or monopolists, who claim that there is some unified set of principles that can explain family life as part of social life in general. The former would recognise the diversity of sociological approaches but would argue or suggest that all or most of these perspectives taken together could deal with most of the questions raised by family life. Here, since the discipline of sociology is perceived as having relatively fuzzy boundaries, such accounts may admit insights from history, social psychology, philosophy, and so on. The latter would seem to take a more exclusive understanding of the sociological enterprise, arguing for a single unifying perspective rather than a diversity of approaches.

The very 'fuzziness' of the sociological perspective presents some additional difficulties. From time to time, claims are made to the effect that sociological explanations are 'really' to do with something else, such as psychoanalysis or evolutionary psychology, arguing that propositions that are apparently about society or social processes are reducible to propositions based upon individuals. Similarly, with rational choice theory we have a blurring of the boundaries between sociology, economics, political science and some versions of individual psychology. In all these cases, it would seem, there is a search for some general principles of explanation that are clearly wider than any particular institution or set of practices and also, possibly, wider than the discipline of sociology itself.

This contrast may seem a little abstract or esoteric with little real significance for everyday life. I shall argue that this is not the case and that these tensions, often latent in sociological discussions of family life, have wider significance and consequences. In the first place, the kind of contrast that I have suggested has its echoes in many other areas of social enquiry; one has only to consider the fierce and often acrimonious debates around the 'sociology of science'. Here the question would seem to be about the ways in which and the extent to which particular disciplines may erect 'keep out' signs to warn sociologists and others against trespassing. Second, and closer to home, these apparently esoteric debates often enter into or lie behind political claims about the nature and significance of family life in a modern society.

In this chapter, I shall look at both these arguments. I shall consider, first, the claim that there is something special or unique about 'the family' and family life. I shall consider, briefly, what these claims might refer to and the consequences of these claims for the sociological analysis of family life. Second, I shall consider the alternative claim that family life is simply a subset of social life in general and that the principles and theories developed in the analysis of the latter can be readily applied, with little or no modification, to the analysis of the former.

Faced with a contrast of this kind, a common move would be to aim for the middle ground and to argue that there is an element of truth in both these claims but that they need to be combined. It is easy enough to propose such an argument but more difficult to demonstrate how it might work in practice. I shall consider two possible ways of combining the specific and the general, one derived from my own attempts to map 'family practices' and the other derived, perhaps unexpectedly, from the writings of Everett Hughes. I shall conclude with a discussion about why this exploration is important.

The family as a specific group

To talk about 'the sociology of the family' implies that there is a specific and identifiable entity called the family. It implies that there is something specific, distinct or unique about this entity and that it cannot be reduced to something else through sociological or any other kind of theorising. The family, in this account, can be treated as an independent variable having consequences for other areas of social life or individual well-being.

However, there is not a consensus about what constitutes the specificity of family life. Rather, there are a variety of different although sometimes overlapping claims about this special or unique character. In the first place, there are claims that point to the extra-social character of family life and that argue that it has its origins in something that is either partially or wholly outside society. Thus the family may be seen as having its basis in certain fundamental biological processes that lie behind the apparent variety of patterns of family living. These fundamental processes not only define the origins of family life but also explain particular processes within it; neo-Darwinist evolutionary psychology might be seen as an influential modern body of theorising here. Thus two modern Darwinists write:

> If the government is to win its game of Happy Families, it needs to understand the rules – most fundamentally, why blood is thicker than water. Family psychology was forged in the context of shared genetic inheritance. To the blind forces of natural selection, altruism towards kin is just one way of replicating genes: help those who share your genes and you help the genes.
>
> Cronin and Curry 2000: 154

Modern Darwinism claims to explain a very wide variety of social phenomena, not simply family life. Yet here we see that the family has a very distinct connection with principles of altruism and, in some senses at least, may be seen as the basis of social life itself.

Overlapping these biological or evolutionary psychology arguments are a range of broadly psychoanalytical accounts that describe the necessary dependencies and anxieties established through the relationships between parents and children over a long period of time. These accounts have a multiple importance in that they point to fundamental processes that arise out of the ties and dependencies in family triangles, show how patterns of behaviour may be reproduced over generations and often show the consequences of early experiences for areas of life apparently far removed from the family. Behaviour at work or the processes of artistic creation may be understood with at least a partial reference to these early family processes.

Some more specifically sociological accounts may also point to the specific or unique characteristics of the family, chief among which are the various functionalist theories. There is, as is well known, a considerable variety of such theories, but they all have at the core some kind of argument along the lines of 'the functions of the family are a,b,c …' (Morgan 1975). The argument may be extended to claim that only the family can perform these particular functions or, since evidence of the functions being shared by other social institutions would seem to be readily available, the argument may be made more specific by claiming that only the family can perform these particular functions in combination. Thus it may be relatively easy to show that the socialisation function, for example, may be performed by other institutions outside the family (schools, peer groups, etc.) but that only the family performs the socialisation alongside other functions such as, in the Parsonian model, the stabilisation of adult personalities (Parsons and Bales 1956; Parsons 1964; Morgan 1975). Other social institutions may play their part in fulfilling the two functions separately, but only the family performs these irreducible functions in combination.

Somewhat on the margins of functionalist analysis are some Marxist or feminist accounts of the family. Here the analysis will be qualified by some such phrase as 'under capitalism' or 'in a patriarchal system', suggesting some sources of historical variation and future transcendence. The focus is on the way in which the family reproduces capitalist or patriarchal sets of relations. However, this analysis is on the margins of this group of theories in that, ultimately at least, the family is a dependent rather than an independent variable and that it is shaped by ideological processes and the class or gender formations that provide the basis of these ideologies.

It is clear that some of these accounts may be readily identified or merge with political or moral understandings. In the case of some feminist or Marxist accounts these evaluations will be largely negative, but the more popular accounts will argue for the centrality and the importance of the family, often implicitly or explicitly drawing upon biological, psychological or functional analyses in support of these arguments. Again it is important to stress that there is not one unified or coherent moral or political account of the family. For example, one version will argue for the distinct character of family life and against any attempts by the state or other bodies to control or modify it. Others will point to the ways in which family life has been undermined in modern society and the adverse consequences for social order and for individuals that follow on from this. In this version, political action is necessary to provide positive support for the family. This would seem to be close to the arguments in favour of supporting family life advanced by New Labour.

It is important to recognise that these moral and political arguments often have their roots in or appeal to widespread popular understandings of the nature of family living. While such popular accounts may not refer to 'the family' in the abstract terms identified above, they may make claims about, for example, the special nature of biological parenthood or the primacy of family claims over other claims. In practice, as we shall see, these everyday moralities are much more complex than this brief account might suggest. It is quite possible, for example, to believe that 'the family comes first' while adhering to the principle of 'family hold back' (the idea that the rules of hospitality require that family members put the needs of their guests before their own needs) on particular occasions where families meet. Both popular phrases refer, in different ways, to the family as a moral entity. The idea that there is something special about family relationships as opposed to other kinds of social relationship would seem to be fairly widespread, even where it is coupled with a realistic recognition that family relationships can be a source of pain as well as of joy.

Within this framework, therefore, the task of family sociology is to explore the variety of expressions of family life in different societies or social groups or the different ways in which the basic biological or psychological facts are woven into social life as a whole. In addition, sociological accounts may explore those social processes that threaten or support family life and the consequences of dysfunction or maladjustment in family life for other areas of social life. Sociology therefore becomes a set of tools for understanding family life but which recognises the importance of the family as an ongoing concern and possibly as something that, ultimately, lies outside the reach of sociological explanation.

Family sociology as applied sociology

With the second orientation, the emphasis is clearly upon 'the sociology' rather than 'the family'. Family relations are simply a subset of a wider class of social relations and should be analysed in these terms rather than in terms of any supposed unique properties. Examples of this mode of theorising might come from exchange theory or rational choice theory. For example, discussing the 'family economics' approach, Gary Becker writes:

> I contend that the economic approach is uniquely powerful because it can integrate a wide range of human behaviour.
>
> Becker 1996: 109

> Indeed, I have come to the position that the economic approach is a comprehensive one that is applicable to all human behaviour.
>
> *ibid.*: 112

Thus, for example, one may speak quite literally of a 'marriage market'. One may argue that Becker's work on the family exists on the margins of sociology and economics (although his *A Treatise on The Family* has recently been hailed as one of sociology's most influential books (Clawson 1998), and it is likely that the sociological approaches that are most likely to take this particular orientation will often aspire to the elegance and purity of economic theory.

However, we may possibly find similar orientations in some versions of ethnomethodology, interactionism and political sociology. There are fundamental processes of social interaction and, beginning from this premise, one may treat the family as one particular site or arena in which we may view and understand these processes. In human groups and interaction, people form and break alliances, create boundaries and distinctions between insiders and outsiders, make more or less rational calculations on the basis of the information and resources available to them, carry out conversations, engage in bargaining or negotiation, and use or respond to the use of power. All these may be seen as fundamental human processes, the foundations, although in different ways, of social theory. The family becomes one of a range of small human groups and family processes, and relationships may be understood in terms of these wider understandings of human interaction.

In practice, it is unlikely that researchers or theorists are wholly indifferent to the specifically family dimension of what they are studying. However, the playing down of the family in the course of more fundamental sociological analysis may be justified on the grounds that sociological theorising needs to make some simplifying assumptions in order to progress, and such assumptions might entail by-passing any specific or special feature of the social institution under examination. What this means is that the research must explore some of the basic principles of human or social interaction first before building in more specific features of the social institution in question.

There are several merits associated with this strategy. First, it serves as a corrective against some of the reifying tendencies implied when people talk about 'the family'. Second, it would sometimes seem to establish more readily the credentials of a distinctly sociological approach, one that does not appear to depend upon extra-social factors such as biology or psychology. The social analyst here recognises both the distinct character and the limitations of his or her scholarly discipline. Sociology, in this version, may not so much be making any grand totalising or imperialistic claims but may be arguing for the distinct, if limited, character of its theoretical traditions, methodology and expertise. The sociologist will seek to work clearly within this tradition and to be relatively agnostic about the ultimate status of the object under investigation, at least for as long as he or she is conducting sociological enquiry. (For similar discussion in relation to social anthropology, see Gluckman 1964.) Finally, and perhaps more simply, this orientation means that analysts do not have to search around for new theories or modes of enquiry when they turn their attention to family life. The theoretical tools are already to hand.

We may sum up the contrast in these terms. In the first case, which may sometimes be described as family studies rather than family sociology, the family is regarded as a special group and family relationships have a distinct character that they do not share directly with other social relationships. In order to fully understand the family, we may need to draw upon insights from other social disciplines such as biology and psychology. In the second case, the family is treated as one of a range of human groupings and family relationships as part of a wider class of social relationships. The practitioners here will, for the most part, seek to deploy distinctly sociological theories.

Put in these rather stark terms, most people will argue in favour of some kind of position between these extremes. However, this exercise is a useful one in beginning to ask questions about how the bracketing of the words 'sociology' and 'family' is achieved and whether it is possible to develop approaches that give equal weight to both sides of the equation. In short, we are asking questions about what intellectual operations are actually involved when sociologists turn their attention to family life. These questions are important in terms of the 'politics of the family': the status of family life within social life as a whole; and the politics of sociology, the various claims to special competence on the part of practitioners of the discipline.

Family practices

Elsewhere, I have attempted to tackle this dilemma through my use of the term 'family practices' and my attempt to elaborate on the usages of this term (Morgan 1996, 1999). The term itself, 'family practices', clearly echoes and draws upon other usages of the term 'practices' in the sociological literature. It is clearly a sociological term, one not likely to be found in everyday speech, and one therefore likely to encourage an attention to wider issues of sociological theorising and language. It seeks to get away from the use of the term 'the family', with all its reifying potential. Part of the argument is that the designation of a set of activities as 'family practices' is in part a consequence of the perspective or intervention of the researcher and that practices so described could also be described in some other way. Thus the 'family practices' identified as associated with meals and meal times could also be defined as consumption practices, gender practices, generational practices, and so on.

However, while the term 'practices' does direct attention to wider theoretical usages within the general body of sociological writings, the continued use of the term 'family' does reintroduce a note of specificity. Family practices are not, it may be argued, any old practices. While it is true that the activities signified by the use of this term might be described in some other way, the use of the term 'family' is not entirely accidental or arbitrary. The use of the term in part reflects a theoretical decision on the part of the observer to describe them in these terms, but the justification for this does not lie purely within the realm of sociological theory. The justification lies in the ways in which social actors describe and account for their practices, the range of circumstances under which they use the term 'family' (or equivalent terms such as 'relations') or where they would consider such a usage relevant. There are two considerations here. First, there is the recognition that the term 'family' is frequently used or implied. Second, the use of the term 'family' reflects the fact that family matters are not just routinely topics of conversation between individuals but are also often seen as matters of serious or moral concern. This is also reflected in the fact that 'family' is also a matter for public debate, although such public discourses are not necessarily always congruent with these more everyday usages and understandings.

Thus there is an interdependence in the term 'family practices', the one qualifying the other. The term 'practices' points to wider generalities beyond the specific activities signified while also undermining the dangers inherent in talk of 'the family'. However, the continued use of the term 'family' anchors these practices in activities that the actors themselves would routinely regard as being distinct, special and of importance in their daily lives. In so far as 'family practices' involves not merely the doing of certain activities in relation to specified others but also the description of or accounting for these activities in 'family' terms, these practices are linked in various ways to the moral order. The 'moral turn' in family studies (Finch and Mason 1993; Sevenhuijsen 1999; Silva and Smart 1999; Ribbens McCarthy *et al.* 2000;) does not reflect an attempt to link the family to moral absolutes but rather a recognition that family practices involve the moral evaluation of choices and a recognition that these matters are of consequence in the daily lives of individuals. This is partly, although not wholly, a reflection of the fact that they so often deal with questions of birth and death, ageing and human need and frailty (Turner 1993). This particular and growing emphasis in family studies may also be linked to more philosophical discussions of the ethics of care and the way in which this may be specifically identified with family practices.

Licence and mandate in the family

Rather than continue this discussion of 'family practices', I wish to explore some further sociological terminology in order to develop the general argument being presented here. It is likely that this discussion of 'licence and mandate' could be included in the more general discussion of family practices, but it is not my intention to take this particular argument very far. Rather, I want to show how the uses of these terms may help us to understand not only family practices themselves but also the process of theorising about these practices.

In some ways these terms, derived from the writings of Everett Hughes, are particularly appropriate for our purposes. Everett Hughes had little to say, directly or indirectly, about family life; his best-known writings dealt with work, occupations and the professions. In the large volume of his collected essays under the title *The Sociological Eye* (Hughes 1971), there are no essays dealing with family matters, and the term does not appear in the index. Yet many of his ideas – 'dirty work', for example – have been found to have a wider applicability, and the same is true of his use of the terms 'licence' and 'mandate'. Indeed, the fact that these terms when used by Hughes had no reference to the family whatsoever makes them, paradoxically, particularly appropriate for this discussion, which is about the meeting of the terms 'sociology' and 'family'.

The term 'licence' is, in part, a statement that one is qualified in a particular field. To have a licence or to be licensed is to have permission (granted by the state or by some wider licensing body) to practise in a particular profession or occupation, to deploy certain recognised and evaluated skills. Licence, in fact, has two meanings according to Hughes. First, there is the legal permission. Second, there is the degree of leeway that is accorded the person so licensed in terms of practice and, in some cases, in terms of lifestyle (Hughes 1971: 375). The term 'licence' represents a stage in a historical process whereby a set of individuals make certain claims about their right to practise and to exclude others not properly qualified and where, in turn, these claims are recognised and codified and subject to processes of control and surveillance.

To some extent, the idea of mandate spreads outwards from this granting of a licence. Within a particular occupation or professional group, practitioners will develop some sense of collective identity and will claim a mandate to define proper conduct in relation to the particular work for themselves and for others The idea of mandate spreads outwards from the body of esoteric knowledge, which is the basis of a claim for licence and which is elaborated among those so licensed. Thus physicians, to use one of Hughes' favourite examples, will not merely practise medicine or surgery but will also make claims of a more general nature to define the nature of health and disease and the delivery of medical care (*ibid.*: 376). It will be noticed, in recent debates about the National Health Service for example, that doctors do not confine their public statements to more or less technical questions of the identification of particular conditions and their treatment but will also feel mandated to raise questions about the funding and the administration of healthcare in society generally.

The distinction between licence and mandate is perhaps a little slippery at times, but this is inevitable given the interdependence of the two terms and the sets of practices that they denote. What they both convey, with slightly different emphases, are sets of exchanges or claims between a particular group (usually an occupational group or an embryonic professional group) and the wider society. This wider society may be quite specific, as in the case of certain licensing agencies or state institutions, or it might be more general, such as 'public opinion'. Second, these exchanges come to define what this group may or must do (while excluding others) to warrant its adoption of a particular occupational or professional title. Finally, partly because detailed specification is frequently impossible or undesirable, the persons so designated are accorded a degree of leeway in their day-to-day activities, their lifestyles and occupational cultures and their rights to intervene in matters outside the formal boundaries of the occupation. It should be stressed that this refers to a continuing set of exchanges so that, for example, doctors or teachers who pronounce on more general political matters may be seen as going beyond their particular mandate. What Hughes is stressing is that such occupational divisions and titles are not merely technical or functional, a matter of who does what, but are essentially bound up with wider societal values: 'Such licence and mandate are the prime manifestations of the *moral* division of labour'(*ibid.*: 288).

Hughes stresses throughout his discussion of professions and occupations that those activities that are thus licensed are rewarded with money or some other kind of return in goods or services. For this reason, it might be supposed that there is a considerable difference between the activities with which he is centrally concerned and the practices of family life, where activities are not only frequently not the subject of monetary reward but where such considerations might actually seem to be inappropriate. However, it is fairly easy to think of activities where many of the considerations to do with licence and mandate still occur but where questions of financial reward might be minimal. We could, for example, develop this analysis to the amateur practitioners of particular skills (sport, acting, music making, etc.) or the activities of numerous kinds of volunteers. Even if we were to argue that such an extension of the terms of reference of the ideas of licence and mandate was metaphorical, it could still be argued that metaphors are often good to think with and may provide us with new insights into family or intimate life.

In the case of family practices, we may see licence and mandate operating in a variety of ways. First, they may apply to particular family titles, such as father, mother, child, grandparent, sibling, etc. Second, they may apply to whole families where they are acting as some kind of collectivity. This may apply to families where there is a strong sense of corporate identity or lineage; the British royal family may still serve as an example, although one that is facing numerous challenges. We may also see collections of family members who together claim to speak on behalf of family life as a whole. An example here may be the recent movement of men called 'The Promise Keepers'. Here men – fathers, husbands and so on – make a claim to speak on behalf of the family as a whole.

However, it is likely that the most relevant application of Hughes' terminology would be at the level of individual family-based titles. In some cases, these titles may have some wider legal underpinnings: the implications of the Child Support Agency for the financial obligations of fathers and the construction of ideas of fatherhood is a recent British example. The more formal institutional basis of family titles often becomes apparent where there is some departure from the norm, as in cases of child neglect, a child's failure to attend school, a parent's failure to pay maintenance, and so on.

However, it would be wrong to confine our attention to the more formally stated and sanctioned statements of parental obligations. Much of the licence attached to the performance of family obligations or duties exists at a less formal level and is subject to day-to-day negotiation, direct or indirect (Finch and Mason 1993). This also points to another important difference between the professions that are at the centre of Hughes' concerns and the practices of adult family members. The former practise on the basis of some licensed and recognised training and expertise. While there have been numerous attempts to 'professionalise' aspects of family living (Reiger 1985), and some kind of instruction for future married couples or parents is often recommended, it cannot be said that these have the same weight as the training of members of established professions. An individual's 'failure' as a family member is not usually the subject of formal legal sanctions but more a matter of informal sanctions within the wider network of family and neighbourhood and the moral reputation of the individual concerned. The same applies to questions of mandate within the family, where there may be a variety of claims and counter-claims along the lines of 'because I am your father', 'because we are sisters', and so on. The fact that many of these claims and counter-claims, these everyday negotiations, are presented in terms of 'ought' bears witness to Hughes' argument that licence and mandate are part of the moral division of labour in society.

There are two aspects of Hughes' analysis that seem to be of particular relevance for families. The first is to do with his notion of guilty knowledge, a feature he would argue of many professions and occupations (Hughes 1971: 286). His example here is the obvious one of the priest, but it is clear that many other occupations have a licence to obtain and to keep secret or guilty knowledge about others, whether they be parishioners, clients or customers.

The extent and the ways in which this may be applied to family life can be readily appreciated. There are several reasons why this notion of guilty knowledge may be especially relevant in a family context. In the first place, there is the close physical proximity or 'bodily density' (Morgan 1996) of some family members, sometimes over a considerable period of time. There is the fact that, in family contexts, individuals often coexist at different stages of their individual lifecourses. Thus, adults cohabit with immature children, and these children and adults may share dwellings, space or life experiences with the very old or people going through periods of chronic sickness and disability, and so on. There are the wider distinctions between the public and the private and the fact that these so often revolve around family and domestic life. Many of these related aspects of guilty knowledge have become the subject of public debate around questions of domestic violence and sexual and physical abuse in recent years. However, it is important to recognise that this guilty knowledge does not simply reside in these more dramatic examples but is built into the more mundane and routine experiences of family living as well. Family photographs may represent the semi-public visualisation of some of the more benign features of guilty knowledge within families: 'Gosh, I looked a fright!' or 'There's Uncle Barry making a fool of himself as usual'.

One particularly important and possibly distinctive feature of this guilty knowledge is the fact that it is often reciprocated. Parishioners confess to priests and not *vice versa*, and doctors have knowledge of their patients that is not usually reversible. However, just as parents have knowledge about their children's past behaviour and habits, so too do children have knowledge and insight into their parents' routine practices. Married or cohabiting couples have guilty knowledge about each other, although not necessarily the same knowledge.

The question of licence and guilty knowledge within the family points to processes of some considerable complexity. A parent, for example, will have knowledge of the minor deviations of a child, now grown up. The licence accorded to the parent here will often require the concealment of this knowledge, although there may be ritual occasions when the licence may allow, or possibly oblige, the parent to share this knowledge with others, whether family members or not. Part of the licence therefore includes some tacit understandings about when concealment is appropriate and when revelation may be permitted. Again, we are concerned with the fluid boundaries between public and private as anxieties over 'kiss and tell' memoirs or the reminiscences of nannies of prominent people remind us.

It should be recognised that such guilty knowledge is not necessarily confined to sets of relationships routinely characterised as family relationships. It certainly extends to all kinds of couple relationships, including gay and lesbian couples and many kinds of friendship. It may also apply to mates at work or people, such as students, who share accommodation over a period of time. It almost certainly applies to individuals brought together in institutions such as prisons, hospitals or military barracks. However, it is likely that family life is characterised by having a particularly dense and complex nexus of guilty knowledge for the reasons already outlined. Further, recognition of this guilty knowledge may be part of what many individuals understand family life to be 'all about'.

The other aspect of Hughes' discussion that is of relevance here is his argument that licence often includes the licence to do dangerous or risky things (Hughes 1971: 289). John Gummer, at the time the Conservative Secretary of State for the Environment, publicly fed a hamburger to his daughter as a dramatic illustration of his attempt to persuade the British public that beef was safe to eat. Of course, the extent to which this was actually a dangerous thing to do is a matter for continued debate; the point here is that the licence was assumed in the context of a parental relationship. However confident his belief in the safety of British beef, it would not have been appropriate for the same minister to persuade somebody else's child to eat a hamburger. Parents may take their children on skiing trips, canoeing expeditions or other outdoor activities without themselves necessarily having had training as teachers of these outdoor, and sometimes dangerous, activities. This contrasts with professional teachers and coaches, who may do similar things with children and who will be called to account in the event of an accident. At a more psychological or interpersonal level, risk and danger may be built into the routine socialisation and disciplining of children or the everyday bodily pleasures and contacts that exist between parents and children, or siblings, within a family context.

It should be noted that these notions of risk are themselves the subject of negotiation, sometimes within families and between family members but also, and perhaps more frequently, between individual family members and outside agencies. If, as Beck has argued (1992), risk is a characteristic feature of modern society, then perceptions of risk are often particularly significant in the context of routine family living. After all, this begins in pregnancy, when the risks attached to smoking, alcohol consumption and inappropriate diets are widely debated and disseminated. Later in life, parents are often held responsible, formally or informally, for the crimes or misbehaviour of their children. Some forms of child rearing or disciplining (too strict or too lax or inconsistent) may be perceived as being particularly risky in terms of the child's life chances and experience in the wider world, yet parents continue to be licensed to take these self-same risks and may be condemned, or feel that they are condemned, if they fail in this respect.

Turning more specifically to questions of mandate, it can be argued that the mere statement of a family title may be enough to proclaim a mandate. 'Speaking as a mother ...' may be heard not only as a statement about oneself but also as a claim to have one's own experiences and opinions taken seriously. 'Standpoint theory', it might be suggested, is not simply a debate in feminist epistemology but something that is routinely practised by women, and men, on numerous everyday occasions. Note that the claim is not simply self-referential but that it also seeks to mark out areas of public or interpersonal life where the person in question has a right to speak. In the case of the title 'mother', the possible field may be very broad: genetically modified foods, pornography, local speed limits and many other aspects of modern life may come under the ambit of the particular mandate being claimed. A humorous example may be taken from *David Copperfield*:

> 'What makes you suppose there is any young lady in the case, Mrs Crupp?' said I.
>
> 'Mr Copperfull,' said Mrs Crupp, with a great deal of feeling, 'I'm a mother myself.'
>
> Dickens, 1903 edition: 315

Other family titles (consider 'speaking as an aunt') may not have quite the same ring to them. However, in some cases such claims may be part of an attempt to renegotiate a stigmatised identity. Thus the claim may be 'speaking as a single mother', or 'speaking as a step-parent'. Gay and lesbian couples may make similar claims to have their lifestyles and experiences taken seriously, thereby providing further challenges to conventional divisions between the public and the private. What these various claims would seem to suggest is the way in which certain family-based identities at least underline a demand to be taken seriously, to be seen as an adult if not always as a responsible adult. Conversely, those who have not had certain family experiences or identities may be denied the right to be heard seriously.

Television discussion programmes (*Kilroy*, for example) make considerable use of these claims and counter-claims around family-based identities.

We may also note at this point more collective attempts to define family-based mandates. The mothers of 'the disappeared' in Argentina may be one example from recent history. Movements on the part of non-residential fathers around issues of 'fathers' rights' may form another, contrasting, illustration. While family-based mandates often have a highly localised, specific and transitory character, they may sometimes assume a more organised form. Thus we have groups on the part of step-parents and the bereaved, and church-based groups and movements may draw heavily on family themes in order to claim their particular mandates to speak on public issues. In the case of religious groups and leaders, the mandate in relation to family issues may seem to be particularly strong. This may be a reflection of the tendency, in Western societies, for the religious sphere to shrink to the personal or interpersonal or a particular identification of religion and the family through the fact that both are, in different ways, concerned with matters of life and death. The various claims on the part of political parties to 'speak for the family' are also well known, although the distance between these claims and everyday experience may sometimes be considerable.

As an example of some of the questions concerning licence and mandate in the family, we may consider the continuing debate about a parent's right to smack a child. This has been the subject of some renewed debate in Britain recently, when the government proposed some restrictions on the right of parents to smack while still retaining the idea of 'reasonable chastisement'. Again, the rights and wrongs of this particular issue are not the question here. On the one hand, the state has provided a licence to parents to exercise this 'reasonable chastisement'. Within this general framework, the parent has considerable licence (in the second meaning of the word) in terms of the degree and kind of physical force being deployed and the occasions on which such chastisement might seem appropriate. Even within the proposed revised guidelines, these limits would seem to be flexible enough.

The other side of the coin is that considerable numbers of British parents (70 per cent, according to Walker (2000)) would resist any attempt to abolish the right to hit a child. In short, they are claiming that right as part of the parental mandate, as part of their general understanding about what being a parent entails. Of course, the meaning of such physical chastisement may vary considerably from seeing it as very much a last resort to seeing it as part of a parent's wider responsibility to a child.

It is also apparent that this matter is the subject of debate and disagreement. Opponents of the practice will point to the experiences of countries where the right to smack has been removed. They may also mobilise through bodies such as Children are Unbeatable to bring the practice to an end. This body represents various professional groups (and therefore provides a good example of Hughes' own use of the term 'mandate') but also includes individuals who, presumably, claim to speak as parents. Paradoxically, therefore, they may be claiming one particular mandate in order to limit another.

More generally, this continuing debate about smacking in Britain reflects wider concerns about the degrees of freedom or leeway that are accorded parents in a modern society. These are the questions that run through debates about child abuse, its identification and control, children's education and the circumstances under which children are taken into care. Questions of licence and mandate may not be as clearly codified as we might find in codes of professional ethics or good practice. Nevertheless, they are present and become apparent on those occasions where some family practices are opened up for public scrutiny.

I hope that I have said enough to suggest that there is considerable potential in applying Hughes' ideas to the study of family life. Naturally, there are differences. Mention has already been made of the financial (or other similar) rewards that are part of professional or occupational licenses and that have little overt or direct relevance in the study of family life. Furthermore, in family life, there would seem to be a greater degree of fluidity and potential for everyday negotiation. Little is formally codified or written down, and where this is the case it often only becomes apparent when things go wrong at the time of a divorce, say, or in cases of child neglect or abuse. Indeed, it may well be the case that a reflection on the tensions and ambiguities around licence and mandate may be a useful way to think through some of the complexities associated with features of modern family living such as step-parenting. The competing claims, or competing perceptions of such claims, between biological and step-parents are about the attempts to renegotiate questions of licence and mandate within modern family living.

It is possible that we may see the insights going both ways. Just as it may be possible to gain insights into family life from concepts originally developed to explore occupational or professional life, so too may our understanding of professional cultures be illuminated from insights derived from the apparently more fluid and negotiated practices of everyday family living. But that, as they say, is another story.

Conclusion

I have argued that there is something problematic in the bracketing of the terms 'sociology' and 'family', as in the textbook or course title 'Sociology of the Family'. The dilemma is whether to stress one side or the other or, if we argue for both, how the interplay between the two terms might be characterised. To stress the former might seem to mean the removal of all that is special or unique about family living, in the eyes of family participants as well as policy makers or moral entrepreneurs. To stress the latter would seem to underwrite certain political agendas that treat the family as special and, indeed, central to human life. In some cases, indeed, this may entail stressing the extra-social character or origins of family life.

The exploration of the terms 'licence' and 'mandate' and their applicability to the study of family practices would seem, on the surface, to opt very clearly for the sociology side of the equation. Not only are these terms developed by a sociologist, they are also developed by a sociologist whose chief interest in this context (and in much of his published work) is the exploration of occupational and professional practices. Hughes could never have been described as a family sociologist.

However, it was argued here that this represents the strength of this exploration. It is hoped that the use of the terms and the discussion surrounding them does serve to highlight or problematise certain areas of family life that perhaps have been relatively unheralded in the past. This might include licence to do dangerous or risky things and the idea of guilty knowledge, removed from some of the more psychoanalytical treatments of family secrets. But the other aspect of the use of these terms is that they perhaps throw light on the processes by which the 'specialness' or 'uniqueness' of family life is announced and maintained. For the present, we can remain agnostic as to whether there 'really' is something special about family living. The focus is shifted on to the processes by which this specialness is constructed. And here we look at the claims and counter-claims that family members, as individuals or sometimes parts of collectivities, make around the licensing and mandating of their practices. Thus debates about 'smacking' are not just about the deployment of legitimate (or otherwise) violence but about the boundaries of the family, the nature of parental responsibilities and rights and the exchanges between the family and agencies of the state: in short, about the processes of licensing and mandating.

Furthermore, we may see links here between Hughes' reference to the 'moral division of labour' and the recent 'moral turn' in family studies. As I pointed out earlier, my reference to this moral turn has nothing to do with much of the moralising that characterises much of the discussion about the family (Phillips 1999). However, the 'moral turn' recognises the existence of these moral debates and treats them as topics for enquiry in their own right. Thus it is a proper question to ask why, in modern society, there is a relatively easy slide from discussions of family to discussions of morality (in a way that is less obvious in, say, discussions of economic life) and it is important to listen carefully to the processes of moral debate and argument that take place around family matters. Here the listening is to the everyday experiences of parents, partners and children rather than simply to the pronouncements of moral entrepreneurs.

Similarly, when Hughes refers to the moral division of labour he is making a Durkheimian reference, which underlines the argument that social and moral phenomena are closely intertwined. The divisions of labour in society are not simply a technical matter; they also raise questions of 'ought', questions of rights, responsibilities and entitlements. The processes of licensing and mandating are in part to do with the distribution of moral claims and authority, and this is as true in relation to family matters as it is in relation to any other distribution of rights and responsibilities. In a complex modern, or postmodern, society, any set of moral claims is met with counter-claims, and again this can be seen clearly in debates about the responsibilities and rights of family members. Whatever the precise nature of the claims, we are aware that serious matters are under discussion.

Finally, there is in Hughes' writing a connection between his discussion of licence and mandate and his understanding of what he describes as the 'dual mandate' of the social sciences (Hughes 1971: 452–4). This duality is not unlike the duality with which I began this essay. On the one hand, there is the pursuit of 'general, abstract knowledge', while on the other hand there is attendance to the particulars, the issues of our own time or, perhaps, of some past time. This is partly a contrast between pure and applied or, in his words, between the timeless and the timely. Elsewhere, he contrasts the approach of St Matthew, whose gospel begins with the particularities of genealogy, and that of St John, who begins with abstract principles. Those who are licensed to practise as sociologists have a mandate to pursue both tendencies, if not equally, at least to maintain a sense of tension or dialectic between them. Perhaps, therefore, his own terminology and the exploration of the possibilities of applying it to the study of family life reflect this dual mandate of the sociologist. Put another way, it is possible that this exploration of the themes of licence and mandate in the context of asking how the bracketing of 'sociology' and 'family' is achieved will throw some light on the nature of sociological understanding as well as upon the particularities of family practices.

References

Beck, U. (1992) *Risk Society: Towards A New Modernity*, London: Sage.

Becker, G. (1996/1976) 'The economic approach to human behaviour', in J. Elster (ed.) *Rational Choice*, Oxford: Basil Blackwell, 108–22.

Bernardes, J. (1997) *Family Studies: An Introduction*, London: Routledge.

Clawson, D. (ed.) (1998) *Required Reading: Sociology's Most Influential Books*, Amherst: University of Massachusetts Press.

Cronin, H. and Curry, O. (2000) 'The evolving family', in H. Wilkinson (ed.) *Family Business*, London: Demos.

Dickens, C. (1903) *David Copperfield*, London: Chapman & Hall.

Finch, J. and Mason, J. (1993) *Negotiating Family Responsibilities*, London: Routledge.

Gluckman, M. (ed.) (1964) *Closed Systems and Open Minds: The Limits of Naivety in Social Anthropology*, Edinburgh and London: Oliver & Boyd.

Hughes, E. (1971) *The Sociological Eye*, Chicago: Aldine Atherton.

Morgan, D.H.J. (1975) *Social Theory and The Family*, London: Routledge & Kegan Paul.

—— (1996) *Family Connections: An Introduction to Family Studies*, Cambridge: Polity Press.

—— (1999) 'Risk and family practices: accounting for change and fluidity in family life', in E.B. Silva and C. Smart (eds) *The New Family?* London: Sage, 13–30.

Parsons, T. (1964) *Essays in Sociological Theory* (revised edition). New York: Free Press.

Parsons, T. and Bales, R.F. (1956) *Family: Socialization and Interaction Process*, London: Routledge & Kegan Paul.

Phillips, M. (1999) *The Sex-Change Society: Feminised Britain and the Neutered Male*, London: Social Market Foundation.

Reiger, K. (1985) *The Disenchantment of the Home: Modernising the Australian Family, 1880–1940*, Oxford: Oxford University Press.

Ribbens McCarthy, J., Edwards, R. and Gillies, V. (2000) 'Moral tales of the child and the adult: narratives of contemporary family lives under changing circumstances', *Sociology* 34(4): 785–804.

Sevenhuijsen, S. (1999) 'Caring in the third way', Working Paper No. 12, Centre for Research in Family, Kinship and Childhood, University of Leeds.

Silva, E.B. and Smart, C. (eds) (1999) *The New Family?* London: Sage.

Turner, B.S. (1993) 'Outline of a general theory of human rights', *Sociology* 27(3): 489–512.

Walker, P. (2000) 'Spare the child', *The Guardian*, 19 January, 17.

8 Policy and rhetoric

The growing interest in fathers and grandparents in Britain

Lynda Clarke and Ceridwen Roberts

Introduction

Family life in Britain has changed dramatically in the last thirty years. Demographic, social and economic changes have affected the living arrangements and family experiences of both parents and children. The changing nature of relationships and diversity of family types, increases including in family break-up and solo living, as well as the relative importance of friends and families are often seen as indicators of family instability. Family break-up may be extremely important for changing family roles but the nature of family life has also changed in other less obvious ways. More families have two parents in paid employment than in previous generations and, while most mothers work part-time, the proportion of mothers who return to full-time work after maternity leave is increasing (Dex 1999). There are also other important changes in domestic life and the role of families. Family activities in the last twenty-five years have become much less home-centred and more individualistic and commercial. For example, the traditional activities of sewing and cooking, child rearing and care for the elderly have lost their central unifying roles. These domestic activities have become less valued, and labour-saving devices and pre-prepared foods are used to cut down on time spent on these onerous tasks, or help is 'bought in' to assist with these roles. Much more time is spent now on so-called 'leisure activities', which involve participation in organised activities outside the home, often with peers and not as family groups (*Nestlé Family Monitor* 2000).

The implications of these family changes for the family roles of both fathers and grandparents are potentially vast. For example, where both parents are working or where family breakdown has occurred, grandparents may be expected to care for grandchildren or to contribute to their support in financial or emotional terms. Fathers, likewise, will be directly affected by family break-up as children almost invariably stay with their mothers, and the role of the non-resident father will be different in nature to that of resident father. The role of fathers has been influenced also by the growing expectation that fathers should be actively involved in childcare and that they may be the primary carers of children when mothers work. Additionally, for many men their fathering is increasingly carried out in the more ambiguous role of stepfather. Likewise, changing attitudes to fatherhood and parenting in general will influence the role of fathers.

There have been other demographic changes that affect family roles. As a result of population ageing, new and extended roles for older adults have been created, and today more older people are experiencing grandparenthood and even great grandparenthood than ever before. However, older people are not only living longer, they are also living healthier lives for longer. Attitudes towards older people's independence and autonomy are also changing. Supporting their children and grandchildren may therefore be at odds with older people's own desires to continue in paid employment or to pursue leisure interests.

In this chapter, we will explore the growing interest in fathers and grandparents in Britain. We will critically analyse how these family relationships and roles have been examined by British family researchers since the initial wave of interest in the 1980s and how the policy developments have related to the research base. We will argue that, while there has been explicit recognition of the importance of these family members in the lives of children, the policy responses have been simplistic and the rhetoric has not recognised the complexity and diversity of family life. We will begin by exploring the public policy context of fatherhood in Britain and then turn to examining grandparenthood.

Public policy and fatherhood

We would like to start by suggesting that the current policy and research interest in fathers and fatherhood may be perceived as an Anglocentric preoccupation that may not be shared to the same extent in other nations. The current focus in the USA, Britain and Australia on fatherhood research and policy is not so evident in other European countries (Clarke and Roberts 2001), despite the early interest in fatherhood in several Nordic countries, notably Sweden (Björnberg 1998). Currently, fatherhood involvement is not a central issue among policy makers and family researchers in Europe, particularly in southern Europe, although this is beginning to change (Giovannini 1998; Fthenakis 2000). A possible reason for this national pattern of preoccupation with fatherhood lies in the high prevalence of family breakdown in northern European countries and the consequent policy implications for economic support of lone mother families. Thus we will review the history of policy interest in fathers in Britain before turning to the research evidence on the involvement of fathers.

Academic interest in fatherhood research in Britain dates back to the late 1970s and early 1980s (McKee and O'Brien 1982; Lewis 1986), but it did not really penetrate the public policy and academic research domain, partly because the funders of research were not enthusiastic. Later an independent policy interest in fathers arose, which was overwhelmingly created by the increase in lone parent households and the issue of growing public expenditure on lone parent families. The phenomenon of lone motherhood emerged in the 1970s but has grown dramatically since the early 1980s. Lone mother families constituted 7.5 per cent of all families in 1971 but doubled as a proportion of all families during the 1980s – from 10.7 per cent of all families in 1981 to 19.8 per cent in 1991, reaching 22 per cent of all families in 1996 (Haskey 1996, 1998).

The Child Support Act was introduced in a hurry in 1991 after looking at the systems to make absent fathers pay for children that were in operation in the USA and Australia (Barnes *et al.* 2000). The Child Support Agency (CSA) came into existence in April 1993 with the express purpose of collecting maintenance from absent fathers. This was the only major policy instrument in early 1990s Britain in relation to fathers and fathering. It was not concerned with fathers in general, only with non-resident fathers who did not perform economically and with making these fathers pay the costs of supporting their children rather than the state. There was almost no analysis of who fathers were and what were their circumstances before this policy system was introduced. The ensuing protest and tremendous rows about the CSA and its operation were perhaps due to this lack of groundwork. The child support legislation produced more mail for parliamentarians than any previous legal change. It produced an even heavier mailbag than the poll tax in the 1990s, according to a senior civil servant who was closely involved with the child support policy (personal communication). The backlash against child support policy that started in 1993 was led in the main by separated and re-partnered fathers, although mothers anxious to break all links with, and be 'independent of', former partners were also vocal critics. The child support legislation has now been reformed (summer 2000), taking account of the complaints about the old legislation made by fathers in second families and lone mothers. It may not perform better, but it is more transparent. The government has in effect abandoned the principle that first families are first and in the new system has made allowances for new responsibilities that men may have to new families – both the children that men subsequently father in second and subsequent families and to any stepchildren brought into their lives through new partnerships. The amount of maintenance to first families is reduced *pro rata* for any children (step or natural) in subsequent families of men. Child support applies to all fathers regardless of legal status, but rights over children are conferred only by marriage.

Another very important strand in the development of policy interest in fathers has been the concern with crime. Growing under the Conservative government, and continuing under Labour, has been anxiety about crime and social disorder among young people, especially young men. In the mid-1990s, critics of the government were laying the blame for social disorder at the door of fathers, or at least the absence of effective fathers (Dennis and Erdos 1993). These writers argued that groups of young people were growing up completely unsocialised by fathers or male elders, out of control and living in so-called 'ghetto' settings – large inner city estates with poor housing and education, and no work prospects. Eventually, because of continued interest in crime and disorder and 'young men out of control', the debate did result in the introduction of severe measures designed to keep unruly youths off the streets at night and compel parents to be responsible for these children. Without confronting the real causes and consequences of this phenomenon using the research evidence that existed, the unruliness of youth was often attributed to the physical absence of the fathers. In the policy arena, the Labour Party seemed unwilling or unable to tackle the place of fatherhood or men in the creation of 'feral sons'. The Crime and Disorder Bill (December 1997) imposed a curfew on these 'feral young men', and compulsory parenting orders placed responsibility on their parents, where non-compliance incurs fines or imprisonment

Against this context, there was a growing awareness in the 1980s that divorcing parents might not be advantageous for children. This interest in parenting was rather attenuated, however, as there were no policy reviews or developments in this area. The Tory government developed a 'back to basics' campaign, which aimed to bolster family values – deter family break-up, stop young women having children alone and on benefit and encourage responsible parenting. It did not focus on fathers directly.

Even when the Labour government came to power in May 1997, the announcement of support for families did not mention the importance of fathers in family lives. Their role in family support was spelt out only in relation to proposals to reform child support. Tony Blair's speech at the Labour Party Conference in September 1997 announced the creation of a first ever Ministerial Group on the Family, which would be chaired by a high-status minister, the Home Secretary. This transferred the focal point (as far as it had existed before) of family policies away from the Department of Health, long accustomed to looking after women and children, and health and social science issues for families, to the Home Office (see also Chapter 3.3). The Family Policy Unit in the Home Office was established in 1998 and, significantly, received a funding stream to finance family support work in the voluntary sector, not renowned for its expertise in this area. It has financed various small practice initiatives for fathers but mainly on a local basis. Its main funding has been allocated to the creation of a new National Family and Parenting Institute (NFPI), providing £2 million over three years to monitor and promote 'good parenting'. The NFPI's brief is to act to improve knowledge and understanding of the role of parents in British society. It is mapping parent initiatives and examining what parents need and want from state support. The NFPI was envisaged as a route to government for parents, briefing the government about parents' desires. The government has also given £1 million to Parentline Plus – basically a telephone helpline for parents staffed by volunteers. The institute's principal task is to direct parents to other support organisations and, as this develops, it will build up expertise about local initiatives for parents. The main funding concerned only with fathers is to Fathers Direct, establishing an information network for fathers and support for practitioners and those working with men, although it is also planning to disseminate research findings and obtain funding to commission a 'fathers' audit' in Britain.

The Labour government also tackled another area in relation to fatherhood, that of the rights of unmarried fathers. As the growth of non-marital childbearing has increased (38 per cent of babies are now born outside marriage), so too have the numbers of unmarried fathers with no formal parental rights to children in law. The early interest of the government resulted in a quick consultation, which was automatically oriented towards the view that fathers who jointly registered should have the same rights as married fathers. It is now proposed to introduce the legislation for this in the Adoption Bill.

Finally, there is the issue of policy towards fathers in general – as opposed to 'deadbeat or dead broke' dads, unmarried or absent dads – which has been rather lacking. There has been movement in the area of parental leave to bring Britain more into line with the provisions experienced by many of its European partners (Department of Trade and Industry 2000). This was given media impetus in 2001 with the arrival of Leo Blair (the Prime Minister's fourth child). The EC recommendation has been incorporated at the lowest possible benefit level for families because there has been considerable pressure to avoid the general provision of parental leave from the business community. The incorporation of this has highlighted wider issues for fathers and fatherhood, and the European Working Time Directive (2000), which regulates hours worked, has recently been introduced. This is particularly important given that Britain had the longest working hours for fathers in Europe, which has often been cited as a major limiting influence on fathers' involvement with their children (Clarke and O'Brien 2002).

Research evidence on fatherhood

During the 1980s, British family research was influenced by the paradigmatic shift occurring across the social sciences away from a mother-centred and feminist approach to theory and data collection towards a consideration of the perspectives of fathers and children. As Michael Rutter reminded researchers in his landmark book, *Maternal Deprivation Reassessed*, 'children have fathers too!' (Rutter 1972). There was dissatisfaction with research that emphasised the mother–child relationship and neglected the place of the male parent. Writers argued that the adult dimension of family life was known mainly through the eyes of mothers and wives and that the perspective of the male experience was left unexplored (McKee and O'Brien 1982). Although there have always been isolated studies of fatherhood in the social sciences in Britain (e.g. Taconis 1969), the range and extent of projects in the late 1970s and early 1980s signified a move away from a mother-centred focus. A new generation of researchers broadened the study of families to incorporate fathers (Beail and McQuire 1982; McKee and O'Brien 1982; Lewis 1986) and children (Jenks 1982; James and Prout 1990; Clarke 1992).

This first wave of fatherhood research from psychologists and sociologists was primarily, although not exclusively, ethnographic and embedded in a 'discovery' mode, with the intention of giving paternal accounts of family life a hearing at the centre of the stage – a father-centred paradigm. First-hand accounts of men's family life and lifecourse transitions, for instance becoming a father or caring for children alone, indicated that men could experience these events in an emotionally intense manner, showing behaviour that did not fit into the stereotype of the distant, disengaged father. A common theme in this work was to uncover more about the *meaning* of being a father – a search for the phenomenology of fatherhood. The legacy of this early work still remains, but is now recast into a more robust methodological framework suggested by researchers at the time:

> It is not enough for research to merely turn from mothers to fathers, since this can only be a short-term and remedial strategy. Theoretical and empirical sophistication must be accomplished so that studies encompass all family interaction and dynamics, including mothers, fathers and children, and extending to the wider kin and community.
>
> McKee and O'Brien 1982: 23

Since this early work, family researchers in a range of disciplines have become more father-sensitive and have been studying fatherhood through different methodologies. It was in this climate that the Family Policy Studies Centre managed to obtain funding for its review of research on fathers in Britain (Burghes *et al.* 1997). This was a seminal piece of work in Britain, notably because of the breadth of the review and because it included the first demographic analysis of fatherhood in Britain. This was possible because a panel dataset had asked men about fertility histories for the first time in Britain. Funding was difficult because of a lack of policy interest in fatherhood, and previous policy had been determined without any knowledge of the demography of fatherhood. Further demographic analyses of fatherhood have been undertaken, including a comparison with American fathers and absent fathers (Clarke *et al.* 1999).

Subsequent contributions to the study of fatherhood come from a variety of disciplines: social policy (absent fathers – Bradshaw *et al.* 1999); sociology (family forms – Ferri and Smith 1999; time with children – Gershuny 2001); psychology (Lewis 2000); and child psychiatry (biological and social vulnerability of fathers – Kraemer 1991, 2000; impact of father absence on children – Cockett and Tripp 1994). Measuring the involvement of fathers has been a preoccupation of the psychologists, whereas the impact on children of poor involvement or absence of fathers has been the main concern of other social researchers. The current preoccupation in Britain with 'social exclusion' has shifted social research emphasis to considering the effects of unemployment and poverty for families but, interestingly, not a separate consideration of the effects of different types of father involvement. Fathers tend to matter only when they are deemed inadequate or absent. Accordingly, there has been a recent funding focus on 'vulnerable' fathers. New projects include young fathers (Speak *et al.* 1997; Quinton and Pollock 2000); unemployed fathers (Warin *et al.* 1999); fathers in a welfare setting (Ghate *et al.* 2000 – involving fathers in family network centres); and those whose families do not fit the majority pattern – cohabiting fathers, non-resident or stepfathers (Bradshaw *et al.* 1999; Pickford 1999; Lewis 2000).

The research evidence on the impact of fathers on child development is more advanced in the USA than in Britain (Clarke and O'Brien 2002). Fathers who are 'involved' with their children have been associated with various positive outcomes for those children, but a recent review of the evidence on British fathers and fatherhood noted the widespread confusion and disagreement on the contribution that men make to contemporary family life (Lewis 2000).

Most research examining the impact of fathers in families has been on the effect of father absence or divorce on children (Rodgers and Pryor 1998). In general in Britain, unlike in the USA, there has been to date a lack of mainstream interest in and also hard evidence for the consequences of fathering, or lack of it, for child outcomes, as well as a lack of concern with fathers in fragile families (poor or fatherless families). Whether fatherless families are at high risk of crime and delinquent behaviour – from a lack of an adequate male role model or dispenser of discipline – or whether it is a function of poverty is still being debated in Britain. There has been some research and debate about whether fathers are disenfranchised when they are not providers (unemployed), and it is claimed by some that many of the problems of social exclusion have their origins in the problems of fathers and boys (*Hansard*, House of Lords debate, 24 January 2001). They claim that fathers matter because there is 'overwhelming statistical evidence' that boys with a poor or non-existent relationship with their fathers are more likely to be violent, do less well in school and be bullies or be bullied, and they are three times more likely to be involved in serious or persistent crime (Graham and Bowling 1995).

A distinction has been made between the institution of fatherhood and the practice of fathering (Jensen 1999; Morgan 2000). This has some overlap with the longstanding distinction between ascribed and achieved fatherhood. There is also an increasingly vociferous argument proposing the evolutionary or 'selfish gene' perspective, which states that social fathering cannot be the same as biological fathering and may be risky for children (Daly and Wilson 1998).

As described above, the link between fatherlessness and crime has been debated in the policy arena for some time (FPSC Crime and the Family Conference 1994; Graham and Bowling 1995). There is still a tremendous emphasis in our discourse on family processes rather than the structure of the family. It is the parenting process rather than the context, be it one or two parents, that counts. As yet, the link between structure and process has not been satisfactorily explained. In other words, how much easier is it to provide effective parenting in our society when there are two of you to undertake this task, and both of you have an investment in that child? One of the issues is that there is a higher incidence of child abuse (hitting) by men in families where they are not related biologically to the children (Daly and Wilson 1998). It is not clear whether this is related to the fact that these families are poorer or to the lack of taboos around the behaviour between adults and children in such families. The poverty and structure (family type) explanations are difficult to disentangle and are further complicated by an environmental relationship. For example, the incidence of petty theft, vandalism, school exclusions and poor, fatherless or unemployed families is highest in deprived areas – inner city social housing estates, the British equivalent of 'ghettos'. The issue of inadequate parenting or fathering has been associated with poor families and poor neighbourhoods, and these are being addressed in research and government policy as well as specific issues, such as teenage parenting and the poverty of lone mothers.

One study attempting to measure the impact of parental input (including involvement by fathers) in different family types in a working-class community found that positive educational outcomes for children were associated with material well-being, educational aspirations, maternal praise and parental employment patterns. Children performed best when mothers were in employment, but the gains were less strong when both parents worked full-time. Paternal praise was also important for positive educational outcomes in two-parent households (O'Brien and Jones 1999; Ryan 2000). Several studies of father involvement and associated outcomes in adolescence and later life have been undertaken in Britain. One survey of teenagers found that low father involvement and high peer victimisation contributed significantly and independently to low levels of life satisfaction in adolescent boys (Flouri and Buchanan 2002). There was also evidence of a buffering effect of father involvement in that it protected children from extreme victimisation.

In summary, from a review of the research on fatherhood in Britain (Clarke and O'Brien 2002) we would conclude:

- Father involvement in terms of taking responsibility for children has been identified as being particularly important by the psychological, social and policy literature, but it has been under-investigated.
- Fathering is a multi-dimensional role and can take diverse forms. Given that fathers must balance and prioritise their roles, fatherhood in practice may be very different to stated expectations or desires.
- The context of fathering is also important. Demographic and social factors, especially those relating to employment and the nature of the relationship between the mother and the father, are important. The

accepted norms surrounding fatherhood will differ between different groups (socio-economic class, ethnic group).
- The quality of the relationship between father and child is as important as, or more important than, its frequency.

An important point was made early on in the academic debate in Britain but is worth re-emphasising because it tends to be overlooked. In 1982, Martin Richards commented that 'fathers should not be regarded merely as alternative mothers'. Fathering has multiple dimensions and encompasses a great diversity of styles and relationships. How fathers decide what to prioritise in their lives, how much time they devote to children and how much effort to expend on fathering vary according to a number of factors, both individual and social. Some recent work has urged a 'contextual' approach to the study of fathering, which takes into account fathers' circumstances and how they balance the different dimensions of their role, for example economic provision and childcare (Burghes *et al.* 1997). The pressures of being the major breadwinner and the demand also to be 'involved' as a hands-on carer or 'new dad' have given rise to confusion among fathers about their role. This is further complicated when it has to be renegotiated after separation from the children and their mother (e.g. Barker 1994; Simpson *et al.* 1995; Warin *et al.* 1999; Trinder *et al.* 2001).

Research evidence also points to the importance of the mother in mediating a father's relationship with his children, being 'gate-keepers' to the children (Backett 1987; Hutson and Jenkins 1989; Ribbens 1994; Smart 1999; Gilles *et al.* 2000). It has also been argued that it is men's wives who mediate their partners' relationship with his parents and who mediate relationships with grandchildren and grandparents (Cotterill 1994). This leads on to a consideration of research and policy in relation to grandparents.

Public policy and research on grandparenthood

In spite of the general acknowledgement of the importance of family relationships for personal well-being (Graham and Bowling 1995), it is true that we know little about the diversity of the role of grandparenting in Britain, its meaning for older people or the contribution it makes to their quality of life. Very little research on grandparenting and grandparents has been conducted in this country. Conversely, in America there is a well-established tradition of research on grandparents and, furthermore, there is an impressive array of around 600 to 700 support groups for grandparents as well as strong grandparent lobbies in Washington and in individual states (Young and Stogden 2000). The issues surrounding grandparenthood are therefore that much more advanced in the USA, and this is from where much of the research on the subject emanates. Also, the policy debate is much more advanced and in the public domain, to the extent that law suits are being brought by grandparents in order to gain access to or custody of grandchildren.

The role of grandparents has been largely ignored by social researchers and family policy specialists in this country, and there are virtually no groups specifically promoting the rights of grandparents. It is only in the last couple of years that estimates of numbers of grandparents and the level and type of contact between grandparents and grandchildren have been made. From a quota sample of grandparents undertaken by Age Concern (1997), it was revealed that 29 per cent of the adult population are grandparents, and over three-quarters of people aged 66 or over are grandparents. More recently, in their work looking at kin exchange beyond the household, Grundy *et al.* (1999) established a framework of all kin exchanges, including grandparental exchanges. From this nationally representative study, we know that around 70 per cent of middle-aged and older people are grandparents (Grundy and Clarke 2000).

The government's first Green Paper on *Supporting Families* recognised the role of the extended family and grandparents in supporting parents and children and providing stability (Home Office 1998: 18–19). However, the only evidence quoted on the role of grandparents is from a small market research survey and the recommendation to service providers to encourage grandparents to play a positive role in the lives of their families was somewhat vague and simplistic. Brief mention is made of the use of older people and grandparents by schools and as volunteers in the community, for example as 'grandparent mentors' in secondary schools. The specific service provisions to facilitate grandparent–grandchild interaction are threefold. First, the social services are urged to work with the extended family when relationships in the nuclear family are under stress and to consider grandparents as an 'effective placement' when children have to be looked after by the local authority. Second, health visitors are encouraged to involve the wider family; and, third, housing departments are advised to 'give due weight to the housing needs of grandparents ... for example by allocating homes so that wider families, particularly those with dependent children, are wherever possible living near to each other'.

The paper quotes a survey by Age Concern as showing that most grandparents are already involved in the care of their grandchildren. This survey showed that '92 per cent of grandparents have regular contact with their grandchildren. They are the most important source of day-care of children: 47 per cent help look after their grandchildren. Most children see their grandparents as important figures in their lives'. There is no recognition in this document of the diversity of the role of grandparenting in Britain, what grandparents do for their families or how happy they are with their role. Most importantly, there is no mention of grandparental rights or access to children after the divorce of their parents.

Apart from the classic kinship studies of the 1950s and 1960s by Townsend and Young, very little research has been conducted specifically on grandparenting and grandparents in this country. Until recently, what we knew about grandparents was drawn from a few qualitative studies focusing on specific issues and some quantitative work on older people and kin exchanges from a general perspective. Such studies included work on becoming a grandparent, negotiating the grandparental role in the family, grandfatherhood and grandparents' material help for families with young children (Cunningham-Burley 1985, 1986, 1987; Wilson, 1987). Finch and Mason (1993) also undertook both a survey and a qualitative examination of family obligations and responsibilities, which included grandparents. These studies have all provided useful clues about specific facets of being a grandparent but were not designed to be generalised or, in the latter case, was not aimed at exploring the grandparent role in particular.

A number of studies, although not investigating grandparenthood directly, have provided useful insights into the social life and kin support of older people in certain locations or for particular groups of people. Phillipson (1998) returned to the urban areas of the three major studies of older people in the 1940s and 1950s (Bethnal Green, Wolverhampton and Woodford) to examine the change and continuities in the lives of older people. He found that kinship ties remained central to these older people but that they were more likely to live alone and to have important 'personal communities', in the shape of friends, than fifty years ago. The impact of family change on older people has also been examined in a qualitative study, in the shape of inter-generational ties and transfers in step-families by Bornat *et al.* (1998). They report that family break-up and reconstitution bring some older people, their adult children and stepchildren closer together but may lead to older men living in relative isolation, while ties between mothers and daughters may be strengthened.

Some evidence of grandparental input into families can be gleaned from questions on patterns of contact and support from extended family members. For example, the British Social Attitudes Survey (BSAS) kinship module of 1995 (McGlone *et al.* 1998) and a module on young people in the 1998 BSAS included grandparenting, but only from the grandchild's perspective. A qualitative study of grandparents that explored the role that grandparents felt they played in the lives of their grandchildren was also undertaken by Age Concern (1998). Findings confirmed that this role was important for many older people in Britain.

Research looking at issues around grandparenting has therefore been greatly lacking. However, the last few years have seen growing interest in the topic of grandparenthood in Britain, and a number of studies have recently been funded. The 1998 BSAS (Dench *et al.* 1999) represents a first look at grandparenting using a nationally representative sample. The survey asked grandparents about their relationship with one randomly selected grandchild, and *vice versa*. Most of the respondents regarded their relationships with grandchildren as extremely important, and 64 per cent of the grandparents agreed that 'grandparenting is a very rewarding aspect of my life'. The survey covered a number of issues, including the level of involvement of grandparents with their grandchildren; satisfaction with the grandparenting role; grandparenting when family breakdown has taken place; and support provided for working mothers. It provides a general and valuable overview of attitudes towards various aspects of the grandparenting experience but does not look at any one issue in depth.

More recent research on the role and meaning of grandparenthood in Britain, funded under the ESRC 'Growing Older' programme, conducted national quantitative and qualitative studies (Clarke and Cairns 2000, 2001a). This project interviewed 850 grandparents in a first-stage study and then followed up forty-five grandparents in depth to probe the role of grandparenting in general, how the role is negotiated with children and how this is affected by family break-up. Financial, emotional and practical help with grandchildren were explored, as well as the satisfaction of the grandparenting role as far as the grandparents were concerned. It found that there is great diversity in the operation of grandparenting roles, which vary both between and within age groups, genders and family types of the grandchild. There is general agreement on the importance of grandparent status, but how this is played out varies greatly. It found that grandparents differ in the amount of help they give to their children and grandchildren. Some are happy to give any amount of help, but many grandparents have a clear idea of the limits of the help they are prepared to give to grandchildren, although many are willing to offer more help in times of trouble, especially family breakdown. There was evidence of both onerous undertaking of childcare and financial support by grandparents, including becoming custodial grandparents, as well as difficulties and great distress when contact with grandchildren was lost or withheld (Clarke and Cairns 2001b).

Family breakdown: the effect on grandparents

Grandparents have been called the 'other victims of divorce', because their relationship with their grandchildren can be seriously compromised by either removal or restriction of access to the children (Kornhaber 1996). In the United States, grandparents have the right to sue for visitation rights to their grandchildren where parental death or divorce has occurred and in some states in cases of step-parent adoption (Drew and Smith 1999). As mentioned previously, there is also an active grandparents' rights movement in North America, and legislation on grandparents' right to petition for visitation privileges to children has developed alongside research into the difficulties experienced in the acquisition of access in situations of family crisis (Derdeyn 1985). In Britain, since the 1989 Children Act, grandparents can apply to the courts for permission to contact their grandchildren. However, even when a contact order has been obtained by the grandparent, there is little that holds the parent to abide by the court ruling. Parents who do not do so can be held in contempt of court and serve twenty-eight days in prison. However, few grandparents would wish to take such an action and risk their grandchildren being placed in care. Additionally, it is likely that this action would only increase the anger of the parents and jeopardise the opportunity to see the grandchildren in the long term (Drew and Smith 1999). The impact of divorce on grandparents is potentially wide-ranging and devastating, particularly where access to grandchildren is removed. The grandparent–parent relationship discussed above is important here. When separation or divorce has occurred, maintaining friendly relations with former children-in-law may be crucial, particularly if this parent gains custody of the grandchildren. Gladstone (1989) described how parents can facilitate or prevent contact between grandparents and grandchildren, and Fischer (1983) found this to be the main component determining grandparental access to grandchildren following divorce.

Again, however, most of the research in this area is American. Issues covered include the impact of divorce on contact with grandchildren; satisfaction with the grandparent–grandchild relationship; and the physical and emotional health of the grandparent.

Other small-scale qualitative studies have recently been undertaken. Drew and Smith (1999) carried out a study to assess the impact of divorce on the grandparent–grandchild relationship. Findings showed that, in particular, grandparents who reported a loss of contact with grandchildren had emotional and physical health problems related to this loss. The study provides valuable insights into the affect of separation or divorce on grandparents. However, it is limited in that the sample of grandparents was small and self-selected. The grandparents were contacted through the Grandparents' Federation, so respondents may perhaps have experienced more problems than others with grandchildren affected by family breakdown. Another study recently completed in this country looked at the negotiation of the grandparenting role within the family (Tunaley 1998). The work was carried out a part of a wider study, funded by the telecommunications company British Telecom, of communication across three generations. Grandparents' relationships with other family members in eighty-seven three-generation families were explored. The results revealed that while grandparents played an active role in their families, both parents and grandparents asserted that they should not 'interfere' in their children's and grandchildren's lives. Again, the study was based on a small sample. A small qualitative report has also been produced by the London Borough of Lewisham Policy and Equalities Unit (Oliver 1998) to assess the needs of grandparents who provide childcare for their grandchildren. Similarly, a report has been produced by Plymouth City Council social services (Pitcher 1999) assessing the needs of custodial grandparents.

Conclusions

In summary, this chapter has explored the growing interest in fathers and grandparents in Britain. It has argued that, while there has been explicit recognition of the importance of these family members in the lives of children, the policy responses have been simplistic and the rhetoric has not recognised the complexity and diversity of family life.

In Britain, unlike in many other countries, policy towards families has not been developed from research-based knowledge. It has involved service- and practice-based initiatives led by rhetoric and pressure groups. The *Supporting Families* Green Paper virtually ignores the role of fathers in a 'healthy' family life, but the Ministerial Group on the Family and the Family Support Grant have developed several initiatives and intervention projects to support fathers. However, these were not developed from an evidence base on fatherhood in general but from pressure from two groups – absent fathers and fathers who wanted legislation and support for more shared care (the 'new' men).

We are at the cusp of an expansion of interest in fathers in Britain, although the main concern is with the consequences of fatherlessness for children. There is no coordinated policy or research interest in fatherhood and fathers *per se*. In the government's 1998 Green Paper, the first ever government consultation paper on the family, it is stated that 'Fathers have a crucial role to play in their children's upbringing', but this is not until halfway through the document, and most of the references to fathers are in relation to child support. Public policies and media attention still focus on the negative aspects of fatherhood. An economic view of fathering continues to dominate policy and research, and funding for research has been notoriously difficult to obtain. There is still confusion about the part that men play in contemporary families, but rigorous study and debate has begun. The fact that a lengthy recent debate in the House of Lords centred on boys and fatherhood is most encouraging: 'We should be seeking ways to channel all that is valuable in a boy's masculinity into positive directions that will help him take up his complementary and constructive role in a two-sex society' (Lord Quirk, *Hansard*, 24 January 2001). We would agree that the important role that fathers play in family lives in Britain has yet to be mapped and would emphasise that fathers are different to mothers. The task facing us is to measure how different!

The government's Green Paper did recognise the role that grandparents have, and could have, in family life but was too simplistic in its ideas about what grandparents could do for their children and grandchildren. The recommendations are somewhat naive about the issues involved and do not address the complexity of family life and relationships. The real issues of the diversity of grandparents, the heterogeneity of how grandparenting is played out in families and the difficult position of grandparents – both in practice and in law – were ignored. Also, some of the more complicated issues, for example formalising grandparental contact after family breakdown, were not considered.

References

Age Concern (1997) news release, London: Age Concern.

—— (1998) *Across the Generations*, London: Age Concern.

Backett, K. (1987) 'The negotiation of fatherhood', in C. Lewis and M. O'Brien (eds) *Reassessing Fatherhood*, London: Sage.

Barker, R.W. (1994) *Lone Fathers and Masculinities*, Aldershot: Avebury.

Barnes, H., Clarke, L., Paull, G. and Walker, I. (2000) 'Child support reform and low income families', Family Policy Studies Working Paper 10. London: Family Policy Studies Centre.

Beail, N. and McGuire, J. (1982) *Fathers: Psychological Perspectives*, London: Junction Books.

Bornat, J., Dimmock, B. and Peace, S. (1998) 'The impact of family change on older people: the case of stepfamilies', research results: ESRC Population and Household Change programme. Swindon: Economic and Social Research Council.

Björnberg, U. (1998) 'Family orientation among men: a process of change in Sweden', in E. Drew, R. Emerek and E. Mahon (eds) *Women, Work and the Family in Europe*, London: Routledge.

Bradshaw, J., Stimson, C., Skinner, C. and Williams, J. (1999) *Absent Fathers?* London: Routledge.

Burghes, L., Clarke, L. and Cronin, N. (1997) 'Fathers and fatherhood in Britain', Occasional Paper 23. London: Family Policy Studies Centre.

Clarke, L. (1992) 'Children's family circumstances: recent trends in Great Britain', *European Journal of Population* 20(4): 309–40.

Clarke, L. and Cairns, H. (2000) 'The demography of grandparenting', paper presented to the British Population Studies Conference, Utrecht.

—— (2001a) 'Grandparents and childcare: the research evidence', in B. Broad (ed.) *Kinship Care*, London: Routledge.

—— (2001b) 'The demography of grandparenthood in Britain', paper presented to the European Population Conference, Helsinki.

Clarke, L., Cooksey, E. and Verropoulou, G. (1999) 'Fathers and absent fathers: socio-demographic similarities in Britain and the United States', *Demography* 35(2): 217–28.

Clarke, L. and O'Brien, M. (2002) 'Father involvement in Britain: the research and policy evidence' in R.D. Day and M. Lamb (eds) *Reconceptualising and Measuring Fatherhood*, New York: Lawrence Erlbaum.

Clarke, L. and Roberts, C. (2001) *Fatherhood in the New Millennium*, York: Joseph Rowntree Foundation.

Cockett, M. and Tripp, J. (1994) *The Exeter Family Study; Family Breakdown and its Impact on Children*, Exeter: University of Exeter Press.

Cotterill, P. (1994) *Friendly Relations? Mothers and Daughters in Law*, London: Taylor & Francis.

Cunningham-Burley, S. (1985) 'Constructing grandparenthood: anticipating appropriate action', *Sociology* 19(3): 421–36.

—— (1986) 'Becoming a grandparent', *Ageing and Society* 6: 453–70.

—— (1987) 'The experience of grandfatherhood', in C. Lewis and M. O'Brien (eds) *Reassessing Fatherhood: New Observations on Fathers and the Modern Family*, London: Sage.

Daly, M. and Wilson, M. (1998) *The Truth about Cinderella: A Darwinian View of Parental Love*, London: Weidenfeld & Nicolson.

Dench, G., Ogg, J. and Thomson, K. (1999) 'The role of grandparents', in *British Social Attitudes Survey*, London: Institute for Social and Community Planning.

Dennis, N. and Erdos, G. (1993) *Families without Fatherhood*, London: Institute for Economic Affairs.

Department of Trade and Industry (2000) *Work and Parents, Competitiveness and Choice*, London: DTI.

Derdeyn, S.P. (1985) 'Grandparent visitation rights: rendering family dissention more pronounced?' *American Journal of Orthopsychiatry* 55(2): 277–87.

Dex, S. (ed.) (1999) *Families and the Labour Market: Trends, Pressures and Policies*, York and London: Joseph Rowntree Foundation/Family Policy Studies Centre.

Drew, L.A. and Smith, P.K. (1999) 'The impact of parental separation/divorce on grandparent–grandchild relationships', *International Journal of Ageing and Human Development* 16: 67–78.

Ferri, E. and Smith, E. (1999) *Parenting in the 1990s*, London: Family Policy Studies Centre.

Finch, J. and Mason, J. (1993) *Negotiating Family Responsibilities*, London: Routledge.

Fischer, L.R. (1983) 'Transition of grandmotherhood', *International Journal of Ageing and Human Development* 16: 67–78.

Flouri, E. and Buchanan. A. (2002, in press) 'Life satisfaction in teenage boys: the moderating role of father involvement and bullying', *Aggressive Behaviour* 28(2).

FPSC Crime and the Family Conference (1994) proceedings edited by C. Henricson. London: Family Policy Studies Centre.

Fthenakis, W. (2000) 'The role of fathers in Germany', in *Fatherhood in the New Millennium Conference Proceedings*, London: Family Policy Studies Centre.

Gershuny, J. (2001) *Changing Times*, Oxford: Oxford University Press.

Ghate, D., Shaw, C. and Hazel, N. (2000) *Fathers and Family Centres: Engaging Fathers in Preventive Services*, York: Joseph Rowntree Foundation.

Gilles, V., Ribbens McCarthy, J. and Holland, J. (2000) *Pulling Together, Pulling Apart: The Family Lives of Young People*, London: Family Policy Studies Centre/Joseph Rowntree Foundation.

Giovannini, D. (1998) 'Are fathers changing? Comparing some different images on sharing of childcare and domestic work', in E. Drew, R. Emerek and E. Mahon (eds) *Women, Work and the Family in Europe*, London: Routledge.

Gladstone, J.W. (1989) 'Grandmother–grandchild contact: the mediating influence of the middle generation following marriage breakdown and remarriage', *Canadian Journal of Ageing* 8: 355–6.

Graham, J. and Bowling, B. (1995) *Young People and Crime*, Research Findings No. 24. London: Home Office.

Grundy, E. and Clarke, L. (2000) 'Grandparents and grandparenting in Britain today', paper presented to Grandparenting in the 21st Century Conference, March.

Grundy, E., Murphy, M. and Shelton, N. (1999) 'Looking beyond the household: intergenerational perspectives on living kin and contacts with kin in Great Britain', *Population Trends* 97.

Haskey, J. (1996) 'Population review: families and households in Great Britain', *Population Trends* 85, 7–14.

—— (1998) 'One-parent families and their dependent children', *Population Trends* 91: 5–14.

Hutson, S. and Jenkins, R. (1989) *Taking the Strain: Families, Unemployment and Transition*, Buckingham: Open University Press.

James, A. and Prout, A. (eds) (1990) *Constructing and Reconstructing Childhood.* London: Falmer Press.

Jenks, C. (1982) *The Sociology of Childhood*, London: Batsford.

Jensen, A.-M. (1999) 'Property, power and prestige – the feminisation of childhood', in M. du Bois-Reymond, H. Sunker and H.H. Kruger (eds) *Childhood in Europe: Approaches, Trends and Findings*, New York: Peter Land.

Kornhaber, A. (1996) *Contemporary Grandparenting*, Thousand Oaks, Calif.: Sage.

Kraemer, S. (1991) 'The origins of fatherhood', *Family Process* 30: 377–92.

—— (2000) 'The fragile male', *British Medical Journal* 321: 1609–12.

Lewis, C. (1986) *Becoming A Father*, Buckingham: Open University Press.

—— (2000) 'A man's place is in the home: fathers and families in the UK', *Foundations*, York: Joseph Rowntree Foundation.

McGlone, F., Park, A. and Smith, K. (1998) *Families and Kinship*, London: Family Policy Studies Centre.

McKee, L. and O'Brien, M. (eds) (1982) *The Father Figure*, London: Tavistock.

Morgan, D. (2000) 'Gender practices and fathering practices', in B. Hudson (ed.) *Fathers and the State*, Cambridge: Cambridge University Press.

Nestlé Family Monitor (2000). London: Nestlé.

O'Brien, M. and Jones, D. (1999) 'Children, parental involvement and educational attainment: an English case study', special issue of *Cambridge Journal of Economics* on the family, 23(5): 599–621.

Oliver, C. (1998) *Labour of Love: The Experience of Grandparents as Informal Carers*, London: London Borough of Lewisham Policy and Equalities Unit.

Phillipson, C. (1998) 'The family and community life of older people: social networks and social support in three urban areas', research results: ESRC Population and Household Change programme. Swindon: Economic and Social Research Council.

Pickford, R. (1999) *Fathers, Marriage and the Law*, London: Family Policy Studies Centre.

Pitcher, D. (1999) *When Grandparents Care*, Plymouth: Plymouth City Council Social Services.

Quinton, D. and Pollock, S. (2000) 'The transition to fatherhood by young men: influences on commitment', ESRC REGARD website.

Ribbens, J. (1994) *Mothers and Their Children: A Feminist Sociology of Childrearing*, London: Sage.

Richards, M. (1982) 'How should we approach the study of fathers?' in L. McKee and M. O'Brien (eds) *The Father Figure*, London: Tavistock.

Rodgers, B. and Pryor, J. (1998) *Divorce and Separation: The Outcomes for Children*, York: Joseph Rowntree Foundation.

Ryan, M. (2000) *Working with Fathers*, Department of Health report. Oxford: Radcliffe.

Rutter, M. (1972) *Maternal Deprivation Reassessed*, Harmondsworth, Middlesex: Penguin.

Social Trends (2000) London: Stationery Office.

Simpson, B., Walker, J. and McCarthy, P. (1995) *Being There: Fathers after Divorce*, Newcastle: Relate Centre for Family Studies.

Smart, C. (1999) 'The "new" parenthood: fathers and mothers after divorce', in E.B. Silva and C. Smart (eds) *The New Family?*, London: Sage.

Speak, S., Cameron, S. and Gilroy, R. (1997) *Young Single Fathers: Participation in Fatherhood – Bridges and Barriers*, London: Family Policy Studies Centre.

Taconis, L. (1969) 'The role of the contemporary father in rearing young children', *Educational Research* 2(2): 83–94.

Trinder, L., Beck, M. and Connolly, J. (2001) 'The contact project: first year report.' Joseph Rowntree project (ongoing), University of East Anglia.

Tunaley, T. (1998) 'Grandparents and the family: support versus interference', paper presented to the annual conference of the British Psychological Society, 15 December.

Warin, J., Solomon, Y., Lewis, C. and Langford, W. (1999) *Fathers, Work and Family Life*, London: Family Policy Studies Centre.

Wilson, G. (1987) 'Women's work: the role of grandparents in intergenerational transfers', *Sociological Review* 35(4): 703–20.

Young, M. and Stogden, J. (2000) 'The new old age', in H. Wilkinson (ed.) *Family Business*, Demos Collection 15. London: Demos.

9 Caring, earning and changing

Parenthood and employment after divorce

Bren Neale and Carol Smart

Introduction

Recent government policy on family life has stressed the importance of paid work as a means of improving the life chances of family members. The new ethos, which focuses mainly on lone parents, supports the idea that mothers can and even *should* work to improve the circumstances of their families. This is at odds with a more traditional view, which suggests that mothers should be full-time carers (although there has never been an unequivocal policy that has supported lone mothers outside the labour market). As Land and Lewis (1998) argue, there has been a shift from defining lone mothers as mothers to defining them as workers:

> We are offering a New Deal for Lone Parents receiving Income Support, which will help them to improve their families' lives, by helping them to overcome barriers to work through advice, … training and help with finding a job.
>
> Ministerial Group on the Family 1998: 22

Researchers have argued against the reliance on an implicit model of economic rationality, which underpins many of the recent policies affecting lone mothers and benefit recipients (Ford 1998; Duncan and Edwards 1999). This model has tended to assume that people are motivated principally by economic gain, but lone mothers themselves give a range of reasons for not being in paid work that go far beyond economic criteria.

Alongside this encouragement to mothers to enter paid work, fathers are being encouraged to take more responsibility for the care of their children through the introduction of flexible 'family-friendly' working hours, parental leave and good conditions of part-time employment (Ministerial Group on the Family 1998; Burgess 1998). Fatherhood, no less than motherhood, is being redefined by policy makers to incorporate 'carer' as well as 'worker'. Current evidence does not as yet suggest any wholesale change in the way that fathers are practising their parenting (see Backett 1987; Ribbens 1994; Burghes *et al.* 1997; Warin *et al.* 1999; Gillies *et al.* 2000), but the infrastructure for these changes is being put in place.

While such policies have a broad currency, they have particular salience for separated and divorced parents, who face the challenge of finding new ways to support themselves and their families. Such parents were the focus of a recent study that sought to explore the negotiation of post-divorce parenthood (reported in Smart and Neale 1999). We carried out two rounds of interviews with sixty separated or divorced parents to see how things might have changed for them over an eighteen-month period. We also obtained further data on the families three years later when we returned to interview their children (Smart *et al.* 2001). The predominantly White sample[1] included an equal number of mothers and fathers (these were not former partners but were drawn from different families). While our research did not focus on employment and financial issues, parents inevitably take these factors into account in negotiating their parenthood. Moreover, it is at times of family transition that taken-for-granted assumptions about child-care and resources are re-examined and new ways of parenting actively negotiated (Smart and Neale 1999). Divorce can signal changes to styles and patterns of parenting as the parents' life trajectories diverge. For example, fathers may become more or less committed to childcare, while mothers may reduce or increase their commitments to paid work (Maclean 1991). These patterns are not reducible to one-dimensional explanations, for they are the products of a complex interplay of localised factors. But we would argue that, in the context of divorce, it is hard to understand the position of mothers *vis-à-vis* employment without taking into account the position of fathers in relation to the labour market and their inclination to engage in childcare and support their children financially. We also need to understand the patterns of earning and caring that developed at the point of entry into parenthood, since this dramatically affects the opportunities and constraints that parents subsequently face.

In this chapter, we attempt to develop a more nuanced understanding of how caring and earning imperatives are interrelated following divorce and the diverse rationales that parents adopt for their actions. We suggest that while mothers and fathers can balance these imperatives in a complex variety of ways, they remain gendered in as much as mothers are more likely to start from an imperative to care, while fathers start from an imperative to earn. At the point of entry into parenthood, most parents continue to adopt conventional patterns of earning and caring, which influence their subsequent actions. We explore below the ways in which parents maintain or move beyond these conventional patterns and the moral considerations that underpin their negotiations.

Conventional divisions of labour

COLIN HANKS: It wouldn't have been practical [for me to have the children]. She didn't have a job at the time and she was looking after them full-time, because she's always been that sort of mum. I wouldn't have been able to look after them ... it wouldn't have been right, even if I hadn't been working.

JIM WALTERS: If I'm honest, it's wonderful [being a part-time parent] ... I'm a workaholic ... [and] there is a lot of conflict in trying to follow a profession and being a parent, which isn't there now.

These quotations reflect a conventional division of labour, whereby mothers are responsible for childcare while fathers, as wage earners, are responsible for financial provision. This division of labour between caring and earning has inevitably over-determined post-divorce employment patterns. But equally important, these arrangements have been incorporated into modern identities of masculinity and femininity. Both of these fathers were constrained by the strong carer identity of their former wives as well as their own worker identities. Yet while work was of central importance in the lives of these fathers, they had taken their children's needs into account in their career strategies. Colin had turned down promotion because this would have meant moving away and seeing less of his children, while Jim delayed a change of career because he would have been less able to fulfil his provider role.

The mothers in our sample who had given up work at the point of entry into parenthood continued this pattern, at least in the short term:

ANN BLACK: He always took it for granted I would keep [them], obviously he's working, he couldn't afford to give up work, so he weren't prepared to look after them anyway. I've always looked after them and you assume they stay with me, because I've always been there, I don't work, I gave up work when I had them.

SYLVIA ASHTON: I'm not going to work because it's not worth it. If I went to work, I would have to earn nearly £200 per week to make up. Like I get £117 now but I get me council tax paid and me rent paid whereas if I go to work full-time I go on family credit and all that goes up, so you're no better off ... I'm not going to go out to work like that to leave me kids until they're old enough ... I don't put on [my family], I don't say to them, 'Come and look after the kids' ... I do it myself ... I'll be getting [a job] when Katie starts school.

Sylvia had taken on shift work as a cleaner when her husband became unemployed, but she had stopped when they divorced because she was needed at home. Sylvia was no doubt constrained by her lack of standing in the labour market, but hers was not a purely economic argument. She had made considerable emotional investment in her parenting and was weighing up the merits of working for no gain against the needs of her four young children and her desire not to become dependent on her kin. Eighteen months later, Sylvia returned to her cleaning job at a time when her youngest child had started school and she could depend on her new live-in partner to 'mind' the children until she got home.

Tina's position and rationale for not working were similar to Sylvia's:

TINA HURST: I'm still at home ... there's not very much [work] you can get because [employers] don't collaborate with the school holidays ... I just don't trust people to look after me kids ... [The father] doesn't pay anything ... It wouldn't make any difference [if I got maintenance] because I wouldn't be any better off. [The] social just take it off you anyhow ... All I know is that by doing it from the social I know I'm going to get it, whereas waiting for [the father] I was never sure.

As a long-term recipient of state benefits, Tina had a standard of living that was precariously low. She had to save for months to replace worn-out household items, and she greatly regretted not being able to afford toys for the children. But she clearly valued having a reliable source of income that was under her control rather than having to rely on voluntary and unreliable payments from the father. Because of his violent and oppressive behaviour during the marriage, she also wanted to avoid being bound into a moral contract with him (an issue we explore below).

Just as fathers took their children into account in their strategies for paid work, so these mothers took financial considerations into account in their strategies for motherhood. Sylvia had undertaken some paid work since becoming a mother, and none of these women envisaged remaining disengaged from the labour market in the long term. But their priority was to retain responsibility for the direct care of their children rather than delegating this task to someone else, at least while their children were young.

New divisions of labour

Whatever the constraints on moving beyond conventional patterns of paid work and parenthood, these patterns are slowly being transformed, and it seems that divorce may act as a catalyst for such change. Recent evidence suggests that divorced fathers increasingly want to see their children and that a small proportion want an active share in childcare (Maccoby and Mnookin 1992). Here we explore the rationales of two fathers who opted to share the care of their children:

LEON HOLT: If we'd still been together, I would be doing the usual stereotyped father role ... come in from work, play with them, watch TV, at weekends, have more time to myself ... [to] play golf. I was just there and I probably didn't pay them much attention ... I made a conscious decision ... that I was going to see my children growing up ... I have to plan my working week around them ... I tend to make sure that Wednesday and Friday mornings [when the children stay] I don't have early meetings.

MATT FORD: When they [arrived] we agreed to share the care and we both worked part-time ... In terms of work, I can take it or leave it. Obviously I need the money, but I'm not interested in climbing up the ladder ... Adjusting to the children ... was great for me, I really enjoyed it, and I'd stay at home and look after them. But Susan, who's more into her job, she found it a dilemma. She was much better at taking them out and giving them treats and I was much better at coping with the day to day grind ... So I cut my hours down and she went back to work full-time ... Since the divorce they have lived with me Monday to Friday and they go to her at the weekend.

Matt was unusual in our sample in being the only father to make caring a priority from the point he entered parenthood. The fact that his children were adopted and their arrival carefully planned may well have influenced this process. Subsequently, he was able to sustain his carer status as a matter of course. More typically, Leon made a conscious decision to become a caring parent at the point of divorce and spent time gradually building up trust with his former wife and negotiating shared care. He had always been a good provider and continued in this role, but he was able to combine child-care with his career because he cooperated closely with the mother in a flexible arrangement that operated 'almost as if we were still married'.

Both of these fathers made sacrifices for the privilege of sharing the care of their children. Matt lived modestly and did not envisage setting up home with his new partner until the children had left home, while Leon, with a busy career, had little time to find a new partner. These fathers were prepared for their lives to remain closely bound up with the lives of their former partners in a system of mutual respect and trust. Other fathers in our sample aspired to care for their children in these ways, but as we will show below, the new patterns could not always be sustained.

A small minority of the mothers in our sample had retained their professional jobs upon becoming parents and then sustained these after divorce. These women had long experience of the 'double shift' of earning and caring, and of organising paid childcare:

SALLY BURTON: I thought we would have an equal marriage ... but it just shifted back into a very chauvinistic division of labour ... The way it was divided was that I did all the practical, hard work stuff and he had all the fun ... I would end up running from the office to the child minder and I was absolutely shattered by the end of the day ... He was just free to get on with his job, get back whenever he wanted.

After the divorce, Sally hired an *au pair* to help with her children while she was at work. When she was offered a job in another part of the country near her new partner and parents, she faced a conflict of interest between her own needs and those of her teenage children. Eventually, she declined the offer. She could not take the children away from their father and their own lives, but neither could she bring herself to leave them.

Other mothers in our sample were trying to establish a new sense of self in the aftermath of their divorces. Once their children were of school age, they sought new opportunities for paid work or took up training opportunities to increase their self-esteem and improve their life chances:

JESSICA HUNT: I've gone back to college and I'm working part time … My mum sort of helps me out a bit [with the children], and my ex [spouse] … he has them Sundays, and Monday and Tuesday evenings, so it gives me a chance to get on with things … I know it's a bit selfish of me, but it gives me a chance to get on.

RACHEL COOPER: I work full-time, I come out with £718 after tax … I can't see myself not working. I love my children and I love being around them, but I'm not a homely, motherly person … I've got to make commitments for my children and I do arrange things around my children, not me … like buying clothes, I buy them things first … [but] I've got to have my work and I've got to have my independence. I'm picking a life up for me now, as well as for the children.

Over time, Jessica moved to a co-parenting arrangement with the father, viewing the father's input as important for her two sons. This meant that the father's responsibility shifted from financial support to the more tangible commitment of direct care, while Jessica was no longer dependent on his erratic maintenance payments but could secure her own income. Rachel's situation differed in that she had very little support from the father or other family members. She had to juggle her dual commitments by herself. Her disposable income, after paying for after-school childcare, was hardly more than that of Sylvia's (see above), and her standard of living (in social housing) was also at a comparable level:

RACHEL COOPER: [Their father] hardly sees them … He says 'I don't know [when I'll call] I'm working, I'll get in touch' … It's absolutely awful when you've got a sick child, especially if you work, you've got nobody else you can ring up and say, 'The child's poorly' and can they pick them up … You don't know who to go to in an emergency.

Rachel's decision to take paid work was motivated not by financial gain but by factors to do with the independence, sociability and personal fulfilment of her job (Duncan and Edwards 1999). Both women expressed some guilt about their desire to engage in a 'project of the self' and insisted that their children were still their main priority.

These examples from working mothers show the continuing strength of the imperative for mothers to define themselves as carers, even when their employment has become an integral part of their identity. They also show that whatever patterns are put in place are not fixed but fluid. Parents continually reassess the balance between their childcare and employment constraints and opportunities, taking into account the changing needs of the children, the changing circumstances of the other parent and considerations around kin support and new partnerships.

Implicit moral contracts: bargaining over children and money

After a divorce or separation, issues over children and money are inextricably linked for parents. Yet recent legislation (the Children Act 1989 and Child Support Acts 1991 and 1994) has attempted to separate issues of child contact and maintenance payments. Disputes over contact are now resolved without reference to financial support, while non-resident parents are required to pay maintenance regardless of whether they have contact with a child. The overall legislative and policy framework supports the resident (as opposed to the non-resident) parent. Caring for one's child after divorce brings material and financial benefits, such as entitlement to the family home, maintenance from the other parent and a range of state benefits. Typically, it is the mother, as the resident parent, who receives support and the father, as the non-resident parent with greater personal freedom and earnings potential, who provides it. This seems appropriate given the evidence that resident mothers suffer long-term economic disadvantages in comparison with fathers (Eekelaar and Maclean 1986; Bradshaw and Millar 1991; Hill 2000).

How these benefits are apportioned between the parents depends not on gender *per se* but on the different positions that they occupy in relation to their children:

TINA HURST: My first husband, he took the house, 'cos he had my daughter and I thought that was only fair, and I just took some of my belongings. My mum said, 'Don't you give the house up this time. You're keeping the kids; they need their home ... You lost everything last time'. I said, 'I know, but that was different, he was having the child' ... The situation was reversed. It was easy enough for me on my own to go and find somewhere separate.

However, this differential treatment of mothers and fathers is increasingly interpreted (by fathers at least) as unfair gender discrimination, particularly in a climate where mothers have the potential (whether realised or not) to combine their parenting with wage earning in their own right (Beck 1992). Fathers might argue that mothers should not 'have it all', or that if mothers can now combine caring with earning, then fathers should have this option as well.

Below we explore how divorced parents negotiate their respective commitments and responsibilities around money and children, illustrating how moral and economic factors are intertwined in a complex variety of ways. Among the parents in our study, it seemed that even the most harmonious parental arrangements were underpinned by implicit moral bargaining over the children and money. This bargaining took a variety of forms:

ANN BLACK: He gets paid on the Thursday, so he comes up with me money, then he'd take them up to his mum's on Saturday …

INTERVIEWER: How would you feel if he weren't paying?

ANN: It's a hard thing to say, but he wouldn't see the kids … If he doesn't pay for the children, he doesn't see them. Whether that's wrong I don't know, but that's how I see it at the moment … I shouldn't compare the kids with the money, but I suppose I'm getting back at him there for what he did [i.e. ending the marriage].

GORDON FENTON: I started paying £5 a fortnight, which I sent her in cash. I wrote her a note, saying 'there's no point in declaring this' but I wanted to contribute. She sent it back and I sent it back again and then her [husband] … came round to my flat and told me in no uncertain terms not to send presents or maintenance.

In Ann's view, a father who does not pay maintenance would be disqualified from having contact with his child. She justified this on the grounds that her former spouse had reneged on the marriage, but she also acknowledged this to be a morally suspect position that might not be sustainable. By the same logic, a father who pays maintenance can secure a right to his child. This was Gordon's position. His 3-year-old son did not know of his existence, because he had not seen him since he was a baby, had never lived with him nor supported him financially. But Gordon wanted desperately to forge a relationship with the child and tried to do so by sending money to the mother and repeatedly leaving gifts for the child in the front garden, which were signed 'from Dad'. But these gifts and the reciprocal obligations that they symbolised were rejected because the mother and stepfather apparently did not want to enter into a moral 'contract' with him. Gordon was eventually granted formal rights to a relationship with his son through the courts (which he did not manage to consolidate in practice), but he also faced prosecution for harassment.

These examples involved stark choices about the exchange of children and money and whether such an exchange should occur in the first place. Where there is some degree of sharing of the children, or where both share paid work as well as childcare, the negotiations can take a more subtle form. For Diane Roper, the issue was about the conditions under which the exchange should take place and what the transaction signified:

DIANE ROPER: One weekend, when the boys were going to their dad's, I was going away and I asked [their father] if he would wash their uniforms over the weekend and I would iron them when I got back. [My little boy] came home with a letter and it said, 'Never repeat this again, never. You get paid to do it, not me'.

According to Diane, the father in this case viewed his maintenance money as a payment to her to carry out childcare duties. Casting her in the role of a paid servant or employee, he saw himself as exempt from such work, preferring to define his relationship with his children in terms of the privilege of sharing 'quality' time with them rather than the responsibility of washing their clothes. He seemed to resent what he saw as Diane's attempts to offload her responsibilities on to him while she indulged in time for herself, and he seemed to regard maintenance payments not so much as 'support' for his first family but as 'stealing' on Diane's part:

DIANE ROPER: The week he left, he said to the boys, 'mummy is trying to steal all my money, so I won't have enough money to get a place to live and you won't be able to come and see me'.

Where former partners exist in a state of tension or open dispute, the moral bargaining can become increasingly explicit, to the extent that practical considerations or the needs of the children can become marginalised or lost sight of altogether. In this case, relations between the parents deteriorated to the point where all financial support and child contact were severed.

These examples show that there is much to these monetary exchanges that cannot be reduced to simple economic explanations. When fathers pay maintenance they are engaging in more than a utilitarian transfer of cash to support their children's upbringing. They are paying (or, in Gordon's case, attempting to pay, either in cash or in kind) for the privilege of seeing their children, for a share of parental authority and for the mother's day-to-day responsibilities for childcare. If the transfer of money is imbued with symbolic significance, so too is the transfer of the children. Mothers are not simply handing over the children for contact but are giving up some of their time with and authority over their children in exchange for financial support and what they hope will be valued input into their children's lives. In other words, the parents are engaging in, resisting or otherwise negotiating a moral contract over their respective responsibilities and commitments (Mauss 1954).

Negotiating new patterns of parenting

Moving to a new pattern of caring and earning after divorce adds another layer of complexity to these negotiations. In our sample, negotiations were conducted in a variety of ways and driven by varied motives. Parents such as Matt and Leon (above) negotiated the changes in a measured way, based on an ethic of care for the children, respect for their former partners and a willingness to transform their parental identities (Smart and Neale 1999; Neale and Smart 1999). For others in our sample, the changes were undertaken involuntarily or with some ambivalence. For example, some fathers found themselves caring for children because they had become unemployed and therefore had time to spare, or because the mothers had fled the home, become ill or were otherwise unable or unwilling to parent on their own. Two fathers (the former husbands of Sylvia Ashton and Ann Black) applied for social housing on the grounds that their children would be staying with them and then found that the mothers held them to the arrangement. Negotiating new practices in these unforeseen circumstances was difficult, especially where one parent wished to change against the wishes of the other, or where parents were unable to trust each other's motives.

Much like Diane Roper (above), mothers who were willing to share the children could find themselves accused of using their former partners as unpaid helpers. This had been Jessica's experience:

> JESSICA HUNT: He said he wanted custody of the children … I said, 'Look, if you really, really feel that you can look after these kids on a full-time basis, give yourself a weekend with them to see how it feels and then progress to a week and see how you cope' … He absolutely hit the roof, 'cos he's got this thing in his head that he'd be baby-sitting for me.

At the same time, fathers who wanted an active caring role were open to accusations of mercenary motives that went beyond any genuine desire to be with their children. Again, there could be more than a grain of truth in this, especially where parental relationships were acrimonious. Of course, most parents avoid making overt links between children and the material assets that they bring with them, because they are supposed to value a 'pure' relationship with their children. But there were examples in our study of such calculated thinking:

> BILL MERTON: If I have Michael for over 104 days and nights a year, it's classed as shared care so that will be in my favour [i.e. will reduce maintenance payments]. When he comes here I clothe him, I feed him, I treat him … I've worked it out; it's roughly about 150 days I have him … I fit him in around me night shifts … If there's any overtime I've got to juggle it in between … If I had him [to live] here … me mother could stop here while I'm on nights, so that would be worked out … And *his* mother would be classed as unemployed and not as a single parent, which means she'd lose her benefits.

Bill had retained the family home when his wife left, and he was candid about his desire to gain the upper hand by exchanging his financial obligations for caring obligations. After some coercion on Bill's part, his son moved in with him. However, unlike Leon Holt (above), Bill made no effort to plan his work around his child; nor did he reduce his work hours. Eighteen months later, Bill discovered that he was financially worse off. His plans for family help had not materialised, and he was struggling to combine childcare and night shifts:

BILL MERTON: It's bloody hard, you don't know if you're coming or going ... I've had no sleep today ... It's getting to me mentally ... I was led to believe that there was a lot of help ... through social services ... I says, 'Do you have any night services?' and they say, 'Oh no, no funding'. There is no help; it's all pay out, pay out, pay out. I'm struggling as it is financially but I can't get any help with school dinners, free school clothing ... [or] child minders.

I've never had a penny off her [the mother]. She stopped buying him clothes ... She loves it. [She says] 'Are you tired? I've had a lovely night's sleep!' sort of rubbing it in ... I said to her 'How about you seeing our Michael a bit more ... so I can get out ... I can't ... relax, I can't go for a drink or anything, or see me mates or go fishing'. I says, 'I'm just tied to the house'. I says, 'You've got all this freedom ... all I'm getting is Michael and going mental' ... She said, 'Well, I'll have him three nights'.

Eventually, the child returned to live with his mother and Bill's contact with him became sporadic. In this case, the negotiations were driven by a power struggle between the parents rather than by any measured consideration of the child's needs or the practicalities of his care.

As a variation on this theme, a parent's motives for altering a conventional division of labour may be less to do with material gain than with a sense of moral outrage over the divorce and a desire for revenge. Keith Minster, for example, did not want to lose his home or his children after his wife left him. She had been a full-time mother, but Keith explained that he forced her to leave the house without the children and kept contact to a minimum, since he felt that she no longer deserved the children. He was able to take this stance because he had been made redundant and had time to look after the children. Subsequently, however, the difficulties of bringing up two children on his own became apparent and, with the help of his family, he returned to work:

KEITH MINSTER [FIRST INTERVIEW]: The best bits are having them, and that's that. The worst bit is the hard work looking after them – the washing and cooking, getting them ready for school ... It's a lot harder without a doubt ... The kids were miles better off before, having a mum and dad at home ... Two parents looking after kids are better than one.

KEITH MINSTER [EIGHTEEN MONTHS LATER]: I feel happier [now I'm working], it gives me something else to concentrate on ... I couldn't have done it without my [parents] ... I'd have probably been on social security, struggling and losing the house ... I [used to have] a good job, a lot better than I have now ... The money's a lot less.

INTERVIEWER: Do you think about new partners at all?

KEITH: No, no, not at all ... I've tried ... I don't think it's fair really but that's the way it is ... It's different between men and women. A man would regularly take on a woman with two kids but you try forming a relationship with a girl when you're a man with two kids ... The hard times are on a night when they're in bed and you're here by yourself. That's the worst. Lonely. But I've got a big family and I try to get out twice a week.

Although Keith had chosen a carer role, he was doing so in circumstances not of his own choosing. He had not wanted a divorce; nor had he envisaged the hard 'daily grind' of caring. Much like Bill Merton, the transformation in his responsibilities had not been matched by any corresponding transformation in his identity as a parent. He had assumed that he might eventually remarry, find a stepmother for the children and return to full-time work. But he discovered that shifting to a caring role meant that he had little financial security or time to offer a new partner; he felt he had become ineligible as a spouse. He also realised that his children missed their mother. Eventually, the children went to live with their mother and Keith saw them infrequently. Moving on emotionally from the divorce in this way gave him the potential to find a better job and form a second family unit with a new partner.

Whether fathers find childcare rewarding and are able to sustain a change in their role depends very much on what motivates them to care in the first place. Where they are driven by motives other than a genuine desire to be with their children, they may well find that the reality does not match their expectations.

Transformations in fathering cannot take place without a corresponding transformation in mothering and in the identities of mothers. Some mothers in our sample were driven by fathers to modify or substantially give up their caring responsibilities. Perhaps not surprisingly, they felt disenfranchised:

FELICITY LESSING: He started fighting to have an equal share of them and I was saying, 'Look, I gave up my job in order to be their mother and I do my little bit of freelance to keep ticking over but basically my role is to be their mother. I'm more *available* for them and you've got a highly successful career' ... We really couldn't agree about this and we thumped the table ... But he said, 'The children need their father' and I couldn't really disagree ... I'm having to get used to having less time with them ... I feel empty without them.

JENNY SWIFT: I gave up my career to look after the children ... [but] he wanted to cut me out of the children's lives completely and he's just about done it ... I don't really feel like a mother any more ... If you've never ... had children, you wouldn't miss it but if you've had that ... you

> know what you've lost really ... I suppose I've put my energies into different things ... work and hobbies ... That was the only way to survive ... It's just a completely different life to the one I had.

These mothers had no option but to search for other means to sustain them, both emotionally and financially. Felicity rekindled her freelance career, arranging her work round her children so that she could see them whenever possible. She also derived satisfaction from maintaining a co-parenting arrangement, which she felt benefited her sons. Jenny recounted how her former husband had 'snatched' the children and had subsequently retained them after receiving a Child Support Agency assessment. As a result, she lost her maintenance and had to give up her home. She worked hard to maintain a fragile relationship with her son and daughter and eventually negotiated some regular contact with her son. While she derived satisfaction from her work, it remained a substitute activity and she suffered greatly from the loss of her parental identity. What made this easier to bear in the long term was the realisation that the nature of her mothering would have changed in any case as the children grew older.

Gendered imperatives?

The evidence presented in this chapter illustrates the complex array of social considerations that parents take into account when they negotiate their responsibilities after divorce. These factors include the needs and wishes of the children; the nature of parent–child relationships; the circumstances and aspirations of the other parent and the history of the parental relationship; options for childcare; support from and commitments to the wider family; the potential for new partnerships and the nature of new family commitments; financial and housing circumstances; employment opportunities and constraints; and, not least, their parental identity and the way it has been forged over time. Issues surrounding caring and earning are bound up with each other in what are as much moral as economic or contractual negotiations and exchanges.[2]

However, the complex interplay of these factors in negotiating parenthood has not necessarily been taken into account in the development of family policies. To see such negotiations purely in economic or contractual terms[3] gives us only a partial understanding of what matters to parents and why they negotiate their responsibilities in such varied ways. Our data also show that parents do not reason in purely individualistic or single-minded ways. They inevitably take into account the position of others (albeit that this relational reasoning may not necessarily be based on an ethic of care but may be driven by an ethic of justice or retribution) (Smart and Neale 1999; Mason 2000).

In practice, there has always been some flexibility over how caring and earning imperatives are met. Counterposing the idea of the 'atomistic, economic' father with that of the 'caring' mother' would be far too simplistic. At the same time, stereotypes of what mothering and fathering entail are still strongly evident and impact on how masculine and feminine identities are forged and the ways in which they may be transformed over time. The identities of the mothers in our sample appeared to be bound up primarily with their relationship with their children. They were more likely to start with an imperative to care, which they perceived as an enduring commitment, a complex mixture of responsibility and privilege involving caring for and about their children. They also recognised the economic imperatives of raising children and may have extended their role to accommodate this, in the process delegating some of their caring responsibilities to others. But they did not necessarily see the financial aspect of parenting as their direct responsibility. They sought a variety of ways to ensure some financial provision or 'payments in kind' for their family, including reliance on the other parent or wider kin, new partners, the state or local support networks. Even where they did become wage earners, they were likely to continue to see their children as their prime responsibility and to try to fit other commitments around them. A strong element of choice is still associated with a mother's decision to enter or stay in the labour market and, where mothers do enter paid work, the motive may be as much to do with the personal fulfilment of paid work as it is with economic necessity.

In contrast, the identities of most of the fathers in our study remained bound up primarily with their employment. They were likely to start with an imperative to secure paid work, which they perceived in terms of an enduring commitment to provide for the family, as well as offering personal status, fulfilment and economic power. They were also likely to recognise the imperative to care for their children, and some extended their role to accommodate this, even to the extent of reducing their commitments to paid work. But they did not necessarily see childcare as their direct responsibility and sought a variety of ways to secure this care, including relying on the other parent or wider kin, new partners, paid child minders or other community resources. Even where they did care, they were likely to perceive their employment as their core commitment and try to fit childcare around it. A strong element of choice is still associated with a father's decision to care and, where fathers do so, the motive may be more to do with the desire for a privileged, 'fun' relationship with the children than with a willingness to take on new responsibilities.

However, our data also show that there is nothing inevitable about these gendered distinctions. Divorce may well act as a catalyst for change as parents seek new ways to practise family life. The government's new initiatives may also have a transformative effect. Yet accompanying these initiatives there has been a valorisation of 'fathering', seen in terms of the provision of 'quality' time for the children (Burgess 1998) and an implicit devaluing of 'mothering' and the caring work that it has traditionally entailed. However, as Duncan and Edwards (1999) have shown, whatever policy directives are put in place, parents will continue to find a diversity of ways of balancing childcare responsibilities and paid work. After divorce or separation, parents have to make difficult moral choices between competing constraints and opportunities and keep these choices under constant review as the needs and circumstances of family members change. Family policies that take account of the moral considerations that underpin parental negotiations are more likely to be effective than those that focus solely on abstract economic factors or contractual obligations. Flexible policies that allow for the dynamics of family life are also likely to be beneficial and more supportive of parents. Whatever the impact of new government policies on parental decision making, parents may find it easier to sustain their responsibilities if these are not imposed upon them but are the result of personal negotiations, a balancing of needs and genuine commitments.

Notes

1 Our sample did not allow for an exploration of ethnicity or cultural background in relation to the issues discussed here, although empirical evidence suggests that there may well be differences across cultural boundaries. African-Caribbean mothers, for example, are more likely to adopt a dual earner/carer identity than their White counterparts (Duncan and Edwards 1999). We are currently conducting research on the culture of divorce that will explore experiences across a range of ethnic and religious backgrounds.
2 *Cf.* Duncan and Edwards 1999, who in a variety of parenting contexts show the complex ways in which parents balance childcare and paid work.
3 *Cf.* Giddens 1998.

References

Backett, K. (1987) 'The negotiation of fatherhood', in C. Lewis and M. O'Brien (eds) *Re-assessing Fatherhood*, London: Sage.
Beck, U. (1992) *Risk Society: Towards a New Modernity*, London: Sage.
Bradshaw, J. and Millar, J. (1991) *Lone Parent Families in the UK*, DSS Research Report No. 6. London: HMSO
Burgess, A. (1998) *The Complete Parent*, London: Institute of Public Policy Research.
Burghes, L., Clarke, L. and Cronin, N. (1997) 'Fathers and fatherhood in Britain', Occasional Paper No. 23. London: Family Policy Studies Centre.
Duncan, S. and Edwards, R. (1999) *Lone Mothers, Paid Work and Gendered Moral Rationalities*, London: Macmillan.
Edwards. R. and Duncan, S. (1996) 'Rational economic man or lone mothers in context? The uptake of paid work', in E. Silva (ed.) *Good Enough Mothering: Feminist Perspectives on Lone Motherhood*, London: Routledge.
Eekelaar, J. and Maclean, M. (1986) *Maintenance After Divorce*, Oxford: Clarendon Press.
Ford, R. (1998) 'Lone mothers' decision whether or not to work: childcare in the balance', in R. Ford and J. Millar (eds) *Private Lives and Public Responses: Lone Parenthood and Future Policy in the UK*, London: Policy Studies Institute.

Giddens, A. (1998) *The Third Way. The Renewal of Social Democracy*, Cambridge: Polity Press.

Gillies, V., Ribbens McCarthy, J. and Holland, J. (2000) *Pulling Together, Pulling Apart: The Family Lives of Young People*, London/York: Family Policy Studies Centre/Joseph Rowntree Foundation.

Hill, A. (2000) 'Men made richer by divorce', report of British Household Panel Survey data undertaken by Jonathan Scales, Institute of Economic and Social Research, University of Essex, *The Observer*, 22 October.

Land, H. and Lewis, J. (1998) 'The problem of lone motherhood in the British context', in R. Ford and J. Millar (eds) *Private Lives and Public Responses: Lone Parenthood and Future Policy in the UK*, London: Policy Studies Institute.

Maccoby, E. and Mnookin, R. (1992) *Dividing the Child: Social and Legal Dilemmas of Custody*, Cambridge, Mass.: Harvard University Press.

Maclean, M. (1991) *Surviving Divorce: Women's Resources after Separation*, London: Macmillan.

Mason, J. (2000) 'Deciding where to live: relational reasoning and narratives of the self', Working Paper No. 18, Centre for Research on Family, Kinship and Childhood, University of Leeds.

Mauss, M. (1954 [1925]) *The Gift*, London: Cohen & West.

Ministerial Group on the Family (1998) *Supporting Families: A Consultation Document*, London: HMSO.

Neale, B. and Smart, C. (1999) 'In whose best interests? Theorising family life following parental separation or divorce', in S. Sclater and C. Piper (eds) *Undercurrents of Divorce*, Aldershot: Dartmouth.

Ribbens, J. (1994) *Mothers and their Children*, London: Sage.

Smart, C. and Neale, B. (1999) *Family Fragments?* Cambridge: Polity Press.

Smart, C., Neale, B. and Wade, A. (2001) *The Changing Experience of Childhood: Families and Divorce*, Cambridge: Polity Press.

Warin, J., Solomon, C., Lewis, C. and Langford, W. (1999) *Fathers, Work and Family Life*, London/York: Family Policy Studies Centre/Joseph Rowntree Foundation.

10 The individual in public and private

The significance of mothers and children[1]

Jane Ribbens McCarthy and Rosalind Edwards

Current concerns with public and private

Family issues have had a chequered history in sociology in the second half of the twentieth century (see Chapter 7), and while such issues may appear to have been receiving greater attention in recent years, much of this interest has not been framed in terms of 'family' at all. Family sociology has thus tended to shift into a sociology of relationships and intimacy, in the process attracting attention from some prominent mainstream sociological theorists, notably Anthony Giddens (1991, 1992) and Ulrich Beck and Elisabeth Beck-Gernsheim (1995). However, this concern with intimacy neglects relationships between parents and children (Smart 1997; Jamieson 1998), a neglect that has important gendered implications for the sort of sociology we produce. Relationships with their children not only shape women's working lives and life trajectories but also relate to significant social experiences centred on childrearing activities – what feminist writers have tended to refer to as the 'private' sphere.

In this chapter, we want to consider how recent attention paid to the self, and to intimacy between adults, has led to a shift in the theorising of public and private spheres. While we recognise that the concepts of public and private have been used in quite different ways in the literature, a particular concern among some feminist and family academics has been the relationship between, on the one hand, family and the domestic household and, on the other hand, civil society, the state and bureaucracies, and the world of paid work and the market (Wientraub 1997; Landes 1998b; Slater 1998). In feminist literature, these terms have been hotly debated but have served to reveal the ways in which mainstream academic disciplines have been rooted in male activities in the public domain (Stacey 1981).

Recent sociological writing that has reframed ideas about 'the private' in terms of intimacy (Bailey 2000) thus risks marginalising women's lives in sociology in a new way (Ribbens McCarthy and Edwards 2001). This is because the associated neglect of generational relationships, as these occur in the context of contemporary Western constructions and understandings of adulthood and childhood, obscures key aspects of mothers' and children's experiences, shared in child-based social settings. A central issue concerns variable understandings of individuality, collectivity and connectedness, which may be lined up in different ways alongside the concepts of public and private. These variable understandings have important implications for family sociology in particular but also for sociological theorising more generally. This is because public and private in contemporary Western societies are constructed as dichotomous categories (Weintraub 1997; Slater 1998), such that one can only be fully understood by reference to the other. As we go on to argue, such dichotomous thinking may be useful and illuminating at times, but at other times it may be helpful to develop a more layered and complex way of thinking about different social settings and practices.

Our concern in this chapter is not to valorise the two spheres in relation to each other, as some writers appear to do (as discussed by Landes 1998b; Stacey 1998). Rather, we seek to explore the complex ways in which the concepts of 'public' and 'private' have been defined, and to suggest some ways in which this usage has variously highlighted or obscured familial and other experiences that implicate a relational view of self, differentiated by gender, and also by age, class, ethnicity and socio-historical context. In this we are extending the concerns of earlier work (Edwards 1993; Ribbens 1994; Bell and Ribbens 1994; Ribbens and Edwards 1995; Edwards and Ribbens 1998), which has in turn drawn upon a wide range of feminist writings in this area (e.g. Pateman 1970; Rosaldo and Lamphere 1974; Elshtain 1981; Stacey 1981; Benn and Gaus 1983; Gamarnikow *et al.* 1983; Eisenstein 1984; Sassoon 1987; Sharistanian 1987; Walby 1990; Benhabib 1992; Davidoff 1995; Fraser 1997).

There has been a growing awareness of the particular socio-historical context for the differing understandings of self and individuality with which we are concerned here (e.g. Kivisto 1998) and their links with particular political and welfare regimes. In parallel fashion, the academic and political usage of public and private occurs in relation to particular socio-historical contexts, especially with regard to liberal democracies based on notions of individual citizenship (Chamberlayne 1998). This means that there may also be variations between different welfare state regimes, particularly in the extent to which motherhood is 'public' in terms of women's integration into the public sphere through paid work, and whether this employment is full- or part-time, and the concomitant institutionalisation of children in publicly provided organised care settings (Pfau-Effinger 1998; Edwards 2001a).

Kenneth Gergen (1999) argues that Western notions of the individual carry considerable disadvantages for contemporary theorising, and he seeks to develop a basis for a more relational view of self. In this discussion, however, there is no recognition that particular understandings of the self and individuality may be socially distributed in contemporary Western societies themselves (as well as cross-culturally). Other writers (e.g. Gilligan 1988, 1994) have sought to develop a gendered relational view of self within a specifically feminist framework. Yet the notion of the autonomous, self-contained individual predominates in Western cultures and suffuses the psychological, political, sociological and therapeutic literature.[2] Our concern in this chapter, then, is to consider these issues in relation to concepts of public and private, since variable usages of these terms may illuminate or obscure the gendered social distribution of understandings of individuality and connectedness, cut across by issues of class and ethnicity.

In particular, we suggest that certain 'ideal typical' tensions are conveyed by the contrast between 'the public' and 'the private', including:

- individuality versus collectivity and connection;
- an instrumental means–ends orientation versus an orientation to concrete, everyday processes, including the idea that relationships are important in themselves;
- formal (bureaucratic) regulation versus informal fluidity; and
- contractually governed universalistic relationships versus normatively governed particularistic relationships, including the role of care in these.

In this chapter, we are concentrating on the first of these three tensions, but the others are closely associated, since we are concerned to preserve a theoretical space that allows for an understanding of 'the private' that is based on connectedness, everyday practices and processes, informal fluidity and particularistic care relationships. It is the ways in which these different themes may be overlaid that leads to their being experienced as distinct and extensive ways of being.

In our discussion below, we seek to keep in mind two distinct areas of reference in the usage of the concepts. While at times the concepts may be identified with particular (although variable) *physical locations*, such as home, neighbourhood, workplace or government, at other times they are used to identify differences in *forms of social relationships, practices and orientations* that may not always be straightforwardly associated with particular physical locations. These two aspects are interrelated, but they are often treated wrongly as synonymous. Various writers have therefore struggled to find an appropriate language to capture just what it is that the distinction refers to, including Myra Marx Ferree's (1985) different 'value systems', David Cheal's (1991) 'contrasting principles of social organisation' and Dorothy Smith's (1987) discussion of different 'modes of organisational consciousness'. We ourselves have suggested previously that the distinctions amount to different 'ways of being' in the world (Edwards 1993; Ribbens 1994).[3] Here we also refer to 'social practices and orientations' in order to encompass the fact that it is social actors who engage in (that is, who 'do') routine sets of practices that create, invoke and depend upon certain values and expectations. This has considerable resonance with David Morgan's more specific usage of 'family practices' (1996; see also Chapter 7). Whatever term is adopted, all these distinctions carry gendered implications for a considerable range of issues in people's family lives (Ribbens and Edwards 1995; Edwards and Ribbens 1998). In order to understand these, we need to consider the significance of children for the (gendered) development of 'the private sphere'.

The historical construction of 'childhood', 'motherhood' and the development of the 'private sphere'

Childhood became institutionalised as a separate phase of life during the process of Western industrialisation (e.g. Ennew 1986; Hockey and James 1993; Pilcher 1995; Jenks 1996a), including through the construction of the special site of 'home' as the appropriate place for children, their exclusion from paid work and segregation into educational establishments and play sites (Edwards 2001a). Underlying this institutionalisation of separateness are themes of the dependency, vulnerability and incompetence of children (Archard 1993). In contemporary Western societies, the child is constructed in opposition to the adult (see Ribbens McCarthy *et al.* 2000 for further discussion).

This version of childhood is very much bound up with a specific construction of womanhood, in ways that continue to have key social significance for the experiences of men and women in contemporary Western societies, structured around this separateness of children. Here, however, we must note the particular ethnic and class implications of such structures. For example, motherhood has not led to Black women's withdrawal from the labour market, and indeed historically they serviced some middle-class White women's private spheres at the expense of their own (Glenn 1985; Bryan *et al.* 1985). Whatever their class and ethnicity, however, in conservative and liberal welfare regimes especially, mothers have become increasingly positioned as the primary custodians of the vision of 'separated' and idealised dependent childhood.

The differential gendered involvement of parents in caring for children is associated with aspects of the gendering of the concepts of public and private. Those involved in the care of children, especially very small children, have to be able to tolerate disruptions, particularly of time and of emotions. Industrialisation saw the increasing regulation of time and of emotional expression, but small children have scant respect for such issues. 'Patience' can be seen as a primary parenting virtue precisely because it involves an ability to live in the child's timescale rather than the adult one (Ribbens 1994). Yet a major part of the care of young children is concerned with training them into the time schedules and routines of contemporary industrial society. Control of their emotions and their expression may take even longer to put into place, because children's potential for disrupting 'civilised' expectations is associated with a profound discrepancy between the behaviour of so-called adults and children (Elias 1994). Indeed, embarrassment at children's lack of socially acceptable behaviour is a pervasive experience among those responsible for them (Cahill 1990; Ribbens 1994). Anxieties about the ability to appear a 'competent mother' in front of other audiences may restrict women's movements in social settings and public places outside the home (Mauthner 1994; Miller 1999), leading to their concentration in settings that are considered child (family?) friendly.

There is thus a potent combination of ideas about children that signals their inappropriateness for inclusion in the 'adult' public domain and their appropriate placement in a separate sphere where they may experience 'childhood' – epitomised as the home.[4] Such expectations, or even moral injunctions, may well be becoming overlaid, and in tension, with more modernist and (White) middle-class notions of pedagogic childrearing as overseeing and facilitating the development of children as reflexive, rational and forward-thinking individuals (e.g. Walkerdine and Lucy 1989; Dahlberg 1996). Indeed, Anthony Giddens (1991, 1992) poses this form of childrearing as part of a more general move towards a 'democratisation' of the private, which is understood as the intimate and is bound up with individuality, as we discuss further below. However, such (unique) individuality is inevitably compromised or transformed by ascribed characteristics related to family membership (Ribbens 1994), and it cannot be equated with individuality in the public sphere.[5] Furthermore, social and economic differences mean that, for Black and working-class families in particular, it can be either inappropriate to focus on children as a self-project or difficult to maximise a space for innocence and freedom (e.g. Phoenix 1987; Walkerdine and Lucey 1989; Reynolds 1998). But perhaps a crucial point here is that (White, middle-class) others may expect them to meet at least some of these requirements.

The private sphere, values and ways of being

The idealised institutionalisation of childhood, alongside the inappropriateness of children in adult-centred public domains, means that there is something particular about the experience of caring for young children in contemporary Western societies (taking into account cultural variations in ideas about which particular locations are considered inappropriate). A 'proper' childhood is intrinsically tied up with ideals about what constitutes 'good' mothering, whether this encompasses paid work or not (Edwards 2001a). These experiences are associated with specific social practices, ways of being and orientations to relationships. They centre on a sense of connectedness in normatively governed particularistic relationships, which are considered important for their own sake. These relationships are mediated through informal, concrete, mundane, everyday caring activities, which are oriented towards process in the here and now, not outcomes at some future point (e.g. Mayall 1990). These experiences and social practices are not always warm and reflexive and, indeed, connectedness may be a crucial aspect of domestic violence. Different orientations to time and emotions are particularly significant elements of this way of being, however. And since the care of young children is a gendered activity, the concomitant experience and understanding of this way of being is also highly gendered.

Furthermore, these experiences can be shared between women in kinship and friendship networks, especially those centred on children and concentrated on specific social or geographical locations (Bell and Ribbens 1994; Doucet 2000). This overlaying of social practices and orientations, in association with age, generation and gender divisions centred on particular sites, means that this way of being may be experienced at times as a different 'world', albeit one that may be almost invisible to those whose experiences are primarily located in the public way of being. Lucy Bailey suggests that mothers she interviewed likened the entry into motherhood as being 'through the looking glass' (in Lewis Carroll's language), so that they 'entered an inexplicable new world to which different rules applied' (1999: 346).

Some feminist political philosophers, such as Joan Tronto (1993) and Selma Sevenhuijsen (1998 and Chapter 6), have also focused on aspects of these social practices and ways of being in order to make the case for care as a moral activity, based on responsibilities and relationships. This underpins their arguments that the values involved (empathy, attentiveness, responsiveness to need, connection) form an 'ethic of care' that could enrich and better guide formulations of democratic citizenship (rather than the more individualistic juridical and contractarian conceptions in contemporary Western societies).[6] However, Sevenhuijsen specifically rejects an equation of care (solely) with childrearing in the private sphere as shading into valorising maternalism, while Sara Ruddick (1995) equally argues against any equation of mothering with caring. Nevertheless, along with others such as Jenny Hockey and Alison James (1993), we see children as the prototype for other forms of dependency, with these value orientations shading over into other forms of caring.[7] At the same time, it is crucial to recognise that, just as this way of being may not be restricted in practice to the home or to children, not all our orientations to children are necessarily of this type, either ideally or practically. For example, besides the possibility that relationships with children may be coercive, violent or abusive, we may also at times take a very strategic and/or instrumental orientation to our childcare. Indeed, the social and economic differences we noted earlier may mean that, for example, Black mothers need to think particularly strategically about their childrearing in the face of racism (Reynolds 1998 and Chapter 3.4) and in the light of the historical goals of 'survival' and 'overcoming' (Dilworth-Anderson *et al.* 1993).

The perspective on the private with which we are concerned, then, has come to be a largely female experience (or at the very least, female and child-centred experience). In what follows, we treat the public as largely residual in order to elucidate differences in the meanings surrounding the use of the concept of 'the private'. There is therefore a danger that, in seeking to focus attention on the private in our terms, we might be seen as taking the sort of 'revisionist' stance we noted earlier: that is, that we are in danger of glorifying women's primary site of exploitation and oppression (Delphy and Leonard 1992). This is certainly not our intention. We are neither valorising nor depoliticising the private. Indeed, we see it as intensely political both in terms of its relationship to the public sphere and in its being the site of significant practices and orientations that are concerned with major questions around the relationship between individuals, families and other social settings (and thus providing sociology with conceptual challenges). Rather, we are seeking to trace and elaborate understandings of individuality and connectedness in the different ways in which public and private have been discussed, in our concern to retain a theoretical and analytical space for issues of connectedness, particularly around children.

Individuality and connectedness in contemporary social theorising of the 'private'

Part of the ambiguity about how themes of (different versions of) individuality, connectedness and collectivities relate to themes of private and public depends on whether the private is seen in terms of intimacy or family and whether the public is seen in terms of political activity or the marketplace. Themes about different versions of individuality, collectivities and connectedness are crucially implicated in different views of public and private but may be understood in quite different ways in relation to these concepts.

How the individual is theorised and placed within the shifting meanings of public and private is a particularly key issue in analysis. This is paralleled by the question of how community/collectivities are theorised and placed in terms of public and private, and in which there may also be particular understandings of the individual at stake that need to be further distinguished. Thus a collectivity may consist of an aggregation of (autonomous and separate) individuals, while connectedness refers to a collapse of – or, at least, an ambiguity around – the boundaries of autonomy, implying instead a relational understanding of individuality as embedded in webs of relationships. It is failure to pay attention to these nuances that obscures what we regard as important issues.

Thus, in some versions of the public–private distinction, the public domain is about collectivity and the private is understood to be quintessentially individualistic in providing the potential space to know the (autonomous) self. We suggest that such a conception is a particularly masculine vision of the private, and that the consideration of children particularly upsets these themes because childcare is about the connectedness of particular individuals, often in quite social settings. Under this latter view, it is the public that can be seen as individualistic and self-interested. Indeed, for many women, and also for other less publicly powerful groups such as Black men and Black women, the public is less likely to be experienced as about collectivity and empowerment (Hill Collins 1990, 1997) or, indeed, as imparting a secure sense of autonomous individuality from which to be part of the collective empowerment.

One important area in which the concepts of public and private have been used is that of legal and political theory. In this literature (feminist and otherwise), public is considered in terms of the power and laws of the state, set alongside the rights of private (autonomous) individuals. Here too, then, we find that 'the private' is considered in terms of personal privacy, freedom and rights, and it is the individual who is the substantive site where the private may be found: 'The private domain of each adult [male and female] is like a bubble with flexible contours. It follows the agent who is its centre wherever the agent takes it' (Gobetti 1997: 124).

Nevertheless, Jean Cohen argues that the notion of personal privacy is not necessarily dependent upon an individualistic model of the self which denies (women's) experience of interdependence and interconnectedness. She goes on to provide a list of zones of intimacy that require decisional privacy and autonomy in the face of high levels of public regulation and intervention: 'marriage, divorce, sexual relations, procreation, child-rearing, abortion and so forth' (1997: 140). However, this list lumps together issues about intimacy between adults and issues about relationships between parents and children. In so doing, it obscures precisely some of those ambiguities that arise for women (particularly) around issues of individuality and connectedness, i.e. where do we, as individuals, begin and end? This is an issue that has particular meaning in regard to children, who are not understood to be separate autonomous beings (Burman 1994).

Slippages that centralise 'intimacy' in ways that might be quite inappropriate for theorising and analysing many aspects of (gendered, generational) family lives are similarly found in the writings of Anthony Giddens and Ulrich Beck. In Giddens' work, 'the private' is understood as the site for intimacy (1991) and the development of 'pure relationships', as part of the reflexive project of the self, thus marginalising relationships with children (Smart 1997; Smart and Neale 1999). Where children are considered by Giddens, it is primarily in terms of their future capacity for intimate ties, or else in terms of an abstract notion that they be treated as 'the putative equal of the adult' (1992: 191) to create a democratic personal order within the private (1999). The effect of this may be to disguise and obscure the actual (institutionalised) positions in which children and parents are placed, in the process taking adult–adult relationships as the model for adult–child interactions in an abstract line of reasoning that seems to have little bearing on the lived experiences of parents and children in contemporary Western societies.

In the work of Beck and Beck-Gernsheim (notably the chapter written by Elisabeth Beck-Gernsheim), there is greater discussion of the particular, indeed special, significance of children in contemporary industrialised societies: 'The child becomes the last remaining, irrevocable, unique love object. Partners come and go but the child stays ... The child ... is the way of "putting the magic back" into life to make up for general disenchantment' (1995: 37). Nevertheless, this perspective is lost by the final chapter of their book, where love – in terms of erotic love between adults – is discussed as the modern secular religion. Overall, we find a slippage between intimacy and erotic love between adults, parenthood and the requirement to love one's children, and notions of 'family'. When Beck and Beck-Gernsheim use the word 'private', it has variable meanings, including not-work life, personal experience and family. And when Beck (1997) discusses freedom and the 'democratization of the family', his discussion centres on youth rather than children, based on (largely speculative) descriptions of uneasy relationships between parents and young people.

Beck's condemnation of 'the private enslavement of children by their parents in the guise of care' (1997: 161), and Giddens' call for a 'democracy of the emotions' in parent–child relations – based upon a fictive idea of how 'the child' would legitimate parental authority if he or she had access to adult knowledge – both signally fail to illuminate the actual experiences of women with young children in their daily lives. Their analyses marginalise children themselves as present beings, and crucially also marginalise the lives of those caretakers (primarily mothers) whose experiences are centrally focused around childcare and the construction of childhood as an ongoing daily activity. Instead, ideas of a possible democracy of 'the family' import a masculinist language derived from public, political spheres, redefining the nature of 'children' in the process. This is not to deny that such language may not have its uses at times (as we will consider further below), but it is to draw attention to what may also be obscured by such notions.

Furthermore, as Lynn Jamieson (1998) argues, while the modern emphasis on reflexive intimacy may also apply in some ways to contemporary understandings of parent–child relationships (which may be more of a White and middle-class phenomenon, as we noted earlier), intimacy can be about things other than disclosure and pure relationships, and parent–child relationships are about a great deal more than intimacy, encompassing a much greater range of activities and experiences in varied localities. To subsume parent–child relationships, and 'family' practices more broadly, under notions of intimacy is to risk seriously distorting and/or excluding key areas of family relationships (discussed further in Ribbens McCarthy and Edwards 2001).

There may, then, be particular understandings of the individual implicated in some of this (masculinist) sociological theorising of the private as democratic intimacy. Furthermore, notions of 'family' are very closely bound up with ideas about motherhood, such that for many mothers it may be difficult at points to distinguish any sense of their own unique individualities in a domestic setting. Indeed, such issues relate to the work of those feminist writers who have been concerned with the private sphere as exploiting women as individuals (such as through notions of private patriarchy; see, for example, Walby 1990).[8]

Similarly, in considering the public sphere, there are major ambiguities about how far this is seen as the primary site for the individual, or for a more collective orientation. Again, feminist writers line up in various ways with the different strands of the argument. Thus writers such as Nancy Fraser (1998) and Sayla Benhabib (1998) view the public as predominantly about collectivities, discussing prevalent meanings of the public in terms of an orientation towards shared interests, or to concerns that are shared by everyone, or locations or discursive forums that are accessible to everyone. However, this vision of the public as being about collective concerns may still depend upon the particular version of the individual that sees the collective as composed of individuals as disconnected and autonomous beings. It is thus crucially important to distinguish notions of collectivities from notions of connectedness, which embrace a more relational view of the individual.

Beyond dualistic thinking?

The sort of slippages and confusions that we have discussed above in contemporary theorising about public and private, and ideas about individuality, collectivities and connection, perhaps point to the desirability of moving beyond dualisms so that we can develop a more layered sense of different social spaces and associated social practices. Such an approach might help us to avoid some of the theoretical risks associated with the conflation of family, parenting, kinship and intimacy in adult relationships that we have pointed out above (other rationales for transcending the dualism are discussed in Edwards 1993).

For example, some feminist writers have considered distinctions to be made within the public domain (including Pateman 1989; Walby 1990; Fraser 1992; Benhabib 1998). Other writers have sought to illuminate an intermediate social space between public and private. Prue Chamberlayne (1998), for instance, is concerned with 'the social' as providing possible opportunities for the extension of privately based concerns into political activities, while Albert Hunter (1995) poses the notion of 'the parochial' as a communal social order falling between the particular and the universal. Here again, however, we find that issues around women's lives and caring activities may be illuminated or obscured (Ribbens McCarthy and Edwards 1999a), highlighting the need for an explicit gender awareness that pays attention to connectedness around children. Similarly, Raia Prokhovnik (1998) introduces a form of layered thinking around notions of citizenship that includes an emphasis on the non-domestic activities of women outside the public domains of work and politics.

In a different direction, we have suggested another way of going beyond dualistic thinking by distinguishing the personal from the private (Edwards and Ribbens 1998). Such an approach suits our purposes in rescuing the private from a total identification with intimacy and a sense of the self or identity. It also allows us to see the public and the private each as social, since they are concerned with interactions between people in variable locations, and the sets of meanings and experiences that are associated with these. We believe that this is what Dorothy Smith (1987) is trying to capture with her notion of 'modes of *organisational* consciousness', and similarly David Cheal (1991) with his reference to 'contrasting principles of *social organisation*' (emphasis added).

The concept of the personal is intended instead to draw attention to experiences that are constituted around a sense of self or identity, to do with emotions, intimacy or the body. In this sense, the personal may provide a space for considering the more contemporary Western notion of the autonomous individual with an interior life that is experienced as isolated and unknown to others (Gergen 1999). We do not intend to suggest that the personal is individualistic in any essential way, and we are explicit in our view that the personal is also social. What we are trying to capture by this concept is, 'the social as ontologically experienced by the individual; that is, in relation to a person's own sense of being or existence' (Edwards and Ribbens 1998: 14). We are thus trying to distinguish 'the private', as a set of practices and orientations that are shared within social settings and interactions, from that use of 'the private' that centres on interior experience. To introduce such distinctions around the notion of 'the private' alongside those ideas that consider different meanings within the category of 'the public' (discussed above) leads to altogether more complex and layered notions than are possible in a straightforward dichotomy of public and private.

Dualistic thinking as an aid to conceptual insight?

Nevertheless, we believe that dualistic thinking may also serve important purposes at times, since it may help to illuminate what is assumed in, or left outside, particular ways of thinking about families and family life. It can draw our attention to what is assumed in particular taken-for-granted languages and concepts that may be used by academics and applied to empirical family life and domestic settings in ways that have highly significant but otherwise unnoticed consequences. We first raised this in relation to the concept of 'strategy' (Edwards and Ribbens 1991). Here we briefly examine the notion of 'work' to consider what may be gained and lost by the application of an implicitly masculinist, publicly based language to describe the lives of women as mothers.

The concept of 'work' has been used quite explicitly by feminists and others to describe women's activities in the home, most notably since Ann Oakley's (1974/76) pioneering study of housewives as workers. Some of the advantages of this language of mothering as work may include that it reminds us of the drudgery and makes the labour visible; that it resists sentimentalising mothering; that it reminds us of the economic significance of mothering; that it attributes status to mothers (albeit a status based on public values); and that it resists naturalising mothering activities and promotes a picture of learned behaviour requiring skill and knowledge. Indeed, the language of mothering as work seems to have become widely adopted in much public discourse, with ideas of mothering as an important job requiring particular 'parenting skills' for which individuals can be 'educated' and 'trained' in organised programmes.

However, a consideration of what the word 'work' actually means draws attention to the fact that it is a gendered and historically situated concept, such that in contemporary Western societies it has particular meanings based on activities in the public domain, with associated masculine identities (Pahl 1988/92). In this context, we would add, it is also a concept that depends upon notions of the autonomous individual, in the guise of the activities of 'the labourer' whose wages are an individual possession that can only be transformed with difficulty into the relational context of family lives (Burgoyne 1990). Do we, then, risk imposing a publicly based male vision of individualised 'work' on women's lives with their children in private settings? What room is left for mothering as centred on emotion, moral identity and a particularistic relationship that does not constitute a purposive project with clearly identifiable outcomes (see, for example, Boulton 1983; Gieve 1987; Ruddick 1995)? Do we risk seeking to value women's lives in ways that actually distort women's own understandings of their activities, relationships and identities?

For example, both mothers and children in a range of Western societies may define a key aspect of caring for children in terms of 'being there'. This is a subtle and complex notion that includes ideas of potential availability and psychological attentiveness that cannot be encompassed within notions of mothering as 'work' and that depend crucially on a sense of connectedness in the world, counteracting the sense of the isolated individual. Mothers can place a symbolic, physical, practical and expressive stress on this aspect of parenting in providing an ontological security for children (Hallden 1999; Ribbens 1994). Similarly, children and young people can also lay emphasis on the importance of having parents – mothers especially – who are 'there' emotionally and practically if they are needed, seeing this as a demonstration of their care and concern and likewise striving to 'be there for them' as required (Backe-Hansen 2001; Brannen *et al.* 2000; Gillies *et al.* 2001; Montandon 2001). Furthermore, this is in the context of children making distinctions between settings and relationships in their lives that map on to our discussion of public and private, and associated differences of social practices and orientations (for example, in relation to school/teachers and home/parents – Mayall 1994; also see contributions to Edwards 2001b).

This identification of the social orientation of 'being there' points to ongoing and widely understood particularistic relationships and practices in family life across generations in contemporary Western societies, which crucially implicates a sense of connectedness. Unless we keep open a theoretical space that allows us to conceptualise mothers' (and children's) lives in terms other than those of the public domain, however, significant understandings such as 'being there' may simply be rendered invisible, or otherwise obscured and reframed.[9]

Conclusions

The concepts of public and private are undoubtedly exceedingly complex and shifting, but we have argued that they remain important and useful. Much feminist work has been concerned to address public/private distinctions in order to explore and reveal gender subordination (Benhabib 1998), as well as to consider other power dimensions around these distinctions, such as race/ethnicity (Hill Collins 1997; Fraser 1998). However, we have been arguing that there has also been another important strand of feminist work that has sought to explore aspects of the private in more detail and to show some alternative social practices, orientations and ways of being (however contingent) in women's positioning and experiences within the private. Aspects of this can be seen in Selma Sevenhuijsen's (1998 and Chapter 6) work on a feminist ethic of care, based on care as a moral relational activity involving connected responsibility and responsiveness. We have suggested that this issue of connectedness, particularly centred on childcare, mothering and caring more generally, is a key aspect of such alternative social practices and ways of being. An important issue, then, is the question of how themes around collectivities, individuality and connectedness map on to, or cut across, distinctions between public and private, and how far the use of the concepts may illuminate or obscure such issues. We have argued that the private has become equated with the personal and the individual in recent theorising about the nature of family/intimate relationships in a way that excludes what we see as some crucial feminist concerns about the nature of these relationships and their social character as this relates to gender and generation. Some contemporary theorists, both mainstream male writers and feminist writers, have thus lost sight of the private in our terms, either through a concentration on the personal or through a concentration on the public.

Clearly, there are issues about whether, on the one hand, the public/private distinction has outlived its usefulness, such that it is time to move on to less dichotomised ways of theorising different social locations and experiences, or whether, on the other hand, dichotomised thinking may have its uses at times. Whatever position is taken, we need to be alert to the possibilities of confusing and conflating important themes, and thereby obscuring key aspects of contemporary social lives around gender, generation and other major social divisions. Our concern here has been to draw attention to the risk that recent theorising about the private has seen the predominance of a White, Western, middle-class masculinist view based upon a particular understanding of the individual. In the process, we may be losing sight of issues of connectedness around children and the associated relational view of individuality that is a crucial aspect of many women's lived experiences and that has been the key theoretical space opened up by a particular strand of (predominantly) feminist writings on the private. In developing and theorising our understanding of the complex interplay between public and private, it is crucial not to close off the insights to be gained from this particular perspective on the private in understanding and analysing families.

Notes

1 This chapter draws on an earlier discussion of these issues that we presented to the second TSER Seminar of the Thematic Network, Working and Mothering: Social Practices and Social Policies, Frankfurt, April 1999 (Ribbens McCarthy and Edwards 1999b). We would like to acknowledge the very helpful comments received from those attending.
2 The important notion of 'enmeshment', used in Western family therapy, for example, may be argued to be inappropriate for ethnic minority family members, because it depends upon this version of the individual (Dilworth-Anderson *et al.* 1993; Hardy 1993).
3 As we have explored elsewhere, there are also resonances with Tonnies' distinction between *Gemeinschaft* and *Gesellschaft* (Ribbens McCarthy and Edwards 1999a).
4 Educational establishments occupy an ambiguous position in this scheme of things, being concerned primarily with an orientation towards the child becoming an adult fit to take her or his place in public life. They are also implicated in an increasing institutionalisation of childhood, which can work in tandem with children's familialisation – see discussion in Edwards 2001a.
5 Yeatman (1986) offers a more complex discussion again, distinguishing between a universalistic notion of the individual (located in the public sphere) and a particularistic notion of the (unique) individual (located in the domestic sphere).
6 See also Patricia Hill Collins (1990) for a similar sort of ethic of care derived from African-American women's experiences. She discusses it mainly in relation to knowledge validation, but she makes links to citizenship in the form of an empowering 'voice' for Black women.
7 See Zelitzer (1985) and Beck and Beck-Gernsheim (1995) for a discussion of the values and ideals that may have become increasingly focused on children and parenting in contemporary Western societies.
8 Although Walby (1994) also poses the public as patriarchal but of a more collective kind and latterly distinguishes between degrees of exploitation in different countries and regions.
9 The notion of 'fairness' may constitute another example of a concept that is central to family lives and is crucially shaped by understandings around children and adults but cannot easily be translated into the more public languages of ethics and justice (Ribbens McCarthy and Edwards 2001).

References

Archard, D. (1993) *Children, Rights and Childhood*, London: Routledge.

Backe-Hansen, E. (2001) 'Young people between home and school', in R. Edwards (ed.) *Children, Home and School: Regulation, Autonomy or Connection?* London: RoutledgeFalmer.

Bailey, J. (2000) 'Some meanings of "the private" in sociological thought', *Sociology* 34(3), 381–402.

Bailey, L. (1999) 'Refracted selves? A study of changes in self-identity in the transition to motherhood', *Sociology* 33(2): 335–72.

Beck, U. (1997) 'Democratization of the family', *Childhood* 4(2): 151–68.

Beck, U. and Beck-Gernsheim, E. (1995) *The Normal Chaos of Love* (translated by Mark Ritter and Jane Wiebel). Cambridge: Polity Press.

Bell, L. and Ribbens, J. (1994) 'Isolated housewives and complex maternal worlds: the significance of social contacts between women with young children in industrial societies', *Sociological Review* 42(2): 227–62.

Benhabib, S. (1992) *Situating the Self: Gender, Community and Postmodernism in Contemporary Ethics*, New York: Routledge.

—— (1998) 'Models of public space: Hannah Arendt, the liberal tradition, and Jürgen Habermas', in J.B. Landes (ed.) *Feminism: the Public and the Private*, Oxford: Oxford University Press.

Benn, S.L. and Gaus, J.F. (eds) (1983) *Public and Private in Social Life*, London: Croom Helm.

Brannen, J., Heptinstall, E. and Bhopal, K. (2000) *Connecting Children: Care and Family Life in Later Childhood*, London: RoutledgeFalmer.

Boulton, M.G. (1983) *On Being a Mother: A Study of Women and Pre-School Children*, London: Tavistock.

Bryan, B., Dadzie, S. and Scafe, S. (1985) *The Heart of the Race: Black Women's Lives in Britain*, London: Virago.

Burgoyne, C.B. (1990) 'Money in marriage: how patterns of allocation both reflect and conceal power', *Sociological Review* 38(4): 634–65.

Burman, E. (1994) *Deconstructing Developmental Psychology*, London: Routledge.

Cahill, S. (1990) 'Childhood and public life: reaffirming biographical divisions', *Social Problems* 37(3): 390–402.

Chamberlayne, P. (1998) 'Cultural analysis of the informal sphere', paper presented to the International Sociological Association Conference, Montreal, July.

Cheal, D. (1991) *Family and the State of Theory*, New York: Harvester Wheatsheaf.

Cohen, J.L. (1997) 'Rethinking privacy: autonomy, identity and the abortion controversy', in J. Weintraub and K. Kumar (eds) *Public and Private in Thought and Practice: Perspectives on a Grand Dichotomy*, Chicago: University of Chicago Press.

Dahlberg, G. (1996) 'Negotiating modern childrearing in family life in Sweden', in J. Brannen and R. Edwards (eds) *Perspectives on Parenting and Childhood: Looking Back and Moving Forward*, London: South Bank University/ESRC/Institute of Education.

Davidoff, L. (1995) *Worlds Between: Historical Perspectives on Gender and Class*, Cambridge: Polity Press.

Delphy, C. and Leonard, D. (1992) *Familiar Exploitation: A New Analysis of Marriage in Contemporary Western Societies*, Cambridge: Polity Press.

Dilworth-Anderson, P., Burton, L.M. and Boulin, J. (1993) 'Reframing theories for understanding race, ethnicity and families', in P. Boss, W.J. Doherty, R. LaRossa, W.R. Schumm and S.K. Steinmetz (eds) *Sourcebook of Family Theories and Methods: A Contextual Approach*, New York: Plenum Press.

Doucet, A. (2000) '"There's a huge difference between me as a male carer and women": gender, domestic responsibility and the community as an institutional arena', *Community, Work and Family* 3(2): 163–84.

Edwards, R. (1993) *Mature Women Students: Separating or Connecting Family and Education*, London: Taylor & Francis.

—— (2001a) 'Introduction: conceptualising relationships between home and school in children's lives', in R. Edwards (ed.) *Children, Home and School: Regulation, Autonomy or Connection?* London: RoutledgeFalmer.

—— (ed.) (2001b) *Children, Home and School: Regulation, Autonomy or Connection?* London: RoutledgeFalmer.

Edwards, R. and Ribbens, J. (1991) 'Meandering around "strategy": a research note on strategic discourse in the lives of women', *Sociology* 25(3): 477–89.

—— (1998) 'Living on the edges: public knowledge, private lives and personal experience', in J. Ribbens and R. Edwards (eds) *Feminist Dilemmas in Qualitative Research: Public Knowledge and Private Lives*, London: Sage.

Eisenstein, H. (1984) *Contemporary Feminist Thought*, London: Unwin.

Elias, N. (1939/1994) *The Civilizing Process*, Oxford: Basil Blackwell.

Elshtain, J.B. (1981) *Public Man, Private Woman*, Princeton, NJ: Princeton University Press.

Ennew, J. (1986) *The Sexual Exploitation of Children*, Cambridge: Polity Press.

Ferree, M.M. (1985) 'Between two worlds: German feminist approaches to working class women and work', *Signs*, 10.

Fraser, N. (1992) 'Rethinking the public sphere: a contribution to the critique of actually existing democracy', in H.A. Giroux and P. McLaren (eds) *Between Borders: Pedagogy and the Politics of Cultural Studies*, New York: Routledge.

—— (1997) *Justice Interruptus: Rethinking Key Concepts in a Postsocialist Age*, New York: Routledge.

—— (1998) 'Sex, lies and the public sphere: reflections on the confirmation of Clarence Thomas', in J.B. Landes (ed.) *Feminism: The Public and The Private*, Oxford: Oxford University Press.

Gamarnikow, E., Morgan, D., Purvis, J. and Taylorson, D. (eds) (1983) *The Public and the Private*, London: Heinemann.

Gergen, K.J. (1999) *An Invitation to Social Construction*, London: Sage.

Giddens, A. (1991) *Modernity and Self-identity: Self and Society in the Late Modern Age*, Cambridge: Polity Press.

—— (1992) *The Transformation of Intimacy: Sexuality, Love and Eroticism in Modern Societies*, Cambridge: Polity Press.

—— (1999) 'The family', Reith Lecture, Week 4, BBC Radio 4, 28 April.

Gieve, K. (1987) 'Rethinking feminist attitudes towards motherhood', *Feminist Review* 25: 38–45.

Gillies, V., Ribbens McCarthy, J. and Holland, J. (2001) '*Pulling Together, Pulling Apart': The Family Lives of Young People*, London/York: Family Policies Study Centre/Joseph Rowntree Foundation.

Gilligan, C. (1988) 'Remapping the moral domain: new images of self in relationship', in C. Gilligan, J.V. Ward and J.M. Taylor with B. Bardige (eds) *Mapping the Moral Domain: A Contribution of Women's Thinking to Psychological Theory and Education*, Cambridge, Mass.: Harvard University Press.

—— (1994) 'Listening to a different voice: Celia Kitzinger interviews Carol Gilligan', *Feminism and Psychology* 4(3): 408–19.

Glenn, E. (1985) 'Racial ethnic women's labor: the intersection of race, gender and class oppression', *Review of Radical Political Economics* 17: 86–108.

Gobetti, D. (1997) 'Humankind as a system: private and public agency at the origins of modern liberalism', in J. Weintraub and K. Kumar (eds) *Public and Private in Thought and Practice: Perspectives on a Grand Dichotomy*, Chicago: University of Chicago Press.

Hallden, G. (1999) 'The child as project and the child as being: parents' ideas as frames of reference', *Children and Society* 5(4): 334–46.

Hardy, K.V. (1993) 'Implications for practice with ethnic minority families', in P. Boss, W.J. Doherty, R. LaRossa, W.R. Schumm and S.K. Steinmetz (eds) *Sourcebook of Family Theories and Methods: A Contextual Approach*, New York: Plenum Press.

Hill Collins, P. (1990) *Black Feminist Thought: Knowledge, Consciousness and the Politics of Empowerment*, London: HarperCollins.

—— (1997) 'The more things change, the more they stay the same: African-American women and the new politics of containment', plenary address to the British Sociological Association Annual Conference, University of York, 7–10 April.

Hockey, J. and James, A. (1993) *Growing Up and Growing Old: Ageing and Dependency in the Life Course*, London: Sage.

Hunter, A. (1995) 'Private, parochial and public social orders: the problem of crime and incivility in urban communities', in P. Kasinitz (ed.) *Metropolis: Centre and Symbol of Our Times*, Basingstoke: Macmillan.

Jamieson, L. (1998) *Intimacy: Personal Relationships in Modern Societies*, Cambridge: Polity Press.

Jenks, C. (1996a) 'The postmodern child', in J. Brannen and M. O'Brien (eds) *Children in Families*, Lewes: Falmer Press.

—— (1996b) *Childhood*, London: Routledge.

Kivisto, P. (1998) *Key Ideas in Sociology*, Thousand Oaks, Calif.: Pine Forge Press/Sage.

Landes, J.B. (ed.) (1998a) *Feminism: The Public and The Private*, Oxford: Oxford University Press.

—— (1998b) 'Introduction', in J.B. Landes (ed.) *Feminism: The Public and The Private*, Oxford: Oxford University Press.

Mauthner, N. (1994) 'Postnatal depression: a relational perspective', unpublished Ph.D. dissertation, University of Cambridge.

Mayall, B. (1990) 'A joy or a hassle: child healthcare in a multi-ethnic society', *Children and Society* 4(2): 269–90.

Mayall, B. (1994) *Negotiating Health: School Children at Home and at School*, London: Cassell.

Miller, T. (1999) 'Negotiation and narration: an exploration of first time motherhood', unpublished Ph.D. dissertation, University of Warwick.

Montandon, C. (2001) 'Home and school constraints in children's experience of socialisation in Geneva', in R. Edwards (ed.) *Children, Home and School: Regulation, Autonomy or Connection?* London: RoutledgeFalmer.

Morgan, D.H.J. (1985) *The Family, Politics and Social Theory*, London: Routledge & Kegan Paul.

—— (1996) *Family Connections: An Introduction to Family Studies*, Cambridge: Polity Press.

Oakley, A. (1974/76) *Housewife*, Harmondsworth, Middlesex: Penguin.

Pahl, R. (1988/92) 'Work and employment', in L. McDowell and R. Pringle (eds) *Defining Women: Social Institutions and Gender Divisions*, Cambridge: Polity

Press. [First published in 1988 as 'Editor's introduction: historical aspects of work, employment, unemployment and the sexual division of labour', in R.E. Pahl (ed.) *On Work: Historical, Comparative and Theoretical Approach*, Oxford: Basil Blackwell.]

Pateman, C. (1970) *Participation and Democratic Theory*, Cambridge: Cambridge University Press.

—— (1989) *The Disorder of Women: Democracy, Feminism and Political Theory*, Cambridge: Polity Press.

Pfau-Effinger, B. (1998) 'Gender cultures and the gender arrangement – a theoretical framework for cross-national gender research', *Innovation* 11(2): 147–66.

Phoenix, A. (1987) 'Theories of gender and black families', in G. Weiner and M. Arnot (eds) *Gender Under Scrutiny: New Inquiries in Education*, London: Hutchinson.

Pilcher, J. (1995) *Age and Generation in Modern Britain*, Oxford: Oxford University Press.

Prokhovnik, R. (1998) 'Public and private citizenship: from gender invisibility to feminist inclusiveness', *Feminist Review* 60: 84–104.

Reynolds, T. (1998) 'African-Caribbean mothering: reconstructing a "new" identity', unpublished Ph.D. thesis, South Bank University.

Ribbens, J. (1994) *Mothers and Their Children: A Feminist Sociology of Childrearing*, London: Sage.

Ribbens, J. and Edwards, R. (1995) 'Introducing qualitative research on women in families and households', *Women's Studies International Forum* 18(3): 247–58.

Ribbens McCarthy, J. and Edwards, R. (1999a) 'Gendered lives, gendered concepts? The significance of children for theorising "public" and "private"', paper presented to the BSA Annual Conference, Glasgow, March.

—— (1999b) 'Individuality and connectedness in the lives of mothers and children: maintaining a perspective on public and private', in *Theoretical Perspectives on Working and Mothering*, Report of the Second TSER Seminar of the Thematic Network, Working and Mothering: Social Practices and Social Policies, Frankfurt, April.

—— (2001) 'Illuminating meanings of "the private" in sociological thought: a response to Joe Bailey', *Sociology* 35(3).

Ribbens McCarthy, J., Edwards, R. and Gillies, V. (2000) 'Moral tales of the child and the adult: narratives of contemporary family lives under changing circumstances', *Sociology* 34(4): 785–803.

—— (2001) 'Understandings of "fairness" in re-making "families": parenting and family life after re-partnering', paper presented to the British Sociological Association Annual Conference, University of Manchester.

Rosaldo, M. and Lamphere, L. (eds) (1974) *Women, Culture and Society*, Stanford, Calif.: Stanford University Press.

Ruddick, S. (1995) 'Preface: "Maternal Thinking" Revisited', in S. Ruddick *Maternal Thinking: Towards a Politics of Peace* (2nd edn). Boston: Beacon Press.

Sassoon, A.S. (ed.) (1987) *Women and the State: The Shifting Boundaries of Public and Private*, London: Hutchinson.

Sevenhuijsen, S. (1998) *Citizenship and the Ethics of Care: Feminist Considerations on Justice, Morality and Politics*, London: Routledge.

Sharistanian, J. (ed.) (1987) *Beyond the Public/Domestic Dichotomy: Contemporary Perspectives on Women's Public Lives*, Westport, Conn.: Greenwood Press.

Slater, D. (1998) 'Public/Private', in C. Jenks (ed.) *Core Sociological Dichotomies*, London: Sage.
Smart, C. (1997) 'Wishful thinking and harmful tinkering? Sociological reflections on family policy', *Journal of Social Policy* 26(3): 301–22.
Smart, C. and Neale, B. (1999) *Family Fragments*, Cambridge: Polity Press.
Smith, D.E. (1987) *The Everyday World as Problematic: A Feminist Sociology*, Milton Keynes: Open University Press.
Stacey, J. (1998) 'Transatlantic traffic in the politics of family values', paper presented to the Centre for Family and Household Research, Oxford Brookes University, 13 May.
Stacey, M. (1981) 'The division of labour revisited, or overcoming the two Adams', in P. Abrams, R. Deem, J. Finch and P. Rock (eds) *Practice and Progress: British Sociology 1950–1980*, London: George Allen & Unwin.
Tronto, J. (1993) *Moral Boundaries: A Political Argument for an Ethic of Care*, London: Routledge.
Walby, S. (1990) *Theorising Patriarchy*, Oxford: Basil Blackwell.
—— (1994) 'Methodological and theoretical issues in comparative analysis of gender relations in Western Europe', *Environment and Planning A* 27: 1339–54.
Walkerdine, V. and Lucey, H. (1989) *Democracy in the Kitchen: Regulating Mothers and Socialising Daughters*, London: Virago.
Weintraub, J. (1997) 'The theory and politics of the public/private distinction', in J. Weintraub and K. Kumar (eds) *Public and Private in Thought and Practice: Perspectives on a Grand Dichotomy*, Chicago: University of Chicago Press.
Yeatman, A. (1986) 'Women, domestic life and sociology', in C. Pateman and E. Gross (eds) *Feminist Challenges: Social and Political Theory*, Sydney: Allen & Unwin.
Zelitzer, V.A. (1985) *Pricing the Priceless Child: The Changing Social Value of Children*, New York: Basic Books.

11 Elective families

Lesbian and gay life experiments[1]

Jeffrey Weeks

Families by choice

'Family' is a powerful symbolic term, embracing a variety of meanings. It is also a highly ambivalent and fiercely contested term in the contemporary world, the subject of endless polemics, anxiety and political controversy. It is surely of great significance, therefore, that the term is now in common use among many self-identified 'non-heterosexuals': lesbians, gay men, bisexuals, 'queers', 'homosexuals'. The self-descriptions may vary, but the sense of living outside, even against, traditional heterosexual norms is shaping a distinctive attitude among non-heterosexual people to intimate relationships, in which the claiming of the term 'family' has become an important rallying point. Increasingly, the term is being deployed by many people to denote something broader than the traditional relationships based on lineage, alliance and biology, referring instead to kin-like networks of relationships based on friendship, choice and commitment (Weeks *et al.* 2001). Such networks may include selected blood relatives. They may or may not involve children. But whatever the particular patterns, they have a cultural and symbolic meaning for the people that participate or feel a sense of belonging in and through them. We are seeing the development and public affirmation of 'families of choice' (*cf.* Weston 1991), the sort of 'life experiments' that Giddens (1992) sees as necessary in late modern societies.

There are several interlocking elements in this emerging discourse. In the first place, the use of the term suggests a strong perceived need to appropriate the sort of values and comforts that the family is supposed to embody, even if it regularly fails to do so: continuity over time, emotional and material support, ongoing commitment, and intense engagement. For many others, friendship circles are spoken of as being equivalent to the idealised family (and infinitely preferable to the real one). We can hear this in some characteristic comments on friends as family (see Weeks *et al.* 2001: chapter 1): 'a feeling of belonging to a group of people who like me' (Simon, a gay man aged 32); 'affection, love if you like – you share the good things, and you share the bad things too' (Dan, aged 71); 'I think the friendships I have are family' (Rachel, a 32-year-old lesbian). These may not be everyone's definition of the ideal family; nor are they anywhere near the legal definition of kin, but the words carry intense conviction among those who have chosen to organise their relationships around new forms of commitment.

Second, this usage illustrates a very important ethos that now pervades the non-heterosexual world: a sense of the freedom and agency that the idea of 'created' relationships brings (*cf.* Henriksson 1995). Paul says: 'I take my family [of origin] for granted, whereas my friendships are, to a degree, chosen, and therefore they're created. And I feel a greater responsibility to nourish them'. This is echoed by Malika, a lesbian in her late twenties: 'In the last few years since I've come out I've learnt that family can be anything you want it to be'.

This emphasis on creativity is crucial to our understanding of what is happening. It suggests a new self-confidence in the non-heterosexual world and an awareness of new opportunities and spaces for choosing ways of being in the world. However, this goes alongside a strong awareness of, and resistance to, the continuing hostility towards homosexuality in the wider world, despite the significant changes in public attitudes that have opened up these new possibilities. Elective families still provide the 'lifeline' that the biological family, it is believed, should provide but often cannot or will not for its sexually different offspring.

People slide easily between seeing the family as a site of hostility and something they can invent: friends are *like* family, or they *are* family. The family is something external to you, or something you do. This ambivalence in language is revealing. We are clearly in transition from one set of norms to another. The language of 'family' used by many contemporary non-heterosexual people can be seen as both a challenge to conventional definitions and an attempt to broaden these; as a hankering for legitimacy and an attempt to build something new; as an identification with existing patterns and a more or less conscious effort to subvert them. The stories that many non-heterosexual women and men tell about families of choice are creating a new public space where old and new forms jostle for meaning, and where new patterns of relationship are being invented.

The new stories about elective families that characterise the contemporary non-heterosexual world provide new truths, which in turn circulate in communities and give rise to claims for recognition and legitimisation as crucial elements of the claim to full citizenship (Plummer 1995). New stories about sexual and intimate life emerge, it may be argued, when there is a new audience ready to hear them in communities of meaning and understanding, and when newly vocal groups can have their experiences validated in and through them. They signal both changing perceptions and changing possibilities. Through them, we can speak of intimate lives in new ways.

In the case of the non-heterosexual world, there is a growing audience in the burgeoning sexual communities themselves (Plummer 1995: 121). And there are many individuals who are willing to vocalise new experiences, which has led to a conscious presentation of the viability of non-heterosexual ways of life. As Lewin observes, as narrators 'construct their stories they engage in a process of explaining their own worlds to themselves, thereby conceptualizing who they are' (1998: 38) – and making sure that their stories are heard, not only among their immediate circles but also in the wider world.

People are offering stories to validate their lives and simultaneously revealing their awareness of the similar stories circulating in the communities with which they identify. They provide examples of 'the reflexive project of the self', which Giddens (1991) has argued is characteristic of the late modern world. Faced by the breakdown of traditional ways of life and older forms of legitimisation, people are forced to shape new values, norms and life patterns. In doing so, they draw on their own experiences and those of their significant others and begin to define themselves anew.

From this perspective, the emergence of the emphasis on 'family' and relationships in the life stories of many non-heterosexuals represents an important shift in the cultural politics of sexual nonconformity. Of course, many of the patterns that have recently come to public consciousness are not in any fundamental sense new (see, for example, Bray 1981; Faderman 1981; Smith-Rosenberg 1985; Boswell 1994). At the same time, however, as we learn to understand a rich and complex history of homosexuality, we also need to recognise crucial contemporary changes in the life stories of those who have been forced to live outside the 'heterosexual assumption' (Weeks *et al.* 2001: chapter 2). These changes are the result of two closely intertwined shifts in contemporary culture: a transformation over the past generation in the possibilities for living an openly non-heterosexual life; and wider changes in the organisation of sexuality and gender, which have given rise to both the so-called 'crisis of the family' and complex transformations of intimate life.

Identities/relationship/rights

Since at least the eighteenth century, and increasingly codified from the nineteenth century (Sedgwick 1985, 1990; Trumbach 1998; Weeks 2000), the execrated category of 'the homosexual' has served to define the parameters of what it is to be 'normal', that is heterosexual. The fact that the boundaries between the two have always been permeable, as countless personal histories have revealed, made little difference to popular beliefs and prejudices or the legal realities. The divide between homosexuality and heterosexuality seemed rooted in nature, sanctioned by religion and science and upheld by penal codes. It is not surprising, therefore, that distinct social worlds emerged in which at first male and later female 'homosexuals' developed different ways of life. These worlds were generally covert, and always vulnerable, but they provided the context for the solidification of distinct sexual identities and what Michel Foucault (1979) called a 'reverse discourse'. The hostile categorisation became the starting point for positive identification.

Since the late 1960s, with the emergence of a radical lesbian and gay movement (Weeks 1977/90; D'Emilio 1983; Adam 1994), an affirmation of a positive sense of self and of the collective means of realising this has become the central feature of the non-heterosexual world. Finding community, said one of the interviewees in Kath Weston's book, means discovering 'that your story isn't the only one in the world' (Weston 1991: 123). The new stories, embodied in a library of 'coming out' narratives, told of discovering the self, achieving a new identity, finding others like yourself and gaining a new sense of belonging.

Initially, the transgressive element of lesbian and gay politics offered a sharp critique of the family as the forcing house of hostility to homosexuality and the subordination of women. As the Australian gay theorist Dennis Altman put it: 'straight is to gay as family is to no family' (1979: 47), while the French theorist Guy Hocquenghem (1978) encouraged gays to elaborate friendships as polar opposites to kin. The feminist sociologists Michèle Barrett and Mary McIntosh made a similar point in their critique of (White and Western) familialism in their significantly entitled book *The Anti-social Family* (1982). A phrase in the manifesto of the London Gay Liberation Front (1971: 2) speaks for a host of radical challenges to the family in this moment of transgression: 'The very form of the family works against homosexuality'. It is a denial of identity.

However, since at least the early 1980s (see Altman 1982), a different emphasis has come to the fore, giving rise to the new narratives of intimate relationships. They focus attention on the values of everyday life and form the basis of new claims to full citizenship for those hitherto on the margins, especially where relationships are concerned (Weeks 1998). The achievements of the lesbian and gay movement have opened up possibilities for broader claims for validating a wide range of life experiences. The question of identity has not gone away; nor were issues about relationships absent from the early feminist and lesbian and gay movements. But the nature of intimate life has become increasingly central to the lesbian and gay experience, and it is in this context that the idea of distinctive lesbian and gay families has developed.

However, even the most passionate theoretical advocates of the rights of non-heterosexual people to form their own 'families' are careful to emphasise the dimensions of difference: 'In fact, we are Queering the notion of family and creating families reflective of our life choices. Our expanded pluralist uses of family are politically destructive of the ethic of traditional family values' (Goss 1997: 12). In many ways, the use of the term 'family' underlines the poverty of our language in describing alternative forms of intimate life (Weeks 1991; Weeks *et al.* 2001). It also reflects shifts in the general usage of the term. Since the 1970s, critics of the family have increasingly talked not of replacing the family but of recognizing *alternative families* (Weeks 1991), an acknowledgement of the pluralisation of forms of family life. There are various types of family, the argument goes, differentiated by class, ethnicity, geography or simply lifestyle choices, but most fulfil the basic purposes of family. If there are so many types of family, why should the claims of same-sex intimate relationships be ignored (Stacey 1996: 15)?

The appropriation of the language of the family by many non-heterosexuals can therefore be seen as a battle over meaning, one important way in which the sexually marginal are struggling to assert the validity of their own way of life. In doing this, non-heterosexual people are part of a wider struggle over meaning, both participating in and reflecting a wider crisis over family relationships. As Andrew Sullivan (1997) has argued, if the future of marriage is a critical ground of contestation in the wider world, it is hardly surprising that lesbians and gays should focus their demands on it. If parenting is perceived as in major need of rethinking, then why should non-heterosexuals be excluded from the debate? If families get ever more complex as a result of divorce, remarriage, recombination and step-parenting, why should the chosen families of lesbians and gays, composed of lovers, ex-lovers and friends, be denied a voice?

This has become even more important for many non-heterosexuals because of the completely unanticipated return of epidemic in the early 1980s. Weston has suggested that 'Situated historically in a period of discourse on lesbian and gay kinship, AIDS has served as an impetus to establish and expand gay families' (1991: 183). The epidemic revealed how vulnerable non-heterosexuals were without full recognition of their significant commitments – without full citizenship (Watney 1994: 159–68).

Other developments, especially when children were involved, gave the same message. The first debates about the validity of non-heterosexual family-type relations began in Britain and the USA with controversies over the child custody battles of lesbians in the 1970s (Hanscombe and Forster 1982; Rights of Women Lesbian Custody Project 1986; Lewin 1993). The so-called 'lesbian baby-boom' (Weeks *et al.* 2001: chapter 7) and the claims by lesbians and gay men for equal rights in issues concerning fostering or adoption further underlined the continuation of inequality, despite the gains that had been made over the previous decades. Not surprisingly, by the 1990s throughout Western countries, and notably in Scandinavia, the Netherlands, France and the United States, new demands for partnership rights, same-sex marriage, and recognition of new family forms were flourishing, often in relationship to childcare (*ibid.*: chapter 8). As Nardi (1999) has observed, while the use of the term 'family' may be little more than metaphorical when applied to adult friendships, it has a strong affinity with conventional uses when applied to units with children. All these factors have created a new agenda for non-heterosexual politics in which the language of the family has become a key battleground. In this it is part of a much wider change in intimate life in which questions of what constitutes family values are central.

The changing politics of intimate life

Late modernity, Giddens (1992) has argued, is a post-traditional order in which the question 'how shall I live?' has to be answered in day-to-day decisions about who to be, how to behave and whom we should love. In a world where old sources of authority are challenged, where new identities proliferate and individuals seem to be increasingly thrown back on their own resources for values and guidelines for day-to-day actions, we have no choice but to choose (Weeks 1995, 1998). Giddens, among others, argues that potentially this opens the way to a radical democratisation of the interpersonal domain (see also Beck and Beck-Gernsheim 1995). In practice, there are strong cultural inhibitions and material constraints that limit individual opportunities, and the democratic relationship remains an ideal rather than a living reality (Jamieson 1998, 1999; see also Chapters 6 and 15). Nevertheless, there is an increasing flexibility and 'moral fluency' (Mulgan 1997) in intimate life that stretches across the heterosexual/homosexual divide. Many people are cast adrift from the old verities embodied in tradition: they have to invent new forms for themselves.

Non-heterosexual people have had to be the arch-inventors because so few guidelines have existed for those living outside the conventional heterosexual patterns. But the emergence of a new discourse concerned with wider aspects of homosexual existence than simply sexuality and identity can be seen as part of a new set of preoccupations in contemporary cultures as a whole: a recognition of the opening up of all social identities and patterns of intimate life. Diverse identities, and a variety of different ways of life, produce new and more complex patterns of relationships.

'Families of choice' and other chosen relationships, creative adaptations to rapid change based on voluntary association, are characteristic responses to rapid change. The sociologists Pahl and Spencer (1997; see also Pahl 2000) see the growth of 'friend-like relationships' as characteristic of the contemporary *Zeitgeist*. They argue that these forms are not necessarily supplanting kin relationships but are extending and enriching them. As old communities of fate and necessity decline and family patterns change, the flexible patterns of friendship can provide more adaptable structures for both private life and the labour market, providing effective 'bridging ties' to enable individuals to escape from communities of origin. The central aspect of these friendship networks, Pahl and Spencer argue, is that they are voluntary, they are developed over time, not given, and they help to strengthen our individuality. They have to be worked at, and they make us more reflexive about who we are and what we are doing.

This can be seen as part of a wider transformation of the meaning of intimate life that is leading to a new balance between the desire for individual freedom and the possibilities of commitment (Giddens 1992). The contemporary debate about the family regularly fails to recognise this, and instead we are presented with a stark polarity (Weeks *et al.* 1999). On the one hand, the media and conservative moralists offer us an image of mutuality, interdependence and resilience, represented by an ideal type of the family. At its most evocative, this ideal type is seen as a haven of trust, mutual involvement and shared responsibilities that many argue offers the best hope for a communitarian culture (Etzioni 1995). By its very nature, this traditional model is heterosexual, the norm against which all other intimate relationships must be judged.

On the other hand, set against this, many see a search for individual fulfilment that avoids commitment and is the product of an individualistic and hedonistic culture (see, for example, Dennis and Erdos 1993; Dench 1996; Phillips 1999). Inevitably, the triumph of the latter ethos is seen as corroding and ultimately undermining the first.

However, we would argue that the new narratives of intimate life do not necessarily represent a thinning of family-type commitments and responsibilities but a reorganisation of them in new circumstances. At the centre of this is the fundamental belief that love relationships and partnerships should be a matter of personal choice and not of arrangement or tradition. And the reasons for choice are quite clear: personal attraction, sexual desire, mutual trust and compatibility. The empirical evidence underlines the distance from actuality for very many people of this theoretical model (Holland *et al.* 1998; Jamieson 1998, 1999). Yet the same evidence reveals an unprecedented acknowledgement of the merits of companionate and more equal relationships among the same people, even as we fail to achieve them. Although the reality is often complex, the egalitarian relationship *has* become a measure by which people seek to judge their own individual lives. This model of how we should live may be seen as an expression of a new norm, the quest for individual fulfilment in the context of freely chosen egalitarian relationships.

From this point of view, it can be argued that heterosexual and non-heterosexual forms of life are to some degree converging, as Henning Bech (1992, 1997) has suggested in exploring the implications of the recognition of same-sex partnerships. For both sides of the sexual binary divide there is a common interest in trying to find a balance between individual satisfaction and mutual involvement. This is not the collapse of the family or the triumph of unfettered hedonism. It can be seen as the search for a new form of 'emotional democracy'. The new non-heterosexual stories about 'doing family' (Morgan 1999) can be seen as everyday efforts at achieving this ideal.

Connected lives

The stories that non-heterosexuals tell seek to validate the meaningfulness of chosen relationships, where the narrative of the self secures meaning through a narrative of 'connectedness'. This quotation from Peter, a 32-year-old gay man, illustrates this vividly:

> I think that one of the things that socially always happens is that lesbians and gay men are made into individuals with sad lives who are lonely … and I'm really looking forward to there being something that says, 'There are all these lesbians and gay men and they're living completely connected lives and they have got support, they have got community and they're doing things, better than the heterosexual world,

> because they've created this thing for themselves' ... having people talk about their lives is going to be really good and if it's only read by other lesbians and gay men, who maybe see something in somebody's interview that makes them think, 'Oh, God ... that's like my life', it makes us into a real community with real relationships and real lives, not sort of playing at it. So that's why I wanted to do it [be interviewed] because I thought 'That's a good thing to do'.
>
> quoted in Weeks *et al.* 2001: 25

Comments such as this acknowledge the power of the new narratives about intimate life not only in shaping individual choices but also in potentially changing the cultural circumstances in which these choices are made. Through interactions in the social worlds they inhabit, non-heterosexuals shape new ways of understanding their relationships, and acquire the new skills necessary to affirm the validity of different ways of life. The fact that non-heterosexual individuals want to highlight the positive realities of their relationships in comparison with orthodox patterns gives us important insights into the new narratives that are emerging about elective families, and the ways in which these stories are becoming part of a collective identity.

The most commonly told story is one of friendship: a 'friendship ethic' underpins non-heterosexual ways of life (Nardi 1999; Weeks *et al.* 2001: chapter 3), Whatever the vicissitudes of one-to-one relationships, friendships, which by their nature are freely chosen, provide a focus of emotional belonging, an arena where concepts of care, commitment and mutual responsibility can be worked through. Friendship is a also a school for emotional democracy, which in turn underpins an egalitarian ideal in same-sex relationships. It needs no underlining that a commitment to egalitarian relationships is no guarantee that they can be achieved. Same-sex relationships are subject to all the power disparities that configure more traditional relationships (Dunne 1997; Heaphy *et al.* 1999). However, in the absence of structured gendered assumptions and a traditional division of labour, it is inevitable that negotiation of the relationship, with its egalitarian assumption, becomes central to non-heterosexual relationships: 'Everything has to be discussed, everything is negotiable' (Melanie, a lesbian quoted in Weeks *et al.* 2001: 110). That in turn shapes the ethos of same-sex intimate life and the forms of mutual commitment that develop.

Again, we can see parallels between the emerging non-heterosexual norms and wider patterns of negotiating obligations and mutual responsibilities among kin in the wider world (*cf.* Finch 1989; Finch and Mason 1993). In particular, the evidence suggests that where children and other dependents are concerned, a sense of absolute obligation is strong, however complex the parenting arrangements may be (Weeks *et al.* 2001: chapter 7). However, in friendships and one-to-one relationships, commitment and mutual responsibility are seen as necessarily matters to be worked out over time in a process of egalitarian give and take.

Despite similarities and congruences between heterosexual and non-heterosexual patterns, however, it is important to make a final point. For non-heterosexuals, in the absence of pre-given institutional structures of commitment, there is no real alternative to the endless process of self-invention, of 'life experiments'. They are necessary for the achievement of 'connected lives' and of chosen families.

Note

1 A fuller development of the ideas in this chapter can be found in Weeks *et al.* 2001. This book provides detailed empirical evidence for the arguments made above.

References

Adam, B.D. (1994) *The Rise of a Gay and Lesbian Movement*, New York: Twayne Publishers.

Altman, D. (1979) *Coming Out in the Seventies*, Sydney and Eugene: Wild & Woolley.

—— (1982) *The Homosexualization of America, the Americanization of the Homosexual*, New York: St Martin's Press.

Barrett, M. and McIntosh, M. (1982) *The Anti-social Family*, London: Verso.

Bech, H. (1992) 'Report from a rotten state: "marriage" and "homosexuality" in "Denmark"', in K. Plummer (ed.) *Modern Homosexualities: Fragments of Lesbian and Gay Experience*, London and New York: Routledge.

—— (1997) *When Men Meet: Homosexuality and Modernity*, Cambridge: Polity Press.

Beck, U. and Beck-Gernsheim, E. (1995) *The Normal Chaos of Love*, Cambridge: Polity Press.

Boswell, J. (1994) *Same-sex Unions in Premodern Europe*, New York: Villard Books.

Bray, A. (1981) *Homosexuality in Renaissance England*, London: Gay Men's Press.

D'Emilio, J. (1983) *Sexual Politics, Sexual Communities: The Making of a Homosexual Minority in the United States 1940–1970*, Chicago and London: University of Chicago Press.

Dench, G. (1996) *The Place of Men in Changing Family Attitudes*, London: Institute of Community Studies.

Dennis, N. and Erdos, G. (1993) *Families without Fatherhood*, London: Institute for Economic Affairs, Health and Welfare Unit.

Dunne, G.A. (1997) *Lesbian Lifestyles: Women's Work and the Politics of Sexuality*, London: Macmillan.

Etzioni, A. (1995) *The Spirit of Community: Rights, Responsibilities and the Communitarian Agenda*, London: Fontana Press.

Faderman, L. (1981) *Surpassing the Love of Men*, London: Junction Books.

Finch, J. (1989) *Family Obligation and Social Change*, London: Polity Press.

Finch, J. and Mason, J. (1993) *Negotiating Family Responsibilities*, London: Routledge.

Foucault, M. (1979) *The History of Sexuality. Volume 1: An Introduction*, Harmondsworth: Penguin.

Giddens, A. (1991) *Modernity and Self-Identity*, Cambridge: Polity Press.

—— (1992) *The Transformation of Intimacy: Sexuality, Love and Eroticism in Modern Societies*, Cambridge: Polity Press.

Goss, R.E. (1997) 'Queering procreative privilege: coming out as families', in R.E. Goss and A.S. Strongheart (eds) *Our Families, Our Values: Snapshots of Queer Kinship*, Binghampton, NJ: Harrington Park Press.

Hanscombe, G. and Forster, J. (1982) *Rocking the Cradle: Lesbian Mothers. A Challenge in Family Living*, London: Sheba Feminist Publishers.

Heaphy, B., Donovan, C. and Weeks. J. (1999) 'Sex, money and the kitchen sink: power in same sex couple relationships', in J. Seymour and P. Bagguley (eds) *Relating Intimacies: Power and Resistance*, London: Macmillan.

Henriksson, B. (1995) 'Risk factor love: homosexuality, sexual interaction and HIV prevention', PhD thesis, Department of Social Work, Goteborg University, Sweden.

Hocquenghem, G. (1978) *Homosexual Desire*, London: Allison & Busby.

Holland, J., Ramazanoglu, C., Sharpe, S. and Thomson, R. (1998) *The Male in the Head: Young People, Heterosexuality and Power*, London: Tufnell Press.

Jamieson, L. (1998) *Intimacy: Personal Relationships in Modern Society*, Cambridge: Polity Press.

—— (1999) 'Intimacy transformed: a critical look at the "pure relationship"', *Sociology* 33(3): 477–94.

Lewin, E. (1993) *Lesbian Mothers: Accounts of Gender In American Culture*, Ithaca, NY, and London: Cornell University Press.

—— (1998) *Recognizing Ourselves: Ceremonies of Lesbian and Gay Commitment*, New York: Columbia University Press.

London Gay Liberation Front (1971) 'Manifesto', London: Gay Liberation Front.

Morgan, D.H.J. (1999) 'Risk and family practices: accounting for change and fluidity in family life', in E.B. Silva and C. Smart (eds) *The New Family?* London: Sage.

Mulgan, G. (1997) *Connexity: How to Live in a Connected World*, London: Chatto & Windus.

Nardi, P. (1999) *Gay Men's Friendships: Invincible Communities*, Chicago: University of Chicago Press.

Pahl, R. (2000) *On Friendship*, Cambridge: Polity Press.

Pahl, R. and Spencer, L. (1997) 'The politics of friendship', *Renewal* 5(3–4): 100–7.

Phillips, M. (1999) *The Sex-change Society: Feminised Britain and the Neutered Male*, London: Social Market Foundation.

Plummer, K. (1995) *Telling Sexual Stories: Power, Change and Social Worlds*, London: Routledge.

Rights of Women Lesbian Custody Group (1986) *Lesbian Mothers' Legal Handbook*, London: Women's Press.

Sedgwick, E.K. (1985) *Between Men: English Literature and Male Homosocial Desire*, New York: Columbia University Press.

—— (1990) *Epistemology of the Closet*, Berkeley and Los Angeles: University of California Press.

Smith-Rosenberg, C. (1985) 'The female world of love and ritual', in *Disorderly Conduct: Visions of Gender in Victorian America*, New York and Oxford: Oxford University Press.

Stacey, J. (1996) *In the Name of the Family: Rethinking Family Values in the Post-modern Age*, Boston: Beacon Press.

Sullivan, A. (ed.) (1997) *Same-sex Marriage: Pro and Con – A Reader*, New York: Vintage Books.

Trumbach, R. (1998) *Sex and the Gender Revolution. Volume 1: Heterosexuality and the Third Gender in Enlightenment London*, Chicago and London: University of Chicago Press.

Watney, S. (1994) *Practices of Freedom: Selected Writings on HIV/AIDS*, London: Rivers Oram Press.

Weeks, J. (1977/1990) *Coming out: Homosexual Politics in Britain from the Nineteenth Century to the Present*, London: Quartet.

—— (1991) *Against Nature: Essays on History, Sexuality and Identity*, London: Rivers Oram Press.

—— (1995) *Invented Moralities: Sexual Values in an Age of Uncertainty*, Cambridge: Polity Press.

—— (1998) 'The sexual citizen', *Theory, Culture and Society* 15(3–4): 35–52.

—— (2000) *Making Sexual History*, Cambridge: Polity Press.

Weeks, J., Heaphy, B. and Donovan C. (1999) 'Families of choice: autonomy and mutuality in non-heterosexual relationships', in S. McRae (ed.) *Changing Britain: Families and Households in the 1990s*, Oxford: Oxford University Press.

—— (2001) *Same Sex Intimacies: Families of Choice and Other Life Experiments*, London: Routledge.

Weston, K. (1991) *Families We Choose: Lesbians, Gays, Kinship*, New York: Columbia University Press.

Part IV

Modelling families

12 Economic theory, norms and the care gap, or

Why do economists become parents?

Susan Himmelweit

Introduction: economic theory, children and caring

Economic theory has always had difficulty dealing with children, because children cannot be assumed to behave as rational economic agents. All legislative systems have a notion of an age of majority before which children cannot be expected to behave as full citizens. Below such an age (frequently, in practice, there are a whole series of such ages covering different aspects of life), children are not considered mature enough to make decisions and somebody else, whether an individual parent, a guardian or the state, has to make choices for them. Similarly, in economic theory, children cannot be expected to know what is best for themselves and to act consistently in their own best interests; their interests are therefore usually subsumed under those of others. For neo-classical economics, with its commitment to methodological individualism based on rational choice, the failure of children to behave 'rationally' is a major theoretical difficulty, which it tends to sidestep by ignoring the separate interests of children and of those who behave equally irrationally in caring for them.

However, there is good reason for economists to think about children and the care they need. Any economy has not only to produce goods and services but also to ensure that its population reproduces itself. This requires *inter alia* providing for the needs of children and preparing them for their eventual participation in the economy. Children not only have physical subsistence needs; they also require 'care' in a broader, personal, often more time-consuming sense if they are to become full members of society.

Time spent caring is a major factor limiting people's, particularly women's, participation in the formal economy. And when parents work in the formal economy, their children's care must be provided by others, whether by paid childcare workers, in which case it appears as a visible contribution to the output of the formal economy, or invisibly in the unpaid care economy. The care that children (and others, such as the old and the sick) need is provided in both market and non-market settings. This complicates economic accounting but does not mean that economists can ignore care, for caring behaviour has significant effects on the formal economy.

Economists use simple abstract models to try to deal with the complexities of a real economy. If caring is to be taken into account in developing economic theory and policy, it too needs to be put into an abstract model in which its causes and consequences are reduced to a reasonably small number of variables. In this chapter, I shall examine the extent to which rational choice models developed by neo-classical economists can be used to look at caring and will propose an alternative model that I hope captures some of the features of caring that the other models inappropriately ignore.[1] I shall also consider some broad policy implications of this last model.

The rational choice model

The rational choice model of human behaviour makes a complete separation between influences that are internal to the individual at the moment of choice (preferences) and those that are external (opportunities/constraints) (England 1993). The characteristic individual captured by the rational choice model is a shopper who takes her given preferences to the market and makes the best bargains she can at the prices she finds there. The shopping model has been applied, with greater or lesser success, to certain other aspects of economic behaviour. However, it seems an inappropriate model for caring, because carers' motivations are bound up with the relationships in which they find themselves and the processes in which they engage, rendering the separation between internal preferences and external constraints on their behaviour difficult to maintain (Radin 1996; Himmelweit 1999).

However, rational choice models have been used to analyse behaviour as apparently irrational as caring for children. While some of these models incorporate conventional neo-classical assumptions, most modify some of its standard tenets. All such models are part of the methodologically individualist programme in which individual behaviour, determined by individual preferences and circumstances, is the starting point of social explanation. The models vary in the assumptions they make about the nature of preferences, whether they can change and how, if at all, factors external to the individual would influence such change. The differences between these models thus concern the extent to which individualism informs the structure and development of preferences themselves.

Any rational choice model assumes that people choose their actions by their consequences. Specifically, they choose the course of action that they expect will produce their most preferred feasible outcome. Such an approach is individualist, at least in the weak sense that the process of making decisions is carried on independently of society. Social forces may enter by providing the inputs from which the decisions arise: the preferences and the predicted outcomes of possible courses of action. However, the decision maker *per se* is not a social actor.

Many rational choice models are individualist in a *second*, stronger sense: that the preferences used in decision making are exogenous and fixed characteristics of the individual, at least within the timescale of the model. Society then has no effect on preferences and can impinge on behaviour only by providing constraints and determining what the likely outcome of different courses of action will be.

However, the rational choice model of neo-classical economics is also individualist in a *third*, yet stronger sense. Self-evidently, in any rational choice model, choices are made on self-interested grounds. The assumption in most neo-classical theory is more specific: that such preferences are 'selfish', depending only on the decision maker's assessment of her own well-being. The welfare of others does not then influence her decision making.

Finally, to operationalise such models, a further assumption is often added: that well-being depends on the consumption of purchased goods and services alone, so that decisions over the gaining and spending of money can be considered in isolation from other decisions. In practice, this amounts to assuming either that financial considerations are the basis of all decision making or that different spheres of life are separable in their effects.

In this chapter, I look at five different rational choice models of why parents care for their children. The first model I consider is both economistic and individualist in the strongest sense; it assumes that parents care for children because it is in the parents' financial interests to do so. The second model relaxes the economism but still has parents selfishly self-interested. However, their interests are somewhat more broadly defined and include pleasure from caring for children. The third model allows for the possibility of altruism, of children's welfare entering into their parents' preferences. This model is not individualist in the strongest sense outlined above; it relaxes the assumption that self-interested means selfish and allows for interdependencies between different individuals' preferences. The fourth model admits a more significant change in that it allows parents' preferences to change in response to their experience of both their own individual behaviour and the behaviour of others. However, it is still a rational choice model in that preferences are used to decide what to do. A fifth model introduces a new element by allowing alternative 'substantive' or 'moral' rationalities that do not depend on consequences alone to be introduced into rational choice models (Weber 1968; Elster 1989; Duncan and Edwards 1997, 1999).

A final model rejects rational choice as an explanation for all behaviour. Instead of looking at caring behaviour as a choice made in order best to satisfy preferences, it looks at it as the fulfilment of responsibilities that individuals feel are theirs because of their identification as members of a group subject to particular social norms. This explanation is therefore not individualist even in the weakest sense of the term, because it models a process of decision making that is *itself* subject to social forces. The chapter concludes by considering what such an explanation can bring to the analysis of parental caring behaviour in the context of changing gender identities.

Five economic models of why parents care for children

Model 1: children as an investment

The most economistic view of why parents care for their children is that doing so is an investment by parents in their own future well-being. This theory has been used to explain various features of family life in poorer economies, where children are expected to work from an early age. They can be net contributors to the household of birth when they are still quite young and are expected to support elderly parents (Cain 1977). Since children who are better cared for and better educated may be willing and able to contribute more, money and time spent on the care of children when they are young can be seen as an investment. Returns on the investment accrue as soon as children are old enough to contribute to the household themselves and are especially important when the parents' ability to provide for themselves diminishes.

There may be a class dimension in this. Parents who own property can use control over their children's inheritance to ensure that the children fulfil customary expectations and look after their ageing parents. Children may therefore be a more reliable investment for parents who have property to pass on, which should result in better care for such children (or at least usually for the male children, on whom parents expect to rely for financial support in their old age).[2]

The investment model can explain why subsistence farmers in a rural economy tend to have large families, investing in the quantity rather than the 'quality' of their children (Becker 1991). Although most of the costs of caring for children in such households can be expected to be low, the cost of education may be particularly high if education has to be paid for and if it prevents children contributing time to their households. Furthermore, education may not be so economically important for those who expect to inherit their parents' way of life. It may then be a better investment to have more children rather than to spend more on each one's care.

The birth rate will then fall with economic development because of the declining economic importance of children's work and the rising opportunity costs of their care, especially in terms of women's earnings forgone. Furthermore, as the proportion of the population who are dependent purely on wage labour to make a living increases, education makes a greater difference to children's future income. Such increased educational demands, resulting in longer periods of economic dependency, imply that children are less likely to be net contributors to their parents' household before they leave home. As inherited property becomes less important to the majority of the population, and thus parental control over children declines, children become an unreliable source of support for the elderly. Parents in such economies make provision for their own pensions and can look to few, if any, material benefits from having and caring for children.

So although the investment model can explain why parents find large families a less worthwhile investment and so have fewer, better-educated children in developed economies, the problem is that in such economies raising children does not seem to be a worthwhile financial investment at all. Yet even in the most developed economies, people still have and care for children. The investment model does not, therefore, offer a plausible explanation of caring for children in economies in which most parents do not have significant property to leave and children tend to require support until they are ready to leave home.

Model 2: the pleasures of parenthood

One possible explanation for why parents continue to care for children in circumstances in which it cannot plausibly be argued to bring in a financial return is that caring for children is enjoyable in itself. If parents enjoy the process of caring, get pleasure from helping a child take its first steps or enjoy shopping for their children when away on business trips, these will enter into their preferences. They will then make a rational decision to allocate some time and money to these activities. In that case, parents may have children in order to be able to spend their time in such desirable ways, rather like buying a television in order to spend time watching it. One may also obtain enjoyment from owning the television set itself. Similarly, parents may have children because they enjoy the status of being a parent. Just as with consumer goods, both the acquisition and the use of children may be a source of enjoyment. Thus children are consumption goods, rather than the investment goods of model 1.

For most goods, consumption rises with greater economic prosperity, although not necessarily proportionately. The tendency for fertility to decline with increasing development would therefore be a puzzle for this model. However, the puzzle can be solved by distinguishing between two forms of spending on children (Becker 1991). If the enjoyment that parents get from children depends on both the quantity and quality of the children, where 'quality' depends on various costly and time-consuming inputs such as education, then the quality and quantity of children are substitutable consumption goods for parents. Parents choosing to have fewer children but spending more time and money on each child as income rises are simply substituting quality for quantity of children. This may happen because the opportunity costs of having an extra child rises with increasing earning power, particularly for women. Another possible reason is that child quality becomes particularly important for parents as income rises. In pre-capitalist economies there may have been no such negative effect of income on the desire for more children, but with the transition to an economy in which education matters and takes time, rising incomes will raise the opportunity costs of children, thus decreasing desired family size.

Caring for children in this model is just as self-interestedly rational a choice of activity as any other form of consumption. Parents in this model enjoy spending their time caring; they do not do it for their child's sake. So long as the preference for having and caring for children is taken to be an intrinsic characteristic of people who choose to be parents, a model in which parents act rationally on such preferences satisfies all the individualist tenets of standard neo-classical theory.

Model 3: altruism

Someone who cares for another person is generally thought to be concerned for the other person's welfare. The nearest a rational choice approach gets to caring is to make caring individuals 'altruistic', that is to include a component in a carer's preferences for the consumption or utility of the person for whom they care. Individuals can maximise a utility function that depends on another's welfare in just the same way as one that depends only on their own consumption of different consumer goods. Given the constraints of income and prices, the rational individual decides what to do by trading off the extent to which she satisfies her taste for others' welfare against her taste for various other ways of spending her resources.

Behaving in this way is not exactly what we would usually mean by 'altruism'; as Becker (1991: 279) has pointed out, a person acting upon such preferences 'might be called selfish, not altruistic, in terms of utility.' However, this model is no longer individualist in the strongest sense of an individual's preferences depending only on what is happening to herself. But so long as both the formation of preferences and the method of decision making remain independent of society, the model is still individualist in both these two weaker senses.

Altruism can take two forms: an individual may care directly about another's consumption of commodities, or only indirectly about the utility generated by that consumption. In the former case, the altruist evaluates for herself the consumption bundles of those she cares about and gains utility from their consumption. In the latter case, the altruist has 'non-meddlesome' preferences and is therefore not concerned with the actual consumption of those she cares about but simply has a taste for their utility. Altruistic preferences of either form make an individual's utility partly dependent on another's consumption. Such 'consumption externalities', like other externalities, undermine the core 'invisible hand' theorems of neo-classical economics, which celebrate the efficiency of a competitive market economy. Where people are altruistic, market processes alone will not produce efficiency. Instead, altruism will both 'create a need for socially co-operative actions' and 'itself facilitate voluntary social co-operation' (Collard 1978: 17).

'Non-meddlesome' preferences cause fewer problems for neo-classical welfare economics, the basic theorems of which continue to hold in a competitive market in which transfers as well as exchanges are allowed to take place (*ibid.*). Unfortunately, 'a preference for another's utility' is an insufficient characterisation of caring for children, because non-meddlesome preferences imply that parents would do best for their children by simply augmenting their resources, i.e. by giving them money. But one of the reasons that children are perceived as needing care is precisely because they cannot look after themselves unaided in a market economy. Nor, indeed, do the informational requirements of non-meddlesome preferences make them a plausible basis for altruism between adults, because acting to augment another's utility requires knowledge of the other's full set of preferences.

Model 4: developing a taste for childcare

All the models we have looked at so far have treated preferences as given. Although these models are not necessarily individualist in the strongest sense of an individual only caring about their own well-being, they remain individualist in the sense of the preferences themselves being independent of social influences. However, it seems more plausible to see such preferences as ones that can be cultivated, as endogenous tastes affected by previous experience. In particular, the experience of working with children frequently seems to lead people to care for the welfare of those children and enjoy looking after them. Given that parents, especially mothers, spend a great deal of time with their newborn children, such a learning process may explain why parents are particularly concerned for the welfare of their own children and usually prefer to spend time caring for them rather than for other children. Mother–child bonding would thus figure in such a model as an example of rapid endogenous preference formation.

Becker and others have developed rational choice models that allow for the influence of an individual's behaviour on preferences, in particular on the extent of altruism or the enjoyment of caring activities. These models also open up the possibility that social forces might affect preferences (Becker and Stigler 1977; Stark 1995; Becker 1996). At first glance, it would appear that such models have loosened yet one more degree of individualism, in that preferences are no longer exogenous, fixed characteristics of the individual.

However, this is achieved by making a distinction between current preferences and an underlying set of preferences. Whereas people's underlying preferences do not change, past experiences may alter their current circumstances and as a result affect their preferences between currently available options. Thus a smoker and a non-smoker can have identical underlying preferences, but because of the smoker's previous experience of nicotine consumption, his current preferences are different from those of a non-smoker, who has no history of nicotine consumption. Although both might have made the same choice in identical circumstances, that is, to smoke if addicted to nicotine and not to smoke if not addicted, they are in fact not in the same circumstances: one is addicted and one is not, so they will make different choices (Becker and Stigler 1977). Similarly, no difference in underlying preferences needs to be assumed to explain why people with experience of looking after a child are likely to make different choices from those lacking such experience.

Becker explains why the experience of looking after a child frequently leads people to enjoy doing so as a process of building up what he calls 'personal capital', the acquisition of which makes looking after that child in the future a more worthwhile experience. An individual's personal capital is that stock of all past personal consumption and other experiences that affect the given individual's current and future preferences. In being an acquired stock that affects future possibilities, personal capital is similar to human capital, or indeed to any other sort of capital. However, while the use of other forms of capital makes an individual more productive, personal capital makes involvement in particular activities more worthwhile for that individual. So the time spent in building up a relationship with the child is an investment in personal capital – time spent now in order to give the parent preferences that make time spent in the future more productive of utility, perhaps including utility generated by the child's welfare. The mother's underlying tastes have not changed. She, like everyone else, always had underlying tastes that with the right stock of personal capital would give her such utility; and now, through experience, she has acquired the means of producing it for herself.

Similar arguments can be used to explain all cases of endogenous tastes. Where tastes apparently change because of a person's *own* previous behaviour, that person is said to have acquired 'personal capital'. Where tastes apparently change because of a change in the actions of *others* in an individual's social network, Becker talks of the acquisition of 'social capital'. So while personal capital is a stock that is the result of an individual's *own* past actions on their current and future preferences, social capital is the effect on those preferences of past actions by *others*. In other words, social capital represents the influence on an individual's preferences of their peer group, the social milieu in which they live and of their culture more generally.

Gender differences in parenting behaviour can then be explained by reference to women's greater enjoyment of child-centred activities, but in a way that does not rely on inherently different underlying tastes. Consider a man and a woman with a new baby who have equal earning power and equal productivity in domestic tasks. Even if both parents have the same underlying tastes, whichever of them looks after the baby will acquire personal capital in doing so, which means that in the future they will value looking after the child differently. This means that the initial carer will have a different trade-off between time spent on childcare and time spent on other activities from that of their partner. Compared with an equal division of time, both partners' preferences will be better satisfied through the one with experience of childcare increasing the time they spend on it, while the other shifts towards spending more time on the activities in which they may have acquired personal capital. By extension of this argument, there should be complete specialisation, so that one does all the childcare (assuming it can all be managed by one person) and acquires the maximum amount of baby-specific personal capital, while the other acquires other forms of personal capital by specialising in other activities. One only needs a small element of biological difference to explain why women might have a headstart in acquiring the initial tranche of personal childcare capital.[3]

Social capital may also be involved in generating gender differences in parents' preferences. Mothers may identify with and spend more time with other mothers and through this may enhance their appreciation of activities culturally allocated to women. The father's absence from the home may lead him to build up different social capital. He will interact more with a peer group who are little involved with children, so he will feel free to discover the joys of activities other than childcare.

Personal and social capital are not always utility-augmenting. If personal experiences are not fulfilling, then the personal capital generated by those experiences lowers utility. So caring for ungrateful children can discourage parents from caring in the future. Again, social capital might reinforce this. In a society that expected children to show some warmth in return – which did not take committed parenting for granted – the failure of children to live up to these expectations would be a loss of social capital to their parents. This loss would diminish their pleasure and thus result in their withdrawal of care from difficult children.

This model, in which current preferences are allowed to change, does capture some aspects of the developing relationship that caring entails. However, the problem with the continuing emphasis on choice in these models remains. Frequently, caring is not a choice. Because of who she is and the relationships in which she is engaged, a carer sees herself as having responsibilities. She does not necessarily have such a separated view of her own interests to use as the basis of choice (England 1993). Even when she does stand back and ask herself 'What do I want?' it is not in abstraction from the interests of others around here. In neo-classical terms, she is beset by consumption externalities. But more significantly, she spends much of her time doing what she thinks *should* be done, rather than what she would choose to do by assessing the outcomes of her actions for herself or anybody else.

Model 5: accepting moral responsibility

For many parents, perhaps the most important reason why they care for their children is a sense of moral responsibility for those particular children. A mother who gets up to see to a crying child at night does so because she sees it as her responsibility, whether or not she feels empathy for the child at that particular moment. Indeed, parents may love one child more than their others yet still accept an equal responsibility for them all.

Another way to put it is that parents whose sense of moral responsibility leads them to care for their children are doing so because they feel it is the right way to behave, rather than assessing whether it will lead to their most preferred outcome. If parents behave according to their moral beliefs in this way, then parenting requires an explanation quite different from rational choice. Rational choice is above all concerned with outcomes, which for parents could be their own financial benefit, their enjoyment of parenting or the welfare of their child. People may consider outcomes in choosing how best to carry out their moral responsibilities. However, the motivation for accepting that responsibility in the first place is not outcome-oriented (Elster 1989). It is much more like the adoption of an internally imposed rule.

However, even a rational utility maximiser might follow rules, including rules that they think of as moral imperatives, in some circumstances. In complex situations, following a rule can be shown to be a more effective way of maximising an actor's utility than case-by-case maximisation (Vanberg 1994a; Heiner 1988). To obey the rule might reduce decision-making costs. It may be too costly to assess the opportunity costs of all the different ways of caring for each child; it may therefore be less costly to adopt the rule of raising each child as one was raised oneself. Alternatively, conforming to a rule might reduce the likelihood of mistakes. The unknown factors involved in ensuring a child's safety might lead parents to adopt certain rules, such as never leaving a toddler alone in the house.[4]

Furthermore, the need for coordination can also provide a reason why it might be rational to follow certain rules, or norms, if others are doing so (Sugden 1989; Young 1996). If the other children in a neighbourhood are equipped to play football, it is not taking good care of one's own child to ensure that they have a tennis racquet.

Maximising utility is not necessarily a conscious process, so the actor may not be aware that he is following rules in order to maximise his personal gain. Indeed, many such rules may be experienced as moral obligations. Frequently, the term 'convention' is used to signal a rule whose content has no particular moral weight but is a sensible course of action to follow given that others are doing so, such as driving on the left-hand side of the road. The term 'norm' is more usually applied to a rule to which people experience a moral obligation to conform. However, for a rational choice theorist, that people explain their own behaviour as having moral rather than instrumental motivations does not rule out the need to search for a rational explanation of the behaviour (Vanberg 1994b).

Sociologists typically see moral norms as an alternative explanation of behaviour to rational choice theory, rather than something to be explained by it. Max Weber talked about fulfilling moral norms as part of a logic of 'substantive' rather than formal rationality, as people feel impelled to let values, responsibilities and obligations override the calculation of the best means to meet given ends (Weber 1968). Such norms become social if they are shared across at least some members of society and individuals conform to them because they feel subject to social approval and disapproval. The development of sociology on the basis of such ideas led Duesenberry to coin his well-known aphorism that 'economics is all about how people make choices; sociology is all about why they don't have any choices to make'(1960: 233).

If social norms are enforced by social sanctions, then conforming to them may again be just a matter of rational choice.[5] Such social sanctions are commonly seen to be social disapproval and/or loss of reputation, rather than disutilities that are more material. Social norms then have effects through concerns about the opinions and behaviour of others, to which it is assumed people are sensitive. People may gain utility from the respect and esteem of others if they conform to social norms, and the shame or loss of reputation experienced if they do not conform may be a source of disutility.

Finally, whatever form social sanctions take, they may be internalised so that people do not require the sanctions. Instead, they develop a conscience so that expectations of a gain in self-esteem from following norms, or guilt from not doing so, figure in their unconscious calculation of utility.[6] This is the important step that turns social norms into moral imperatives. In her discussion of this theory of the 'socialised actor', Cancun (1975: 5) puts it like this:

> this potentially anarchic individual [the rational utility maximiser] is harnessed to society through the internalisation of norms and values … individual members are motivated to conform to shared norms; they want to do what they are supposed to do.

In all these accounts, norms are followed because it suits people to do so. Conforming to a norm is a utility-maximising strategy that reduces decision-making costs and/or mistakes or achieves coordination. Alternatively, it is a utility-maximising strategy because it values the benefits of enhancing reputation and avoiding social sanctions and/or making people feel good about themselves and avoiding guilt. Either of these explanations of why individuals conform to a norm is consistent with those individuals believing that they are behaving in accordance with the norm because it is their moral responsibility to do so.

However, both these rational choice approaches fail to answer fundamental questions. The economist's explanation of conforming to norms as the best way to maximise utility in complex situations requires a utility function to be defined prior to and independently of the norms themselves. Therefore, such an account of parenting norms must have a pre-existing notion of what parents hope to gain from caring for children, perhaps derived from one of the theories outlined earlier in this chapter. The sociologist's explanation of conforming to norms as a way of avoiding social sanctions and gaining social approval requires an explanation of why people are sensitive to such sanctions and approval in the first place (Elster 1989). Second, it requires an explanation of the content of norms: why certain behaviour is approved of and other behaviour sanctioned, and where particular social norms come from and how they change.

Norms as expressions of social identity

The previous section showed that norms can be incorporated into a neoclassical framework but that by themselves they add little to our previous analysis. To give them substantive content, we need to examine how norms are *embedded* in society. In particular, to account for parental/maternal/paternal behaviour we need a theory that explains how particular norms apply to people in particular circumstances on the basis of their membership or identification with particular groups. It is as parents, wives, husbands, workers, employers, teachers, schoolchildren and friends that people hold certain specific responsibilities to certain specific others and particular expectations are made of their behaviour. For example, only members of some groups may see themselves as under any obligation to have children. Married women, for example, may feel themselves subject to social pressure to have a child, while until very recently the norm for an unmarried woman was not to become a mother.

Norms, like other institutions, differ across societies, but the norms of most societies impose a primary obligation on parents to take responsibility for their children. However, societies vary in how gender-specific parental responsibilities are and in the extent to which they are shared more widely among families and the wider community. Some societies are based on care being delivered primarily within the mother–child relation, others have a nuclear family norm, others rely on an extended family, and some on sharing many responsibilities for the next generation between a whole clan. Such different family forms in turn affect the accumulation of capital, the structure of land holdings and the existence of a landless class and thus in turn the form that production relations take in the economy. Responsibility for children therefore forms one part of an interlocking and mutually sustaining set of norms that together make up a society of a particular type.

So where do such norms come from and why do people conform to them? Social identity theory treats these questions as interlinked: norms are collective ideas about what type of behaviour confirms an individual's membership of a particular social group. Individuals therefore conform to social norms in order, consciously or unconsciously, to validate an identity, their membership of a social group, whose norms are formed by the behaviour characteristic of that group (Cancun 1975).

This means that norms change when people's identities change and norms also change when the behaviour they support is no longer characteristic of the relevant group. If an increasing number of members of a particular group fail to conform to an existing norm, this norm will weaken for all people that identify themselves as members of that group.

And why might people not conform to a social norm? One reason is that a variety of factors influence what people do. In particular, external conditions may change; if acting according to a particular norm becomes more costly, or in other ways more difficult, people are less likely to fulfil it. Furthermore, norms may come into conflict with each other. For example, many mothers talk about a daily juggling of obligations: to employers, children, husbands, parents, friends and so on. Where norms conflict, people must in practice 'choose' between them in order to act, although this act of choice is quite different from the outcome-oriented process of rational choice.[7] Neither rational economic man nor *homo sociologicus* can provide an explanation of how such choices are made, the latter because he does not know how to give any credence to morality, the former because he does not know how to choose at all. A social evolutionary approach does not require that we have an *a priori* theory of how such dilemmas are resolved. However, such an approach could predict with confidence that stronger norms, those that are observed being fulfilled more frequently by the relevant group, and those that are less costly to fulfil, are likely to be the ones that survive in any such competition between norms.

In this section, I shall develop a simple evolutionary, or adaptive, model of caring based on changing norms but unchanging identities, in which the assumption is made that the norms applying to people identifying with a particular group are formed by the predominant behaviour of that fixed group of people. Later, I shall consider what happens if identities can change too. So, for example, if most mothers with jobs are at home before their children come home from school, this becomes a norm for women identifying themselves as working mothers, to which others will then feel some responsibility to conform. Whether they will actually manage to do so will depend on a number of other factors, such as employer flexibility, bus schedules and family income. Furthermore, there is also another norm concerning their family's standard of living and for many mothers there will be some conflict between these two norms: whether to work long enough to ensure that their family can live up to current expenditure norms, or to work shorter hours in order to be at home before the children return.

If the relative cost of conforming to the two norms changes – let us say there is a rise in the cost of living – then some mothers may increase their hours of employment to earn more but come home later. The first ones to change in this way will probably be those for whom the change is more appropriate: perhaps those who have relatives living nearby who can look after the children, or those whose children are older and are therefore more responsible but cost more to keep. The fact that more mothers are not now at home when their children come from school will weaken the 'being there' norm. Conversely, family expenditure norms will strengthen, so that other mothers will now feel a greater responsibility to augment their family income, and so on.

Where this process stops will depend on how responsive the norms are to changing behaviour. If they are resistant to change, sluggish one might say, then norms and behaviour will settle down to a stable equilibrium. After the initial disturbance, old patterns will re-establish themselves, with perhaps just a few more mothers working longer hours, but others will still be more influenced by the 'being there' norm. On the other hand, if norms are more volatile, the initial change may set off a bandwagon, which will stop only when norms and behaviour again converge, possibly only when most women with school-age children are in full-time employment.

Even if prices subsequently fall, reducing the income needed to meet expenditure norms, the old norm of mothers being at home after school will have weakened, and mothers spending more time earning money may no longer consider that 'good mothers' need to be at home. Rather than re-establishing the norm of being at home before their children, these mothers may consider other responses to the fall in prices, for example whether they should work longer hours now that the real value of their wages has increased.

Contrast this with the standard neo-classical approach which takes preferences as given exogenously. It too would recognise that a rise in the cost of living will, other things being equal, increase the amount of time a woman spends in employment and decrease the amount of time she spends at home. However, once the cost of living falls again, on the assumption that her preferences have not changed, the amount of time she spends at home should return to what it was before. The fact that there was a past change is no longer relevant in explaining current behaviour.

This is one important difference between a model in which norms (or preferences) evolve and a model that takes preferences as given. If preferences are fixed, then history is irrelevant to them. The same external conditions will always produce the same behaviour, and the effects of any change in external conditions can be reversed simply by undoing the change. On the other hand, an approach that models how norms adapt can explain how in apparently identical current circumstances different outcomes may result because of a different historical evolution of norms, identities and behaviour – what is usually meant by culture. Furthermore, because changes in the past will have affected current norms as well as current behaviour, such change may well be irreversible.

Changing norms can have lasting effects because the model assumes a positive feedback mechanism, in which, as an initial change works through the system, the further changes that are produced work in the same direction, reinforcing the initial change.[8] This is unlike negative feedback models where change in one direction leads to a correcting effect in the opposite direction, dampening the initial change. Negative feedback models tend to converge to an equilibrium and are commonly used in economic theory, particularly for modelling markets. Positive feedback mechanisms may not converge to an equilibrium or there may be more than one, in which case initial conditions and the path followed continue to have relevance in determining outcomes. Furthermore, even where there is convergence, the outcome may be unstable and subject to bandwagon effects in which initially a few individuals changing their behaviour can result in large numbers eventually following suit.

Whether such a bandwagon rolls will depend on how strongly changes in behaviour affect norms and *vice versa*. If norms are sluggish and do not weaken much when a few people fail to behave as they prescribe, then bandwagons will be hard to start; a norm that does not easily shift will tend to induce dissidents to conform, rather than their behaviour encouraging others. Such a norm and the behaviour it induces will be stable. More volatile norms, where small numbers changing their behaviour may easily induce others to challenge the norm, will lead to instability and bandwagon effects (Hargreaves-Heap 1992).

The feedback process between norms and behaviour described above is particularly strongly positive because norms are socially generated, so the effects on people are interdependent. A change in the behaviour of any one individual, if interpreted by others as supporting or challenging a norm, will affect the strength of that norm and thus the behaviour of others. Behaviour affected by norms in this ways is 'density-dependent' in that the likelihood of any particular individual adopting a particular type of behaviour in a particular situation depends on its density, that is the frequency with which that behaviour occurs in similar situations in a relevant population.

Social norms are not the only possible case of such density-dependent behaviour. Indeed, it could be a result of rational choice, if observing others behaving in a particular way either makes similar behaviour more desirable or gives new information about its desirability.[9] If other mothers are at home with their children after school, there is the basis for an enjoyable social life that would not be available if all other children were in after-school clubs. Conversely, observing other mothers letting their children come home from school on their own might convince a mother that it is safe to let her children do so too. And, as before, such rational grounds for following others' behaviour may be experienced by actors as having moral force, making conforming to the norm seem the right thing to do in the circumstances.

All density-dependent behaviour, whatever its cause, leads to path dependence and so can set up local and cultural differences in caring behaviour, which become entrenched even though the initial impetus in one direction or the other may have been slight. The mathematics of such models can be very complex and lead to results that are much less predictable than those of the equilibrium models of neo-classical economics (Akerlof 1980; Kirman 1993, 1997). Small changes in initial conditions can lead to much larger changes in behaviour in the long run, thus leading to considerable variations in outcome across different countries or cultures.

In the model with norms, the speed at which a norm changes depends not only upon how much each person reacts to a changing norm but also on how much the norm changes in response to the behaviour of members of the group. If all members of a group face similar conditions, then there is less chance of some members, because of their particular circumstances, changing their behaviour and thus challenging group norms. We should therefore expect, for example, that in a society in which all women face similar conditions, the norms governing their behaviour will be relatively strong.

All this points to the importance of the process by which people identify themselves as members of the group to which a norm applies. Norms work through identities, through particular people identifying themselves as subject to the norms applying to particular groups. The father who defaults on his child support payments may be shifting his identification from being a father to being a single man. He may be making this shift consciously and hedonistically, or he may feel forced into this position by an ex-wife who denies him access to his children. Either way, by identifying himself with another group, a different set of norms influencing his behaviour comes into play.

If there are rigid gender divisions in society, women and men will be more likely to develop distinct identities as members of separate groups with their own separate norms. If group identity is strong, there will be less variation in adherence to group norms and therefore less likelihood that dissident individuals will behave in ways that challenge those norms. So a society more rigidly divided by gender would be more successful than a more egalitarian society at enforcing gendered norms of behaviour, especially on a gender whose range of options was so small that they all faced similar conditions and so behaved similarly. On the other hand, if women and men begin to identify themselves in less gender-specific ways, so that both see themselves as workers and parents, rather than as mothers and breadwinners respectively, then they will adopt different, less gender-specific norms.

Conclusion: understanding change in caring behaviour

To understand how change happens, we need to consider what factors can increase or decrease people's willingness to care for others according to our different models. Considering the costs and benefits of caring is easiest. In all the models, other things being equal, parents will care more for children if the costs of doing so fall and if the benefits, financial or emotional, to the parent increase. If the costs of caring increase or the benefits fall, parents will be less inclined to devote their time and energy to caring.

In some models, the way people think about caring may also change and so alter their behaviour. We saw that altruism and pleasure in caring for children is a taste that can be developed. In particular, it can be induced by personal experience, 'building up personal capital' as Becker would say, or by living in a more caring society, in which more 'social capital' accumulates.

Finally in the social identity model, not only do all the above factors affect caring behaviour, but caring norms are more likely to be fulfilled when they are in harmony with other norms and apply to a large group of people facing reasonably homogenous conditions.

We can therefore list some factors that should work in favour of a society caring well for its children. As the tenets of individualism are successively weakened, more of these factors can be incorporated into a rational choice model. Only the model with social norms can incorporate them all:

1 The costs of caring are not too high for individuals, in terms of both direct consumption costs and the opportunity costs of devoting time to caring.
2 Those who care for children personally benefit from doing so in financial and/or emotional terms.
3 Those who care for children are able to build up long-term relationships with those they care for.
4 The benefits to society of caring are recognised, so that those who care for children experience a positive social valuation of the work they do.
5 A reasonably strong caring norm that which is not in conflict with the other norms of society places the obligation to care for children upon a sufficiently large group of people under similar conditions.

This list obviously oversimplifies many of the factors involved. Nevertheless, it can be used to analyse two possible ways of improving the care of children. One, the traditional view, attempts to encourage men and women to fulfil their traditional gender-specific responsibilities better. The advocates of such 'family values' appear to have decided that the best way of establishing a breadwinning norm for men and a caring norm for women is through emphasising gender differences and restricting the choices and identities open to women, thereby decreasing both the opportunity costs of caring for individual women and the variation in their conditions.

However, this is not the only way in which children could be better cared for. Another way would be to encourage men and women to identify with each other across gender boundaries by pursuing a greater equality of experience, through developing norms that required both men and women to contribute financially to their children and to care for them. If the above analysis is correct, it is equality of experience that matters in fostering group identity and shared norms. Widening the numbers who contribute time to caring would also reduce the individual costs to those who do and ensure that the opportunity costs are more spread. Greater shared experience of caring could also result in the community at large recognising better the benefits that it derives from the caring work that parents do, and so being more willing to contribute institutionally and financially to these costs.

To put this in a contemporary context, consider the anxieties that have been expressed in many countries in which gender norms are changing about the care that children receive (Folbre 1994). These anxieties do not always focus directly on gender norms: some are about inadequate diets or educational failings, for example. The analysis above nevertheless suggests that, once we start moving away from a gender-divided society, in which each gender is expected to make its own specific contribution to the care of children, towards a more equal one, we have to go the whole way if children are to be sufficiently well cared for. If caring is determined by norms, and norms depend on the group with which people identify, then any contemporary deficit of care may have to do with being in transition between a gender-divided society and a more equal one.

Effective norms require a well-defined group for them to apply to. In the current transitional situation, women may no longer identify themselves sufficiently as the only ones who should provide all the care that children need, and men may no longer sufficiently identify themselves as the sole breadwinners to provide enough money. Traditional norms of breadwinner father and caring mother may have sufficiently broken down that men and women fulfil neither norm adequately on their own, yet a new egalitarian norm based on equality of caring and financial support may not yet be well enough established. If children are to be cared for while such more egalitarian norms are established, society more widely will surely need to contribute more to the care of its children than it does in most economies; this might also help with those problems children face that are nothing to do with changing gender norms.

Notes

1 For a macro-level sectoral model of how caring fits into the wider economy, see Himmelweit 1998.

2 This gender difference of parental expectations is thought to account for the marked son preference shown in many poor countries and the shocking difference between female and male child mortality rates in rural Northern India until a few years ago (Miller 1981; United Nations Development Program 1995).

3 There is a clear parallel here with Becker's argument for specialisation within the household based on the acquisition of human capital: that it is efficient for one partner to acquire and use household specific human capital and for the other to acquire and use human capital appropriate to the workplace (Becker 1991).

4 If norms are adopted to reduce decision-making costs the resulting decisions will be worse on average (produce less utility) than if taken on a case-by-case basis, but the reduced cost of decision making makes adopting the norm worthwhile. However, conforming to a norm to avoid making mistakes should result on average in better outcomes.

5 It may be rational to observe social norms in such cases, but it is not necessarily rational to participate in enforcing them, which is not a costless exercise for others. Why then do others do so? In order to avoid others imposing sanctions on them, perhaps? But this leads to infinite regress, which suggests that something more is involved in the social construction of norms than just a self-interested calculation of utility, even where that utility includes sensitivity to socially imposed sanctions.

6 The economist who has most successfully introduced such 'sociological' norms into economic theorising is George Akerlof (1980). In his labour market model, individuals maximise utility that is a function not only of their income, but also of their self-respect that depends on whether they are behaving in accordance

with their personal norms, and their reputation that depends on conforming to social norms. Further, these norms are endogenous to the model with their strength depending on the extent to which they are obeyed. Thus people are less likely to believe in norms that are infrequently observed and will suffer less loss of reputation from flaunting social norms that others do not share.

7 Chattoe makes a closely related point in Chapter 14 of this volume: 'what makes a moral belief "moral" is … that [it] changes by a different *social process* from other kinds of belief'. And Glover in Chapter 13 discusses the relationship of rational choice to the juggling of commitments in her 'balance model' of decision making.

8 The norms in Akerlof's model have this characteristic too. See note 6.

9 Economists have modelled the behaviour of other types of people whose behaviour appears to be directly influenced by that of others and therefore is density dependent, such as speculators on the stock exchange, consumers of fashions items or investors in new technology (Schiller 1984; David 1985; Arthur 1989; Bikhchandani *et al.* 1992).

References

Akerlof, G. (1980) 'A theory of social custom, of which unemployment may be one consequence', *Quarterly Journal of Economics* LXXXIV: 749–75.

Arthur, W.B. (1989) 'Competing technologies, increasing returns and lock-in by historical events', *Economic Journal* IC, 116–31.

Becker, G.S. (1991) *A Treatise on the Family* (enlarged edition). Cambridge, Mass., and London: Harvard University Press.

—— (1996) *Accounting for Tastes*, Cambridge, Mass.: Harvard University Press.

Becker, G.S. and Stigler, G.J. (1977) 'De gustibus non est disputandum', *American Economic Review* 67(2): 76–90.

Bikhchandani, S., Hirschleifer, D. and Welch, I. (1992) 'A theory of fads, fashion, custom and cultural change as informational cascades', *Journal of Political Economy* 100: 992–1026.

Cain, M. (1977) 'The economic activities of children in a village in Bangladesh', *Population and Development Review* 3.

Cancun, F.M. (1975) *What are Norms? A Study of Beliefs and Action in a Maya Community*, Cambridge: Cambridge University Press.

Coleman, J.S. (1990) *Foundations of Social Theory*, Cambridge, Mass.: Harvard University Press.

Collard, D. (1978) *Altruism and Economy*, Oxford: Martin Robertson.

David, P. (1985) 'Clio and the economics of QWERTY', *American Economic Review Proceedings* 75, 332–7.

Duesenberry, J.S. (1960) 'Comment on "An economic analysis of fertility"', in *Demographic and Economic Change in Developed Countries: A Conference of the Universities – National Bureau Committee for Economic Research*, Princeton, NJ: Princeton University Press.

Duncan, S. and Edwards, R. (1997) 'Lone mothers and paid work – rational economic man or gendered moral rationalities?' *Feminist Economics* 3(2): 29–61.

—— (1999) *Lone Mothers and Paid Work – Rational Economic Man or Gendered Moral Rationalities*, London: Macmillan.

Elster, J. (1989) *The Cement of Society*, Cambridge: Cambridge University Press.

England, P. (1993) 'The separative self: androcentric bias in neoclassical assumptions', in M.A. Ferber and J.A. Nelson (eds) *Beyond Economic Man: Feminist Theory and Economics*, Chicago and London: University of Chicago Press.

Folbre, N. (1994) *Who Pays for the Kids? Gender and the Structures of Constraint*, London: Routledge.

Hargreaves-Heap, S. (1992) 'Bandwagon effects', in S. Hargreaves-Heap, M. Hollis, R. Sugden and A. Weale (eds) *The Theory of Choice: A Critical Guide*, Oxford: Basil Blackwell.

Heiner, R.A. (1988) 'The necessity of imperfect decisions', *Journal of Economic Behaviour and Organisations* 10(1): 29–55.

Himmelweit, S. (1998) 'Accounting for caring', *Radical Statistics* 70: 3–7.

—— (1999) 'Caring labour', *Annals of the American Academy of Political and Social Science* 561: 27–38.

Kirman, A.P. (1993) 'Ants, rationality and recruitment', *Quarterly Journal of Economics* CVIII: 137–56.

—— (1997) 'The economy as an interactive system' in W.B. Arthur, S.N. Durlauf and D.A. Lane (eds) *The Economy as Evolving Complex System II*, Reading, Mass.: Addison-Wesley.

Miller, B.D. (1981) *The Endangered Sex: Neglect of Female Children in Rural North India.* Ithaca, NY: Cornell University Press.

Radin, M.J. (1996) *Contested Commodities*, Cambridge, Mass.: Harvard University Press.

Schiller, R.J. (1984) 'Stock prices and social dynamics', *Brookings Papers on Economic Activity* 2: 457–510.

Stark, O. (1995) *Altruism and Beyond: An Economic Analysis of Transfers and Exchanges within Families and Groups*, Cambridge: Cambridge University Press.

Sugden, R. (1989) 'Spontaneous order', *Journal of Economic Perspectives* 3(4): 85–97.

United Nations Development Program (1995) *Human Development Report 1995*, Oxford: UNDP/Oxford University Press.

Vanberg, V.J. (1994a) 'Rules and choice in economics and sociology', in V.J. Vanberg (ed.) *Rules and Choice in Economics*, London: Routledge.

—— (1994b) 'Morality and economics: de moribus est disputandem', in V.J. Vanberg (ed.) *Rules and Choice in Economics*, London: Routledge.

Weber, M. (1968) *Economy and Society*, New York: Bedminster Press. [First published in English translation in 1922.]

Young, H.P. (1996) 'The economics of convention', *Journal of Economic Perspectives* 10(2): 105–22.

13 The 'balance model'

Theorising women's employment behaviour[1]

Judith Glover

Introduction

My thesis in this chapter is that one of the factors behind women's decision making relating to 'employment mobility' may be a perceived need to maintain a balance between commodified (paid) work and uncommodified (unpaid) domestic work. By 'employment mobility', I am referring principally to three types of movement:

1 from outside the labour market into paid work;
2 from part-time to full-time paid work;
3 from a lower to a higher post (via promotion).

All of these movements imply an increase in the time taken up by paid work and may also have spatial implications. I suggest that a spatial–temporal increase in the paid work sphere may create pressure on unpaid work and bring about a perceived imbalance in individual women's lives and in the household. The threat or the actuality of this may mean that women 'choose' not to increase their paid work. This will add to the disadvantage that women experience in the labour market, where part-time working is notoriously subject to low pay and where vertical sex segregation is a causal factor in the pay gap between women and men (Humphries 1995). The focus of my chapter is the post-1970s liberal welfare regime in the UK.

I conceptualise the sub-spheres of unpaid work as work that relates to a range of interpersonal roles, including mother, partner/wife, daughter and friend. In addition, there is household work, household management, indirect care and emotional work, as well as *charge mentale* arising from the interaction of these roles. A wish to preserve balance (by not undertaking employment mobility) may therefore be one explanation of women's position in the labour market: their overall representation, their high levels of part-time working and their vertical segregation. Thus the conservation of balance becomes an *object* of women's decision making in the economic sphere.

In the later part of the chapter, I counter the previous emphasis on agency by suggesting various structural factors that may mediate women's decisions about employment mobility and the preservation of balance. The structural factors include the welfare state type, gender roles, the family/household type, cultural norms and values, and different types of occupation. In the light of this, I conclude that women's decision making about employment can be conceptualised as a 'rational choice'. However, this is not used in the way in which neo-classical economics uses the term. Instead of self-interest being at the basis of employment decisions, something more akin to *self-preservation* may underpin these decisions. My overall aim is to add to existing explanations of women's employment patterns in terms of:

- women's relative presence in the labour market;
- women's propensity to work part-time; and
- vertical sex segregation.

Explaining women's employment behaviour

There is a clear move among social scientists to seek to understand women's employment in a way that accepts the complex interplay of push and pull factors and their effect on employment patterns. Recent exponents of this perspective include Connell (1987), Leira (1992), Ferber and Nelson (1993), Duncan and Edwards (1997, 1999) and Pfau-Effinger (1998). These authors are part of a more general movement to integrate the economic and the social, exemplified by Carling (1991) and Granovetter (1992) and, before them, writers such as Polanyi and Weber. This approach to women's employment has been referred to as the 'gender systems' perspective, exemplified by Pfau-Effinger's work (see Chapter 4.1). In trying to understand why patterns of part-time working vary cross-nationally, she argues that women's employment needs to be understood as the interplay between gendered cultures, the gender order (institutions and structures) and action. Gendered cultures include cultural norms about appropriate spheres of paid and unpaid work of women and men, the allocation of responsibility for children and childcare, and dependencies between women and men.

The gender order is conceptualised in two ways: first, via institutions such as the labour market, family/households and the welfare state; and, second, via 'gender structures' such as the division of labour, power relations and emotional work (Connell 1987). Action, says Pfau-Effinger, implies the social practices of individuals as well as collective action.

The point about the approach exemplified by Pfau-Effinger's work is that it is very far from seeing women's decision making about their employment as a deterministic response to social policy: that if, for example, affordable childcare were to be made available, women would take the decision to enter the labour market (Duncan *et al.* 1995). This is clearly removed from the assumptions made by neo-classical economics and rational choice theory: that economic behaviour is based on individual self-interest (see Chapter 12). It also queries neo-classical assumptions about 'choice' found, for example, in Hakim's (1991, 1995) work. Hakim's perspective, firmly in the neo-classical vein, is that many women choose not to pursue the male model of full-time, continuous employment because they prioritise their domestic concerns over their commitment to paid work. Hakim's perspective has come in for a considerable amount of criticism (e.g. Ginn *et al.* 1996), not least because the issue of choice is regarded as unproblematic. For many feminist writers and researchers, women's employment 'choice' needs to be seen as a complex set of constraints (Laurie 1993; Devine 1994; Crompton 1998).

In seeking here to make a contribution to this body of work, I begin with a particular emphasis on one aspect of Pfau-Effinger's (1998) 'gender arrangements': the social practices of individuals. I develop this concept by bringing in the idea of balance between paid work and unpaid domestic work and discuss how this relates to women's decisions about 'employment mobility', referring to the three aspects defined above. All three kinds of employment mobility would imply a temporal increase in commitment but also a spatial one, since all three would probably require geographical mobility, possibly of a major kind. Advancement in many occupations, typically professional ones, is dependent on employees having the ability to be geographically mobile (Crompton and Sanderson 1990). Hanson and Pratt (1991) argue that geography is at the centre of women's employment decisions, for two main reasons: first, that women's commitment to the various spheres of unpaid work leads them to prioritise proximity; and, second, that women's information networks about jobs are more locally based than men's networks. Furthermore, there is evidence that women have less access than men to a household car (Dale 1986) and have therefore to rely more on inadequate public transport. Limitations on geographical mobility are therefore a major cause of both vertical and horizontal occupational sex segregation.

A balancing act

A perceived need to maintain balance in women's lives is a theme that emerges consistently from a range of literature. Explicit references to a 'balancing act' are found in, for example, Spain and Bianchi (1996) and Buxton (1999). Implicit references are in much of the 'two roles' literature (Myrdal and Klein 1956; Oakley 1976; Lewis and Lewis 1996; Home Office 1998). The achievement of balance is seen as desirable for various reasons. For example, Buxton (1999) argues that a 'work–life balance' is good for both employers and employees. This 'partnership' perspective is also found in the UK government's Green Paper *Supporting Families* (1998). Here a balance between 'work and home' is seen as advantageous for carers, those receiving care, employers, the economy and society as a whole. Individual family members, the Green Paper argues, need to work a sufficient number of hours to provide for themselves economically, but they should not work so many hours that caring activities become neglected or the household becomes dependent on state provision. Perhaps optimistically, the Paper addresses itself in gender-neutral language to family members as the source of caring. This theme is echoed in the Department for Trade and Industry's Green Paper *Work and Parents: Competitiveness and Choice*:

> Parents have to juggle holding down a job with being a good parent. The Government wants to make it easier for parents in work to balance these responsibilities.
>
> DTI 2000: 1

In Britain, the Department for Education and Employment has set up a 'Work–Life Balance Unit' (www.dfee.gov.uk/work-lifebalance), which offers advice to employers on how to develop policies and working practices that enable their employees to achieve 'work–life balance'. Furthermore, the UK Chancellor of the Exchequer, Gordon Brown, referred to the balancing of work and family responsibilities when he announced an increase in maternity pay in the 2001 Budget (http://www.hmtreasury.gov.uk/budget2001).

I want here to consider a different perspective on 'work–life balance'. In setting out what I refer to as the 'balance model', I am proposing that many women (and maybe a growing number of men, a point that I take up in my concluding section) may take economic decisions relating to employment mobility on the basis of a perceived need to maintain a balance between paid work and unpaid domestic work. If balance is to be maintained, predictability and routine are crucial. Anything that has the potential to undermine that predictability is risky. My hypothesis is that women know this and take this knowledge into account when they are making decisions about whether to embark on employment mobility. I am proposing that women are likely to foresee, in a 'rational' way, the personal costs of employment mobility. In possession of this knowledge, they are making an assessment of risk: the risk of imbalance. If women decide that the risk is too great, they will not move from unemployment into the labour market, from part-time working to full-time working or into a promoted post. It may be too risky for women to move into a world that has uncontrollable outcomes and where unanticipated events can come about.

However, this does not mean that women are helpless victims of circumstances. Rather, it implies that they are autonomous actors who are shaping their own biographies and making pragmatic decisions on the basis of their calculations of risk and opportunity. If this sort of decision making is happening on a large scale, then the 'balance model' of decision making could be a major explanation of women's economic 'inactivity', of high levels of part-time working and of persistent vertical sex segregation.

How many roles?

The 'two roles' approach, originally posited by Myrdal and Klein (1956), is essentially an additive model in which the roles associated with paid and unpaid work are seen as separate spheres. 'Reconciliation' of these two spheres is often used in the dual roles rhetoric, with the implication that policy has the potential to reconcile them. Oakley (1976) introduced the possibility that the meeting of the two spheres would not necessarily be smooth – indeed, 'role conflict' might result. Haicault (1984, 1994) argues that the coterminous nature of the two roles of paid and unpaid work causes stress, which she refers to as the *charge mentale*. She argues that the continual movement between demands of time and space places unacceptable psychological demands on women. This movement between possibly conflicting demands implies that uncommodified activities are embedded in commodified activities. For example, it is possible to imagine that a commodified work activity (standing on a production line, sitting at a computer, participating in a meeting) is accompanied by wondering or even worrying about the smooth running of one or other of the uncommodified activities.

Himmelweit (see Chapter 12) refers to a 'daily juggling of obligations: to employers, children, husbands, parents, friends and so on'. This theme of role stress is echoed by Sichtermann (1988), who argues that a 'third burden' arises from the 'functional incompatibility' of the two broad spheres of paid and unpaid work: women exhaust themselves trying to do both. Hochschild (1989) suggests three spheres: 'job, children and housework'. There is little suggestion in the dual/triple roles literature that leisure is allocated any time. Sullivan (1997) argues that the complex coordination required in managing schedules in households as well as doing most of the domestic labour results in a fragmentation of any leisure time that a woman does have.

My view is that there are two main spheres, namely paid and unpaid work, but that within the unpaid work sphere there are several sub-spheres, relating broadly to a series of roles. These spheres and sub-spheres interact in complex ways and are not discrete. A non-exhaustive list would include domestic worker, daughter, mother, wife and partner.[2] Household management, 'direct' and 'indirect' care and emotional work (Connell 1987) are associated with these various roles.

Evidence from the Office for National Statistics (1998) in the UK shows that one in five middle-aged women cares for an elderly, sick or disabled relative or friend. Caring activities clearly extend beyond the immediate family. Nor are they restricted to middle-aged women: ONS figures show that 13 per cent of women aged 30 to 44 have caring activities of this sort. Almost one-third of carers provide help for more than twenty hours per week.

Although the UK does not yet have extensive time budget data,[3] existing data indicate only limited change in the domestic division of labour (Anderson *et al.* 1994). Women still do the major share of household work (*ibid.*; Spain and Bianchi 1996; SCPR 1998). This picture of stability is echoed throughout industrialised countries, and there seems to be little difference between liberal welfare regimes such as the USA (see Blumberg 1991) and social democratic welfare regimes such as Sweden (Lewis 1992). Hochschild (1989) refers to this lack of change as the 'stalled revolution': the persistence of women's primary responsibility for childcare and domestic tasks despite a marked increase in women's paid work.

The more general role of household manager is often overlooked in time-use surveys (Haicault 1994). These surveys typically ask only who does what, not who sees what needs to be done, coordinates efforts, shares out tasks, initiates meetings to discuss who does what, does future planning, and so on, all of which are managerial activities (Sullivan 1997). Perhaps ironically, they are highly valued in the labour market. Linked to the role of household manager is the act of caring, which Sevenhuijsen (see Chapter 6) points out is not just a safety net in times of misfortune but a social process that demands ongoing and daily attention. I am relying here on a distinction between 'indirect care' and 'direct care'. 'Indirect care' is care that is managed by the carer but not necessarily done by her. This is in opposition to 'direct care', where a carer (wife, daughter, mother, friend, etc.) meets the caring needs directly by doing the work herself. This distinction is closely related to Tronto's (1993) distinction between 'caring for', which involves the acceptance of *responsibility* for the needs of others whether or not one does the work oneself, and 'taking care of', which highlights practical *competence* in the day-to-day routines of caring work.

If women are in paid work, particularly if it involves long hours and high pay, the majority of the caring activities may be contracted out, either by buying in labour or by using publicly provided welfare provision (depending on the welfare state type). The point that I wish to emphasise is that indirect care also involves a range of management activities, including recruitment of carers, monitoring of quality and making financial arrangements.

Having set out the possible roles that make up, as I see it, the sphere of unpaid domestic work, I now ask what might be the effect if either the sphere of paid work or one of the sub-spheres of unpaid work expanded.

Interdependency: a knock-on effect

The expansion of one or other of the spheres or sub-spheres can happen for a range of reasons. If, for example, a parent becomes more infirm, then the role of 'daughter' is likely to expand. It will not only expand in a temporal sense but also in terms of direct and/or indirect care, emotional work, household management and *charge mentale*. Focusing on the expansion of the paid work sphere, we could foresee that the knock-on effect on the sphere of unpaid work and its sub-spheres could be similar. Again, on the surface the expansion will be temporal, but it could also affect the sub-spheres of unpaid work in various ways. For example, the roles of mother and daughter may change, in that direct care may be replaced by indirect care. However, indirect care implies an increase in household management –

recruitment of paid carers, monitoring the quality of care and making financial arrangements.

The wife/partner role could change in different ways, depending on the 'gender arrangements' in individual households or in broad cultures. The role of household worker would also sustain a knock-on effect from the expansion of the paid work sphere. One possible effect could be the contracting out of housework, subject to a sufficiently high level of financial resources being available. Another effect might be that the husband/partner takes on more of the household worker role. A further knock-on effect of an increase in the paid work sphere could be that emotional work would increase. Relationships with children, parents and partners could well become more demanding, although possibly only for a transitional period. The *charge mentale* associated with the effort of managing these changes is very likely to become weightier.

How does this scenario relate to employment behaviour? It seems likely that some women will make a judgement that employment mobility (in any of its three types) would entail an increase not only in the time devoted to paid work but also in that devoted to unpaid work. A woman's decision – which would clearly have economic consequences both individually and collectively – might well be to maintain the *status quo* and thereby to preserve balance, both in her life and in that of the household.

However, the model as presented here gives the impression that no change is possible: that 'choice' represents only constraints. But gender relations are socially constructed and must therefore encompass the possibility of variation, given particular conditions. I now address the issue of how and in what circumstances the model can change. One way in which this could happen is through structural factors. In the second part of the chapter, I move on to a consideration of the impact of structure on the 'balance model'.

The impact of gendered cultures and the gender order

The 'balance model' is located within a range of social institutions and structures, all of which have the potential to affect economic decision making. I am referring here to Pfau-Effinger's (1998) 'gendered cultures' and 'gender order'. Several social structures have the potential to mediate the occurrence of imbalance arising from the expansion of the paid work sphere, as modelled above. They include:

- the welfare state type;
- the family/household type;
- the possibility of role change and flexibility in terms of domestic labour and emotional work, depending on cultural notions of power relations between women and men;
- the 'culture of acceptability' regarding the contracting out of unpaid work roles on a paid basis;

- the possibility that some occupations allow for the minimisation of conflict between the various spheres and sub-spheres of paid and unpaid work.

First, the welfare state type is a potentially mediating factor. There is a great deal of cross-national work showing that there are sharply differing levels and types of care provision in different types of welfare state (see, for example, Hill 1996 and all four sections of Chapter 4). Some welfare states have care systems that 'kick in' when households cannot or do not provide care for individual members; other types of welfare state do not. Does this mean that the balance model is only relevant to liberal welfare state regimes? In social democratic welfare state regimes (Esping-Andersen 1990) or weak breadwinner types (Lewis 1992; Sainsbury 1999), there is pervasive affordable childcare and care for older people. Since this would substitute for some aspects of the role of mother and/or daughter, balance could be maintained, because the expansion of the paid work sphere would be absorbed by welfare state provision. However, the distinction between what I have referred to as direct and indirect care still needs to be made, since state provision implies only direct care. Management of care (indirect care) still needs to be covered and, as was pointed out earlier, may in fact increase in magnitude as direct care decreases.

It seems probable, therefore, that although the policies of social democratic welfare states would make the maintenance of balance considerably easier, such policies do not necessarily obviate the problem (see Björnberg 1998 and Chapter 4.3). Furthermore, it is important not to fall into the mechanistic assumption that the existence of a policy will bring about a change of behaviour. It is quite possible, indeed probable, that actors act 'irrationally' in the face of policy implementation, as Duncan and Edwards (1997) point out in their discussion of the 'gendered moral rationalities' of lone parents.

Second, in households and societies where values about appropriate gender roles are less traditional (see Pfau-Effinger's (1998) concept of 'gender culture'), the nature of the wife/partner role may be more flexible. Gendered power relations in some households and in some cultures may be considerably more egalitarian than in others (Hochschild 1989). Where an egalitarian ideology prevails on either a micro or a macro level, the expansion of the paid work sphere might then be accommodated with relative ease, with the husband/partner taking on some or indeed all the unpaid work previously done by the wife/partner. However, the design of many men's jobs implies less availability to make a concession towards domestic labour, particularly in a long-hours culture (Fagan 2001). Fagan's analysis of the British Household Panel Survey shows that in 1995, 50 per cent of men worked more than forty-five hours per week and 29 per cent more than fifty hours. The figures for women were 15 and 9 per cent, respectively. Thus there are potentially profound implications for 'malestream' employment cultures if the 'life–work balance' issue is taken seriously and applied to both men and women.

Third, the family/household type is clearly relevant in that different types have different potential for accommodating an expansion in the paid work sphere. In households where there are two or more adults, the role of daughter or mother could potentially be shifted to another member of the family, for example the husband/partner or a sibling. However, not all families are able to substitute one or other of their members. The obvious example here is lone parents. As Duncan and Edwards point out, lone parents have no resident partner with whom to 'trade or bargain' (1997: 35). The assumption that the caring role could shift to a husband/partner may also be faulty. Here Pfau-Effinger's 'gender culture' comes into play: the power relations and the domestic division of labour within the family. The existence of another adult in a household does not automatically mean the sharing of domestic and caring work.

Fourth, there is also the context of cultural norms and values about what is the 'best' or 'right' decision. Pfau-Effinger (1998) refers to cultural norms and values about the 'correct' division of labour, arguing that these may vary quite considerably in different cultures and different welfare state types. They may also vary within countries (Forsberg 1998). Duncan and Edwards (1997, 1999) propose that women's economic decision making is based, at least partly, on what appears to them to be 'morally right'. Thus, decision making is not based on the foreseen consequences alone; people take decisions about caring because they feel that it is the right way to behave (see Chapter 12). They argue that this judgement varies in different social groups, with ethnicity being a particularly important variable.

A fifth factor bearing on the 'balance model' is that the type of job will also affect the degree of interaction between the unpaid work sphere and paid work. Some occupations have structural and institutional aspects that minimise conflict between the various spheres (Glucksmann 1998). Different occupations provide different opportunities for the balance between paid and unpaid work to be maintained, restored or put in jeopardy. There are similarities here with Crompton and Harris's (1998) 'career trajectory' approach, where they argue that different occupations provide different opportunities for 'lifecourse planning'. The structure of a professional medical career is such that an early decision can be taken to specialise in an area that offers better opportunities for unpaid and paid work to articulate reasonably smoothly. Bank managers, on the other hand, have fewer opportunities for such an approach to 'lifecourse planning'.

Advancement in many professions is dependent on employees being geographically mobile (Crompton and Sanderson 1990). The ability to be geographically mobile raises an interesting point, since it links to the distinction between occupational and organisational careers (Althauser and Kalleberg 1981). An occupation with a job ladder and requirements for pre-entry qualifications is categorised by Althauser and Kalleberg as 'occupational': human capital, in the form of pre-entry qualifications, is portable. On the other hand, an 'organisational' occupation is one where experience of a particular organisation is accrued and advancement is obtained within that organisation. The human capital accumulated in this way is not necessarily validated by other organisations. This restricts the ability to move to other organisations to achieve occupational advancement. Thus, if women are unable to fulfil the geographical mobility requirements of a typical occupational career, they may of necessity have to resort to an organisational model, even though they possess the necessary human capital in the form of formal pre-entry qualifications that would allow them to have an occupational career (Glover 2000).

On the other hand, some occupations have characteristics that make the maintenance of balance more easy. The obvious example here is teaching, an occupation whose structure probably gives the best possibility for a smooth articulation of paid and unpaid work. Working hours largely correspond to children's school hours, and after-school/holiday care is unlikely to be needed. Although the other spheres of unpaid work remain, a large amount of indirect care may be removed. As a result, *charge mentale* may be reduced.

A further characteristic of some parts of the education labour market is that the personal capital[4] that is required to gain advancement has a particular feature: the need for a local reputation. Evetts (1989) argues that being known and respected in a relatively contained local area is an important factor in primary teachers being promoted to headships. This means that one spatial consequence of the paid–unpaid work relationship – restriction on geographical mobility – is of little importance in this particular labour market. A contrast with this aspect of the education labour market is the scientific labour market (see Glover 2000). An institutional aspect of the scientific professions, particularly research posts, is that geographical mobility is expected by employers (O'Driscoll and Andersen 1994; Bowden 1995). Short-term contractual work is the norm and indeed may be seen as necessary training. Furthermore, particular specialisms may be scattered geographically.

The distinction between 'task-oriented' and 'clock-oriented' occupations is relevant here (Thompson 1967). Task-oriented employment, typically well paid and high status, in theory offers more autonomy and there is potential for flexibility of work schedules, providing that the tasks are performed satisfactorily. However, Fagan (2001) argues that this degree of autonomy, which has the potential to ease the unpaid/paid work clash, is notional. Although managerial posts are task-oriented, in reality they involve being 'on call' by clients/customers and/or by higher management. The habitus of these jobs has several components that are not conducive to 'work–life balance': hours are not fixed; they can be extended without notice at either end; a 'long-hours' climate is the norm especially in the UK; and geographical mobility and relocation are likely to be expected. The incursion of the private and the personal into the workplace is judged inappropriate, and spatial and temporal rights over individual employees are assumed. The personal capital required to succeed in such a habitus is therefore likely to be very different from that required in lower-level jobs. Evetts' (1994) work on women engineers provides evidence for this: she suggests that women deliberately opt for the technical expert 'practitioner' route because they know that the more time-demanding (and more highly paid) managerial route will not allow them to reconcile their private and public lives with any ease.

There may therefore be quite significant differences between occupational groups in terms of the habitus of higher-level positions. Some occupational groups may have a range of expectations that women who are trying to juggle the relationship between unpaid and paid work may find hard to fulfil without introducing what they judge to be the potential for crisis. The expectations that are most likely to cause this are:

- geographical mobility, whether in terms of relocation or in terms of travel-to-work times;
- day-to-day variation and unpredictability in terms of time and space;
- linear careers, with high-performance times occurring relatively early in the life cycle; and
- an employer's assumption that the private sphere should not impact on the sphere of paid work.

In such occupations, those who achieve advancement will bring with them a 'baggage' of personal capital that matches these expectations. In occupations with less stringent or more flexible expectations, occupational advancement can be achieved with a less demanding amount of personal capital. The greater the mismatch, the more unlikely that women will seek and/or gain advancement and the more likely, therefore, that the level of vertical segregation will be high.

Is the 'balance model' relevant only to women?

Does the model relate only to women, or could it also be meaningful to a growing number of men? In its discussion of the quest for balance in *Supporting Families* (1998), the government addresses parents, not just mothers. Is this a statement of reality or of wishful thinking? Evidence from time budget studies in the UK suggests that there is a slow growth in the number of young men who are participating more in the domestic division of labour (Anderson *et al.* 1994). Could it be that a growing number of young men take economic decisions as a function of the maintenance of balance between the spheres of paid and unpaid work?

There is a need for empirical work here. If it could be shown that a need to maintain the balance between paid and unpaid work was becoming a key factor in men's decision making about employment mobility, then it seems to me that this would be strong evidence for substantial cultural change. It is possible that the 'balance model' could measure change in the gendered domestic division of labour rather better than time budget studies can do.

Is the 'balance model' just a variation of rational choice theory?

Are individuals seeking to retain equilibrium in their lives and those of their households merely maximising personal utility and calculating opportunity costs? In my vision, actors are, as in rational choice theory, stopping before they act in order to count the likely cost. A calculation is being made. What I am saying could therefore be read as being similar to rational choice theory's insistence on self-interest as a basis for economic decisions. However, there seems to me to be an important difference: rather than self-interest, something more akin to *self-preservation* may be at the base of economic decisions about employment mobility. Women may well realise that an unbalanced 'juggling act' carries certain risks, for example in terms of health and personal welfare – and not just their own personal welfare, but also that of the immediate household. The welfare of others therefore influences decision making (see Chapter 12). In the 'balance model', calculations of consequences are being made, but these are not just economic consequences. Economic decision making can also relate to human survival and health, as Nelson (1993) proposes. Nelson's argument comes close to the idea of 'self-preservation' rather than neo-classical economics' 'self-interest'. She asks:

> Does it seem too prosaic or worldly to define economics as centrally concerned with the study of how humans, in interaction with each other and the environment, provide for their own survival and health?
>
> 1993: 34

Hakim (1991) has argued that many women choose to prioritise their domestic concerns over their 'commitment' to paid work. Is the 'balance model' saying essentially the same thing? I think not. First, a different conception of choice is used. This is not free choice; it has agency at its core, but it is a contingent decision, clearly dependent on many other structural and institutional factors. Second, although an economic decision that is made on the basis of weighing up the risks of household instability is a form of rationality, it is not the neo-classical conception of rationality. Third, it is not solely an individual decision: it is a socially negotiated decision taken by an individual in the immediate context of the household, possibly together with other household members, and in the broader context of macro-institutional and -structural factors, such as the welfare state type, gendered cultures and the gender order, together with the structural aspects of different occupational labour markets.

Fourth, as Chattoe (see Chapter 14) points out, traditional rational choice theory is particular about what generates utility; it has a tendency to deny that utility can be anything other than material. The focus on material rather than social goals, says Chattoe, excludes the possibility that utility can come from interaction and joint activity. My argument is that the maintenance of household balance is a primary object of choice. In this perspective, the objective of action is not to maximise utility for oneself but to sustain the viability of a network of relationships that do not come into the realm of choice.

Duncan and Edwards (1997, 1999) argue that it is possible for people to act out of self-interest without acting as 'rational economic man'. Rationality need not be about selfishness (Folbre 1994). In the 'balance model', decisions are rational according to the circumstances as actors perceive them at a particular moment – that is, they are contingent. My approach here has links with Popper's 'situational logic', which takes as its starting point that 'our actions are to a very large extent explicable in terms of the situation in which they occur' (Popper 1945; 1957).[5] It also has links with Sevenhuijsen's idea that 'situated questions of responsibility and agency' guide actors through recurrent moral dilemmas (Chapter 6).

Conclusion

The traditional dual-role perspective contains an over-simple and mechanistic assumption that by freeing one domestic role (that of the mother, for example, by providing public childcare), there will be a concomitant freeing of another role, that of paid worker. The 'balance model' criticises dual-role theory by suggesting that rather than having an additive model composed of two or three spheres, there is a much more complex and interactive situation.

The balance model also provides a critique of dual-role theory's faith in the power of policy to bring about a reconciliation between the spheres. The complexity and interconnectedness of economic decision making suggests that the introduction of so-called 'family-friendly' policy, such as those suggested in the Green Papers on *Supporting Families* (Home Office 1998) and *Work and Parents: Competitiveness and Choice* (DTI 2000), could have patchy effects.

My proposition is, in summary, that women's decision making about employment mobility (moving into the labour market, moving from part-time to full-time employment, moving into a promoted post) is dependent on a wide range of cultural, institutional and structural factors. But at their core is an individual decision that relates to a wish to retain balance in the household. In many ways, this is a rational choice, but not the kind of rational choice that neo-classical economics accepts unproblematically. It is a 'contingent choice', which has been rationally arrived at in the light of a particular set of circumstances as they are perceived by the actors. The term 'contingent choice' acknowledges that women are not helpless victims of circumstances; rather, they are active decision makers. At the same time, it needs to be recognised that the economic decision making of many women is affected (either constrained or freed) by a range of structural factors. These include women's social and economic circumstances, the macro-level social policy framework, the norms and values of the particular culture in which they are located and features of specific occupations. The core of my argument is that the preferences and tastes that define rational economic decision making may relate, at least partly, to the desire or need to maintain balance between paid and unpaid work. From this point of view, some economists' concept of self-interest could be seen rather more as 'self-preservation' – a 'drawing in of horns' in the face of unanticipated and uncontrollable outcomes. But while this cautious approach might make sense to the individual, there are implications for those individuals (largely women) who decide that the maintenance of balance must take priority over employment mobility. These implications relate primarily to the labour market and include such things as male–female pay differentials, and vertical and horizontal sex segregation: features that are the basis of women's disadvantage in the labour market.

Whether the model presents an over-socialized version of the world would have to be tested empirically. Research might show that women's experience of the world – and decision making about employment in particular – is considerably more constrained by structural and institutional features than is the case for men.

Notes

1 This chapter is an edited version of a paper presented to the European Sociological Association in Amsterdam in August 1999. In an earlier version of this paper, presented to the ESRC seminar series 'Parenting, motherhood and paid work: rationality and ambivalence' at South Bank University, UK, on 16 April 1999, I argued that ecological thinking about ecosystems and the maintenance of balance within an ecosystem was useful. In this version of the paper, I have set aside ecological thinking. The latter was a vehicle that originally helped me to conceptualise the 'balancing act' and the knock-on consequences of one sphere taking up more time.

2 I have argued elsewhere that it is important to make a distinction between the roles of wife/partner and mother (Glover 1994). Through secondary analysis of the UK Labour Force Survey I showed that the roles of wife/partner and mother had a statistically independent effect on whether women were in promoted or unpromoted posts. My study looked at two occupational groups, teachers and office workers, but it seems reasonable to suppose that the results are generalisable.

3 The Office of National Statistics is preparing a new sample survey, the Time Use Survey, which should provide more comprehensive data. However, it is not clear that the 'household manager' role will be identified in this data set, although the pilot study was an advance on previous time budget methodology in that it sought to identify tasks that were carried out simultaneously.

4 I am using the term 'personal capital' to mean a 'baggage' of resources that individuals bring to the labour market: resources that constitute a match or mismatch in terms of the habitus of particular occupations. This seems to me to be akin to Folbre's idea of 'assets' (1994: 40). In the UK, men are more likely to

possess personal capital that matches the habitus. The concept of personal capital is defined by Himmelweit (Chapter 12) as 'that stock of all past personal, consumption and other experiences that affect that individual's current and future preferences'.

5 A criticism of the theory of situational logic is that it can appear to be over-deterministic: our situations dictate our actions, not the other way round. In later work, Popper prefers the term 'situational analysis', which he defines as 'a certain kind of tentative or conjectural explanation of some human action which appeals to the situation in which the agent finds himself [*sic*]' (Popper 1972: 178–9). This is an application of what he calls the 'rationality principle': an action is 'adequate to [the agent's] situation as he [*sic*] saw it' (1972: 179).

References

Althauser, R. and Kalleberg, A. (1981) 'Firms, occupations and the structure of labor markets', in I. Berg (ed.) *Sociological Perspectives on Labor Markets*, New York: Academic Press.

Anderson, M., Bechhofer, F. and Gershuny, J. (1994) *The Social and Political Economy of the Household*, Oxford: Oxford University Press.

Björnberg, U. (1998) 'Family orientation among men: a process of change in Sweden', in E. Drew, R. Emerek and E. Mahon (eds) *Women, Work and the Family in Europe*, London: Routledge.

Blumberg, R.L. (1991) *Gender, Family and Economy: The Triple Overlap*, Thousand Oaks, Calif.: Sage.

Bowden, V. (1995) 'Managing to make a difference: a study of career diversity among men and women research scientists', unpublished PhD thesis, School of Management, University of Manchester Institute of Science and Technology.

Buxton, J. (1999) *Ending the Mother War, Starting the Workplace Revolution*, Basingstoke: Macmillan.

Carling, A. (1991) *Social Division*, London: Verso.

Connell, R. (1987) *Gender and Power: Society, the Person and Sexual Politics*, Cambridge: Polity Press.

Crompton, R. (1998) 'Employment and caring: changes in the gender division of labour', plenary address to Work, Employment & Society Conference, Cambridge, September.

Crompton, R. and Harris, F. (1998) 'Gender relations and employment: the impact of occupation', *Work, Employment & Society* 12(2): 297–315.

Crompton, R. and Sanderson, K. (1990) *Gendered Jobs and Social Change*, London: Unwin Hyman.

Dale, A. (1986) 'Differences in car usage for married men and married women', *Sociology* 20(1): 91–2.

Department for Trade and Industry (DTI) (2000) *Work and Parents: Competitiveness and Choice*, London: DTI.

Devine, F. (1994) 'Segregation and supply: preferences and plans among "self-made" women', *Gender, Work and Organization* 1(2): 94–109.

Duncan, A., Giles, C. and Webb, S. (1995) *The Impact of Subsidising Childcare*, Manchester: Equal Opportunities Commission.

Duncan, S. and Edwards, R. (1997) 'Lone mothers and paid work – rational economic man or gendered moral rationalities?' *Feminist Economics* 3(2): 29–61.

—— (1999) *Lone Mothers, Paid Work and Gendered Moral Rationalities*, London: Macmillan.

Esping-Andersen, G. (1990) *The three worlds of welfare capitalism*, Cambridge: Polity Press.

Evetts, J. (1989) 'The internal labour market for primary teachers', in S. Acker (ed.) *Teachers, Gender and Careers*, Brighton: Falmer Press.

—— (1994) 'Women and career in engineering: continuity and change in the organisation', *Work Employment & Society* 8(1): 101–12.

Fagan, C. (2001) 'The temporal reorganisation of employment and household rhythm of work schedules: the implications for gender and class relations', *The American Behavioural Scientist* 44(7): 1199–212.

Ferber, M. and Nelson, J. (1993) *Beyond Economic Man*, Chicago: University of Chicago Press.

Folbre, N. (1994) *Who Pays for the Kids?* London: Routledge.

Forsberg, G. (1998) 'Regional variations in the gender contract: gender relations in labour markets, local politics and everyday life in Swedish regions', *Innovation* 11: 191–210.

Ginn, J., Arber, S., Brannen, J., Dale, A., Dex, S., Elias, P., Moss, P., Pahl, J., Roberts, C., Rubery, J. and Walby, S. (1996) 'Feminist fallacies? A reply to Hakim on women's employment', *British Journal of Sociology* 47(1): 167–74.

Glover, J. (1994) 'Women teachers and white-collar workers: domestic circumstances and paid work', *Work, Employment & Society* 8(1): 87–100.

—— (2000) *Women and Scientific Employment*, Basingstoke: Macmillan.

Glucksmann, M. (1998) "'What a difference a day makes': a theoretical and historical explanation of temporality and gender', *Sociology* 32(2): 239–58.

Granovetter, M. (1992) 'Economic action and social structure: the problem of embeddedness', in M. Granovetter and R. Swedberg (eds) *The Sociology of Economic Life*, Boulder, Colo.: Westview Press, 53–81 [reprinted from *AJS* 91: 481–510].

Haicault, M. (1984) 'La gestion ordinaire de la vie en deux', *Sociologie du Travail* 3: 268–77.

—— (1994) 'Pertes de savoirs familiaux, nouvelle professionnalité du travail domestique: quels sont les liens avec le système productif?' *Recherches Féministes* 7(1): 125–38.

Hakim, C. (1991) 'Grateful slaves and self-made women: fact and fantasy in women's work orientations', *European Sociological Review* 7: 101–21.

—— (1995) 'Five feminist myths about female employment', *British Journal of Sociology* 46(3): 429–55.

Hanson, S. and Pratt, G. (1991) 'Job search and the occupational segregation of women', *Annals of the Association of American Geographers* 81(2): 229–53.

Hill, M. (1996) *Social Policy: A Comparative Analysis*, Hemel Hempstead: Prentice Hall.

Hochschild, A. (1989) *The Second Shift*, Harmondsworth: Viking Penguin.

Home Office (1998) *Supporting Families, London*: HMSO.

Humphries, J. (1995) 'Economics, gender and equal opportunities', in J. Humphries and J. Rubery (eds) *The Economics of Equal Opportunities*, Manchester: Equal Opportunities Commission.

Laurie, H. (1993) '"A woman's 'choice?" Household contexts and women's labour market decisions', paper presented at the Annual Conference of the British Sociological Association, University of Essex, 5–9 April.
Leira, A. (1992) *Welfare States and Working Mothers*, Cambridge: Cambridge University Press.
Lewis, J. (1992) 'Gender and the development of welfare regimes', *Journal of European Social Policy* 2: 159–73.
Lewis, S. and Lewis, J. (1996) *The Work–Family Challenge*, London: Sage.
Myrdal, A. and Klein, V. (1956) *Women's Two Roles*, London: Routledge & Kegan Paul.
Nelson, J. (1993) 'The study of choice or the study of provisioning? Gender and the definition of economics', in M. Ferber and J. Nelson (eds) *Beyond Economic Man*, Chicago: University of Chicago Press.
Oakley, A. (1976) *Housewife*, London: Allen Lane.
O'Driscoll, M. and Anderson, J. (1994) 'Women in science: attitudes of university students towards a career in research', London: Wellcome Trust Unit for Policy Research in Science and Medicine.
Office for National Statistics (ONS) (1998) *Social Focus on Men and Women*, London: HMSO.
Pfau-Effinger, B. (1998) 'Gender cultures and the gender arrangement – a theoretical framework for cross-national gender research', *Innovation* 11(2): 147–66.
Popper, K. (1945) *The Open Society and Its Enemies*, London: Routledge & Kegan Paul.
—— (1957) *The Poverty of Historicism*, London: Routledge & Kegan Paul.
—— (1972) *Objective Knowledge*, Oxford: Clarendon Press.
Sainsbury, D. (1999) *Gender and Welfare State Regimes*, New York: Oxford University Press.
Social and Community Planning Research (SCPR) (1998) *British and European Social Attitudes*, Aldershot: Ashgate.
Sichtermann, B. (1988) 'The conflict between housework and employment', in J. Jenson, E. Hagen and C. Reddy (eds) *Feminization of the Labour Force*, Cambridge: Polity Press.
Spain, D. and Bianchi, S. (1996) *Balancing Act: Motherhood, Marriage and Employment among American Women*, New York: Russell Sage Foundation.
Sullivan, O. (1997) 'Time waits for no (wo)man: an investigation of the gendered experience of domestic time', *Work, Employment & Society* 31: 221–40.
Supporting Families (1998). London: HMSO.
Thompson, E.P. (1967) 'Time, work-discipline and industrial capitalism', *Past and Present* 38: 56–97.
Tronto, J. (1993) *Moral Boundaries: A Political Argument for an Ethic of Care*, New York: Routledge.

14 Computer simulation of family practices

Edmund Chattoe

Introduction

This chapter begins by briefly defining computer simulation and distinguishing it from two related techniques. The following section discusses existing uses of computer simulation in understanding family practices. Three main approaches can be identified: microsimulation for demography and policy analysis; rule-based models in anthropology; and agent-based models of the emergence of social complexity. I will use these three cases to discuss the implications of the computer simulation approach in more detail. In particular, I shall try to show how simulation avoids the excessive simplifying assumptions of other formal approaches like rational choice while managing to make effective use of rich qualitative data. In doing this, I hope to suggest that formality and excessive abstraction need not be synonymous. In the next section, I will list aspects of family behaviour that seem essential to plausible simulation and argue that current modelling explores these only in a fragmentary way. The final section will then illustrate the requirements of an *integrated* simulation of family behaviour using the theory of gendered moral rationalities (Duncan and Edwards 1999) as a case study.

The chapter has two deliberate limitations: first, it is not intended to be an exhaustive literature survey; second, although the proposed simulation is described in sufficient detail that it could be built, it does not yet exist and results will not be reported. Neither of these objectives could be satisfied effectively in the space available, so they have not been attempted.

What is computer simulation?

Theories of social behaviour are traditionally presented in two ways. The older method is to provide a verbal description. This description typically involves claims about cause and effect or social process. A good example is the series of interactions and cognitive processes by which an individual is labelled deviant and may embark on a deviant career (Downes and Rock 1998: 182–209). In contrast to the verbal approach are a variety of formal methods of representing theories. The paradigm case is the representation of decisions as constrained optimisation forming the basis of most modern economics. The verbal approach is typically criticised for its informality. Stages can easily be left out of the chain of reasoning and, in addition, the net effects of a number of interacting factors are often counterintuitive. A simple but interesting example is provided by the work of Schelling (1971). Imagine a world consisting of a regular grid like a chessboard. On this grid live two kinds of people – red and blue. Each kind has a preference for a minimum percentage of immediate neighbours belonging to the same kind. If any individual cannot satisfy this preference, he/she migrates randomly to an empty square nearby. What is the highest tolerated percentage of neighbours of the other kind that will produce a society of discrete clusters, that is where areas on the grid are occupied only by a single kind? (The implications of Schelling's model for cities in 1960s America should be clear!) Intuition suggests that some degree of racism will be needed for such a result; that is, individuals will require the majority of their neighbours to be of the same type if they are not to migrate. In fact, a figure of only about 30 per cent will still produce clustering. Thus clusters occur even when individuals of both types are quite happy to be in a significant minority. The lesson is that even for an extremely simple model, individual interaction can produce counterintuitive macroscopic effects that the verbal description does not make clear. At the other extreme, formal (usually mathematical or statistical) representations of social processes are criticised for the extreme simplifications that they are obliged to make (see Chapter 12 for the case of economics and families). Furthermore, these simplifications are not empirically motivated but typically stem from the need to produce soluble sets of equations (Chattoe 1996). A basic problem with formal models is that they conflate theory constructs with individual behaviour (see Chattoe 2000a).

In contrast to both these approaches, computer simulation involves the representation of a social process as a computer program.[1] In this respect, it is a formal method in that all the assumptions of the model must be spelled out in the program. Unlike a mathematical model, however, the social process is typically represented in an explicit (rather than abstract or theory-laden) form. This means that running the program does not involve solving anything but simply unfolding the simulated social process.

For example, a mathematical model of supply and demand using differential calculus will aggregate consumer preferences into a demand curve, aggregate the supply curves for individual producers and then solve for the aggregate supply and demand curves to determine the price that clears the market. Subsidiary assumptions about the shapes of the demand and supply curves will be required if this process is to succeed. By contrast, a simulation program for market interaction will represent the shopping trips of consumers and the production decisions of individual firms explicitly (Chattoe 1999). Producers with surplus stock will either have to lower their prices or produce less. Consumers will adapt their expectations as they visit different producers and gain information about market conditions.

Constraints on the structure of this program are not imposed by the formal needs of the theory but by the logic of the explicitly represented social process: for example, producers cannot sell stock they do not have. Although the traditional supply and demand curves can be reconstructed by experiment, running the simulation repeatedly with different input costs, consumer preferences and producer prices, they are correctly treated as *emerging* from the individual interactions of producers and consumers rather than as having any independent existence. One could just as easily use the same simulation to generate evolving histories of the social networks arising from repeated interactions, or the levels of consumer surplus arising from different producer inventory strategies.

For the time being, this abstract definition is adequate to distinguish computer simulation from two related techniques, although this will be developed and illustrated further in the next section. The easier technique to distinguish is also often referred to as 'simulation' but could more usefully be described as 'role playing' (Osmond 1979; Jones 1980; Finger *et al.* 1993).[2] This involves a group of individuals adopting *roles*, such as negotiators from different countries in a United Nations committee. The group simulates the interactions that take place from the perspective of the roles they have adopted. This is obviously an interesting approach to teaching, particularly when the material to be learned is not easily codified or when issues emerge in interaction. As such, role playing has been used both in the teaching of family sociology and in family therapy. Nonetheless, it is clear that it is a totally different technique from computer simulation and will not be discussed further.

The other technique is harder to distinguish, because it also uses computer programming to represent social theories. However, it does this in a way that is importantly different. In this *instrumental* use of computers, the analytical character of the original formal theory (particularly its strong simplifying assumptions) remain unchanged. The computer is simply a tool to handle the difficulties imposed by those assumptions. Such techniques are often used in econometrics, where the basic rationality assumptions of the neo-classical market model remain unchanged. For example, it may be very difficult to find the optimum of a complex function analytically. Alternatively, one can use an iterative hill-climbing computer program to find the optimum. However, this use of computers does not question the empirical relevance of the function specified or answer the more general question about whether optimisation is an appropriate representation of social behaviour.

By contrast, the purpose of *descriptive* computer simulations (like the artificial market described above) is to represent explicitly those aspects of social interaction and cognitive process that are felt to be relevant to the explanation of a particular domain.[3] As with any kind of theorising, the challenge is to abstract effectively from the richness of the problem. Having provided this definition, the rest of this chapter will refer to descriptive computer simulation as 'simulation'.

Existing simulations of family behaviour

Simulations of family behaviour can be divided into three broad groups.[4]

Microsimulation for demography and policy analysis

Microsimulation (Gilbert and Troitzsch 1999: 53–73) is a technique in which a real population of individuals is modelled by a statistically representative subset of database records with a number of attributes such as age, job and marital status. These simulated populations are initialised using real data from official statistics in a base year and then have their attributes updated periodically in accordance with measured probabilities for important life transitions. For example, suppose that women aged between 21 and 25 have an 8 per cent chance per year of becoming pregnant. During every simulated year, each record with the correct gender attribute (female) and age range (21–25) will be assigned a random number draw between 1 and 100, and those scoring 8 or less will be considered to have fallen pregnant that year. At the same time, the age of each simulated individual will be increased by 1, so that some women at the top of the age range will move into a new bracket and be subject to a different age-specific fertility rate. As van Imhoff and Post (1998) point out in their recent survey of demographic microsimulation, this approach is important in population projection because of cohort effects and the interactions between attributes. (Simulating a representative population and grossing up is also advantageous in terms of computational economy.) Similar approaches are used in exploring the implications of transfer payments and other forms of family policy. In this way, it is possible to look not only at the total sum of money transferred but also at the distribution to household types (Harding 1996; Redmond *et al.* 1998) under different assumptions about eligibility rules.

Such approaches are deliberately instrumental.[5] Transition probabilities do not explain behaviour in the same sense that social processes do. The fact that 8 per cent of women between 20 and 25 become pregnant each year does not explain why women (or even types of women) actually start families. Such reasons may include deliberate choice, the effect of social norms and attainment of adequate financial or other resources. This is important because estimated transition probabilities are likely to become increasingly inaccurate as a result of social change. For example, starting a family no longer involves marriage as a precondition. This changing norm will alter age-specific fertility rates, particularly as the menopause approaches, but not *vice versa*. Interestingly, researchers developing microsimulation models of transfer payments typically exclude any assumptions about behavioural impacts because policy makers find them contentious. Needless to say, a refusal to model the behavioural effects of transfer payments on labour market participation, for example, does not mean that these effects cease to occur! In practice, the attributes that microsimulation uses tend to be the supposedly objective and quantitative descriptions that can easily be gleaned from surveys. Dynamic social processes like the formation and dissolution of friendships, the transmission of information, normative control through social networks and even socialisation are not considered. This means that these models will fail to produce sensible policy prescriptions to the extent that these social processes do in fact influence real behaviour. Fairly clearly, they do!

As a largely instrumental technique, microsimulation will not have a great deal to contribute to the subsequent discussion. Nonetheless, one important feature of computer programming is illustrated. The fact that the updating of attributes can occur in a number of different ways is important for what follows. The social process of ageing – that one gets older by a year every year without fail until one dies – is different from the probabilistic process of pregnancy and different again from the linking of records that occurs when two individuals partner or start a family. The interactions of these different mechanisms – as when a woman moves from one age bracket to another – may generate aggregate consequences that are very hard to infer from the transition probabilities and updating rules alone. Indeed, this is why microsimulation has proved relatively successful in the policy arena.

Rule-based simulations in anthropology

The emergence of aggregate structure from individual rules is also a concern of simulation in anthropology.[6] Many anthropologists still share a belief that traditional societies are substantially governed by complex and relatively stable sets of norms, taboos, practices, traditions, and so on. Many classic anthropological studies, like those of the Trobriand *kula* ring (Malinowski 1922) and Azande witchcraft oracles (Evans-Pritchard 1937), set out to show how these complexes of beliefs and norms were effective mechanisms for regulating the societies in which they occurred and gave order to the lives of participants. Nearly all of these descriptions were verbal rather than formal. The dangers of this approach, as with all functionalist approaches, are that of neglecting facts that do not fit the explanation and, conversely, of assuming that particular practices were necessary when they were merely contingent. An interesting line of simulation in anthropology thus involves carrying out counterfactual experiments in simulated societies that represent the key features of ethnographic and other data. Small (1999, 2000) has developed a simulation model of society in Tonga, which she has used to explore the complex rules around marriage and status inheritance. To take a single example, sisters in family lines are expected to marry upwards in terms of status. However, this norm cannot consistently be applied to the oldest sister of the highest line, since there is no available male of higher status she can marry. Many societies with this norm also have a separate norm of the virgin sister, that the eldest female of the highest line must not marry or have children at all, or can only marry an outsider. Small draws the obvious conclusion that this additional norm serves to protect the marrying upwards norm by making it consistently applicable. So far, this is a fairly standard functionalist explanation. In addition, however, she is able to show how removing the norm of the virgin sister impacts dynamically on the status of simulated family lines.

This approach has three important implications. First, it breaks the traditional association between formal theories and quantitative survey data. The flexibility of simulation as a method of representing social processes is illustrated by its ability to deal with the richness of ethnographic (or at least qualitative) data. This is important because much current research on the sociology of the family is qualitative and rightly resistant to the misapplication of oversimplified formal theories such as rational choice (see Chapter 12). Second, it shows that simulation can represent not only accounting rules, of the sort used in microsimulation (for example age, where each individual increases by one year every year), but also cognitive rules or *practices*. *If* the virgin sister norm exists in a particular society and is endorsed by its members, this is what happens in the unfolding of the social process. The final implication is a negative one. Unlike microsimulation models, which are deliberately set up not to be descriptive, rule-based anthropological models might be an extremely interesting technique for the study of contemporary family life. Unfortunately for the theorist, society is no longer traditional (if indeed it ever was), and commonly agreed ways of doing things have largely fallen by the wayside. Furthermore, anthropologists have pointed out that rules are actually negotiated and applied selectively, even in so-called traditional societies (Cleaver 2000). Choices between alternatives and the deliberate adoption of practices, roles, opinions and lifestyles are now not just permitted but frequently expected, although rule-based simulation may still have a role as a first approximation. However, modelling based on societal rules will not be sufficient. This leads to the third simulation approach that may be relevant to the study of family practices.

Multi-agent simulations of emerging social order

Multi-agent simulations (Gilbert and Troitzsch 1999: 158–94) relax the assumption of societal rules and represent both the actions of individuals in an environment and the relevant mental content (typically also in the form of *individual* rules) that motivates that action. Agents may thus have beliefs about the state of the world (including other agents), their own capabilities and the dispositions of other agents towards them. These rules can be modified by adaptation processes and transmitted from one agent to another. Two important examples are a simulation of fishing strategies in Mali (Bousquet *et al.* 1994) and simulations of the emergence of social complexity in the Upper Paleolithic period, based on the EOS simulation developed by Doran and others (Doran 1998; Mayers 1995). Bousquet *et al.* demonstrate the different aggregate effects on fish stocks if fishermen take decisions as rational individuals, using socially transmitted information and on the basis of anthropological norms like a tradition that one tribe tends to fish a particular river. This approach illustrates that there is nothing privileged about rational choice. It is an empirical claim about the cognitive processes (whether conscious or otherwise) used by individuals that could simply be false. More importantly, it shows that different adaptation mechanisms may be more or less effective in different environments (Chattoe 1999).

This approach is obviously important for understanding contemporary family practice. It permits not only dynamic behaviour, as the first two techniques do, but it also allows us to represent systems that are both individual and social. Individuals may take decisions, but the decision rules they use, the norms they observe, the data they base decisions on and the emotional consequences of their actions are almost certain to depend on the wider society.[7] It is to these distinctive features of contemporary family life that I now turn.

What do family simulations need to explain?

Largely by implication, I have suggested that the existing simulations do not yet engage with the core of contemporary family research. In this section, I plan to make this claim more explicit by outlining a number of key features of life in contemporary families that seem essential to a plausible simulation. Family life is not just demographic transition; nor does it typically follow society-wide rules (except in special cases like serious law breaking). Although the multi-agent simulations are much closer to what is required in methodological terms, the simulations of Bousquet *et al.* deal with a single aspect of life (fishing) in terms that are still basically individualistic. Similarly, the EOS simulations explore the emergence of only the very earliest forms of social organisation.

The role of social networks in the organisation of social life has long been recognised (Bott 1957). Who we meet and interact with clearly has a crucial role in the information we obtain, the decision processes we learn, the norms we enforce and those we have enforced on us. Families are fundamental cliques in social networks, with cohabitation ensuring frequent exchange of information and (where appropriate) possibilities for intense normative control.[8] The flavour of family life is dictated by such factors as whether spouses (and perhaps children) have significantly different social networks, resulting in potential conflict, novelty and inter-generational contact. The extent and nature of social networks at different stages of the lifecourse is also an important factor in the life world of young parents, the poor and the elderly. Simulations of the *dynamics* of social networks, which investigate the processes by which network links are made and broken (Carley 1999), will be an important component of any integrated family simulation.[9]

Interestingly, social network data are often collected by reference to joint activities, asking respondents to name those they go to the pub with, or talk about politics with, but the implications of joint activities on the evolution of networks seem to have been largely neglected. Furthermore, the process by which joint activities occur – time planning – has also been disregarded (Chattoe 2000c). Opportunities to form network links depend on joint activities, whether they are chance meetings on trains or daily greetings in the office corridors. Conversely, the existence of network links gives rise to a presumption of joint activities. Relationship formation may lead from meetings in public venues to meetings at home and ultimately to cohabitation and joint performance of household activities like shopping. Young children require substantial supervision, and their needs must always be compatible with proposed activities. Families are then characterised by a significant quantity of joint activities, and the nature of those activities (child-centred, individualistic, work-related, fixed, improvised) is also a key aspect of lifestyle. This approach may also cast additional light on the problem of defining families and increasingly fluid social relationships. A father – as opposed to a biological parent – may be someone who does fathering activities in a fatherly way.

One important implication of the combination of forming social networks and planning joint activities is differential association. The people one meets and interacts with are highly unlikely to be a representative sample or serve as a balanced source of information. This is likely to result in social differentiation, as groups with different views or life circumstances fail to encounter each other. Theories of deviance suggest that this is likely to produce normative judgements as different groups try to normalise their experience. This is not the only source of normative interactions, but these are generally of considerable importance in setting the tone of family life. (Consider battles between teenage children and parents, or the revelation of an illicit affair.) In addition, a family group, sharing many activities and strong emotional ties, may form a very extreme subculture. This mechanism is stressed in the underclass debates but also in literature about the dark side of the family, where child abuse may be covered up, rationalised and denied by all members of a family rather than just the perpetrator and victim (Forward 1990).

The multi-agent approach has already shown that the use of different styles of decision making and adaptation must be supported empirically rather than by appeal to the tractability of theory. Choices may be made as a rational individual, under social influence, on moral grounds, by negotiation or under duress. Despite the work of Becker (1991), it seems hard to deny that an important characteristic of family life is that it is negotiated (Finch and Mason 1993; Smart and Neale 1999) and inflicted (Delphy and Leonard 1992; Grabrucker 1988) at least as often as it is calculated. If what makes the family distinctive is the kind of interactions that occur in it (negotiated rather than calculated), we would expect tensions to arise when different spheres come into conflict (Hochschild with Machung 1990; Sharpe 1984), and this is commonly observed to occur. Clashes between different value systems are another important source of normative judgements. Importantly, the idea of contextual value systems goes against the utilitarian presumption that choices are always commensurable, that they can be assigned an all-things-considered utility. This is a strong empirical claim that is not supported by our unpleasant experience of moral and other dilemmas (Walzer 1983: 3–30).

From the simulation perspective, we can operationalise the notion of different value systems by returning to the discussion of microsimulation and the updating of attributes. What makes a moral belief moral is not that it is a value assigned to an attribute called moral (or that it is the moral term in an all-things-considered utility function). What makes a belief moral is that it changes by a different *social* or *cognitive* process from other kinds of belief. If somebody claims that they have a moral belief that eating meat is wrong, but as soon as they hear about a cheap butcher, they rush to buy a steak, we do not credit their claim that the belief is a moral one. In this case, what causes a belief to be judged as moral is its relative stability in the light of shifts in the balance of personal interest.[10] Having said that, we recognise that one moral belief may be overridden by another, as when one eats meat to avoid hurting the feelings of an elderly relative. An important feature of the simulation approach is thus to be able to represent the parallel evolution of different *kinds* of mental state. As time passes, an individual may learn more facts about a phenomenon, their personal valuations and goals may change, they may change the way they take decisions, and they may encounter support or opposition from people they interact with (see Chapter 12). All these factors will affect when a decision is taken and also what that decision is.

Despite the discussion in the previous section, the utilitarian claim that everything can be reduced to commensurable costs and benefits still seems remarkably hard to refute in a convincing way. Even if the raw materials of decision are constantly changing, surely a decision is all things considered at the point when it is taken? Challenging this claim, and allowing simulated families to act in a moral fashion (whether gendered or not), can be tackled in two ways.

The first is to point out that rational choice is very particular about what generates utility.[11] It focuses on choices involving clearly defined end states, typically material rather than social ones. This excludes the possibility that a substantial amount of utility (both positive and negative) comes from normative interaction and joint activity. If we choose a particular course of action, apart from its intrinsic utility, there are also expectations about the reactions of others that we will weigh in the balance. These expectations, even if completely false, may play a major role in our decision. One reason for this is that there is no limit to the negative utility that others can inflict on us if they are sufficiently disgruntled: protracted sulking is the classic example manifested in joint activities. So far, it appears that expectations of social utility are no different from expectations about personal utility. Individuals can still make rational choices on the basis of expectations. But this similarity is deceptive. It is in the nature of normative interactions that other individuals are diverse and changing continuously, so it is almost impossible to make systematic predictions about the ultimate utility of a particular action. Furthermore, the meaning of a particular action cannot be fixed. Giving an adequate account of the action one took can moderate negative moral judgements, and this process is inevitably interactive and dynamic. In a world in which such social utilities are the dominant factor, individuals will not be able to make rational choices and will have to proceed adaptively or by negotiation.

The second factor is illustrated in an interesting way by the simulation approach. Rational choice recognises that individuals do not choose their preferences, but because it assumes a single style of decision, it fails to recognise that we may not choose that decision style either, at least in the short term. In practice, a moral action like diving into a river in an attempt to save a drowning child may be done literally without stopping to count the cost. This kind of connection between perception and action may be represented explicitly in the mental content of a simulated agent as a rule that is only triggered in certain circumstances. In other circumstances, a calculation process may be used. From the perspective of the simulator, all the rules, triggers and different ways of doing things are visible, but to the agent who lives them, this is not necessarily so. The agent cannot simply choose to be calculative in all circumstances. It may be that, over time, an agent whose moral actions lead to profound personal misery adapts psychologically by relaxing certain moral rules, but this is not a choice: it is something that happens to the mental content of the agent as the simulation unfolds.[12] Thus, in the same way that moral beliefs are distinguished from other beliefs by their process of evolution, so psychological aspects of mental content can be distinguished by the lack of control that the agent has over them.

To summarise, then, a meaningful notion of moral action (and of different styles of decision generally) requires a much better-developed theory of cognitive process than that provided in rational choice. I have discussed how multi-agent simulation is capable of modelling such a theory. As it turns out, what makes rational choice implausible is not that it is a formal method *per se* but that its limitations require too many inappropriate simplifying assumptions to ensure tractability. Multi-agent simulation, by contrast, is able to retain the formality without having to make such implausible simplifications. In the next section, I will use the theory of gendered moral rationalities (Duncan and Edwards 1999) and their impact on lone parents as a case study. The intention is to show how the capabilities of the multi-agent approach and the general requirements for a simulation of family behaviour might be integrated into a working simulation focusing on a specific policy issue.

Integrated simulation of family behaviour: gendered moral rationalities

Gendered moral rationalities – shared understandings about the morally correct and socially acceptable course of action – have been used to explore the uptake of paid work by lone parents (Duncan and Edwards 1999), and it is clear how aspects of the discussion of the previous section are relevant to this social domain. Such moral decisions by lone parents are influenced not only by the financial costs and benefits of different options (as traditional economic analysis tends to argue) but also equally (if not more so) on the time costs and benefits. Even if work is more lucrative, it may be impossible to schedule the activities of mother and child in compatible ways given constraints in labour markets and school organisation. Scheduling of child-care encounters frequent difficulties in dealing with school runs and unexpected illness.[13] As well as scheduling constraints, the resulting schedules are also evaluated in emotional and moral terms. The mother may be unwilling to accept a schedule that allows her too little time with the child. Such a schedule may also be censured by others, particularly if it impacts on the behaviour of the child in other social contexts (see Chapter 13).

Finding a compatible schedule determines the social networks that mothers and children are involved in. Scheduling problems may be addressed by taking turns to do a school run for multiple children, exchanging favours in covering for emergencies, and so on. These interactions and common interests are likely to lead to friendships and the formation of a subculture. Women who use the social network in an instrumental way or to pursue unpopular goals may be censured or excluded. Women excluded from the resources of such networks will be at an obvious disadvantage in finding compatible schedules. Women who find themselves in such networks are likely to evolve situational practices that are very different from those of non-working mothers or working women without children. These differences are likely to lead to normative interactions (gossip, snide comments, praise and offers of help) between groups. These interactions will impact on the sustainability of a particular schedule. (Imagine being the only working mother commuting to a distant male-dominated employer and contrast this with a local employer keen to retain women who recruits largely by word of mouth about its flexibility.)

In addition to the effects of household activity plans on creating, sustaining and dissolving social network links, such a system will be continually awash with communication, mediated by joint activities and network links. Information may include job opportunities, gossip, offers and requests for help, and accounts of other ways of doing things and their evaluation. This rich soup helps individuals to monitor their moral position, solve their scheduling problems, and so on.

It is clear that even a highly simplified multi-agent simulation of this process will be quite complex. Nonetheless, many of the ingredients (like models of dynamic networks and activity planning) are already being developed. Furthermore, we can see how such a model starts to capture the richness of a real social domain. Some lone mothers who are not working will be in that position for purely rational and economic reasons; others will be stabilised by a network of moral evaluations from other non-working mothers; and still others will be suffering constraints from compatibility of schedules. In such a complex system, simplistic changes in policy (presuming only a single type of decision-making strategy) may have unexpected or even counterproductive effects: these can be explored, at least tentatively, by simulation experiments.

Conclusion

This chapter was intended to serve three purposes: first, to introduce the reader to aspects of computer simulation relevant to the understanding of contemporary family practices; second, to sketch out what such a simulation would have to explain and how it might look using a case study of gendered moral rationalities; and, third, to illustrate how computer simulation has methodological (as well as practical) relevance through a discussion of the relations between rational decision making and morality. The possibilities of computer simulation make it clearer that the restrictive assumptions of rational choice are not a necessary aspect of all formal modelling but are contingent on a particular approach. Furthermore, by relaxing restrictive assumptions, the simulation framework is both able to make effective use of richer qualitative data and sharpen the research questions that need to be asked in future. The fact that rational choice cannot represent moral behaviour in an environmentally valid way does not mean that real people do not act morally or that moral talk can be discarded as inconsequential. It means that the theory is inadequate and needs either repairing or discarding.

Notes

1. For a more detailed discussion of computer simulation and illustrations of simulations, see Gilbert and Troitzsch (1999).
2. This technique is also referred to as 'gaming', which helpfully makes the distinction clearer.
3. This flexibility is important, as it makes simulation falsifiable. If a simulation is calibrated on some dimensions of the real system, it should also be able to track other dimensions on which it was not calibrated. The distinction between instrumental and descriptive simulation is discussed in more detail in Chattoe (1996, 2000b).
4. This summary of simulation as it pertains to the family is supported by the more detailed discussion of Halpin (1999). Interestingly, he barely mentions the family as a possible application. A fourth simulation technique, spatial simulation, based on cellular automata (Gilbert and Troitzsch 1999: 121–57) has been used to explore various processes of social differentiation (Hegselmann and Flache 1998; Klüver and Schmidt 1999). The Schelling example has already been discussed. These approaches are not discussed here because they have not yet been used specifically for studying families, although they might form a useful component of such a simulation.
5. Demographic studies have also been carried out using the system dynamics approach. See Gilbert and Troitzsch (1999: 27–52) for a discussion of the approach and Di Piazza and Pearthree (1999) for an interesting anthropological example featuring migration.

6 Dyke (1981) provides a useful, although now somewhat dated, survey of the uses of computer simulation in anthropology.
7 A basic attempt to develop a simulation model of contemporary family budgeting practices from interview data is illustrated by Chattoe and Gilbert (1997, 1999).
8 Although this approach allows strategic behaviour to be modelled, it should not be confused with game theory. Although game theory also models strategic behaviour, it is an offshoot of the rational choice approach and thus suffers from the same problems: extreme simplifying assumptions and conflation of theory constructs with the real mental content of actors. These weaknesses often lead to serious logical problems. In some games, a pair of players can act rationally (in the technical sense) only when each has established what the other is going to do!
9 Carley's model is agent-based in that network links depend on individual beliefs about the knowledge held by others. However, her model is applied mainly to pragmatic or task-focused interactions in the workplace, and it is not clear whether the same logic would apply to more social interactions.
10 We express this awareness by saying that we wish we did not care about a particular thing, while still recognising that we do. Although there may be steps that an individual can take to change their moral framework, these are often arduous and unreliable (Glover 1983).
11 The original utilitarian tradition was based on direct personal experiences of pleasure and pain. This was refined by economics into a formal approach expressed in terms of choices over clearly defined end states that has been accused of lacking any empirical content. It may be that the original approach was neglected too readily and captures some important features of everyday life.
12 The presumption that all mental content is transparent and voluntary has been smuggled from empiricism into utilitarianism and from there into rational choice. Empirically, it is not very plausible.
13 In fact, as I argue elsewhere (Chattoe and Gilbert 1999; Chattoe 2000c), financial outcomes are not typically processed in terms of comparing cash amounts but in terms of manageable lifestyles (activity schedules) that they support.

References

Becker, G.S. (1991) *A Treatise on the Family* (enlarged edition). Harvard, Mass.: Harvard University Press.

Bott, E. (1957) *Family and Social Network*, London: Tavistock.

Bousquet, F., Cambier, C., Mullon, C., Morand, P. and Quensiere, J. (1994) 'Simulating fishermen's society', in N. Gilbert and J. Doran (eds) *Simulating Societies: The Computer Simulation of Social Phenomena*, London: UCL Press.

Carley, K.M. (1999) 'On the evolution of social and organizational networks', *Research on the Sociology of Organizations* 16: 3–30.

Chattoe, E. (1996) 'Why are we simulating anyway? Some answers from economics', in K.G. Troitzsch, U. Mueller, N. Gilbert, N. Doran and J.E. Doran (eds) *Social Science Microsimulation*, Berlin: Springer-Verlag.

—— (1999) 'A co-evolutionary simulation of multi-branch enterprises', paper presented at the European Meeting on Applied Evolutionary Economics, Grenoble, 7–9 June: http://www.sociology.ox.ac.uk/chattoe.html

—— (2000a) 'Why is building multi-agent models of social systems so difficult? A case study of innovation diffusion', paper presented at the XXIV International Conference of Agricultural Economists, Berlin, 13–19 August: http://www.sociology.ox.ac.uk/chattoe.html

—— (2000b) 'Review of *Computational Techniques for Modelling Learning in Economics* edited by Thomas Brenner', *Journal of Evolutionary Economics* 10: 585–91.

—— (2000c) 'Good times and old clothes: the importance of time planning and time use in consumption', paper presented at the BSA Annual Conference 'Making Time/Marking Time', University of York, 17–20 April: http://www.sociology.ox.ac.uk/chattoe.html

Chattoe, E. and Gilbert, N. (1997) 'A simulation of adaptation mechanisms in budgetary decision making', in R. Conte, R. Hegselmann and P. Terna (eds) *Simulating Social Phenomena*, Berlin: Springer-Verlag, 401–18.

—— (1999) 'Talking about budgets: time and uncertainty in household decision making', *Sociology* 33: 85–103.

Cleaver, F. (2000) 'Moral ecological rationality, institutions and managing common property resources', *Development and Change* 31: 361–83.

Delphy, C. and Leonard, D. (1992) *Familiar Exploitation: A New Analysis of Marriage in Contemporary Western Societies*, Cambridge: Polity Press.

Di Piazza, A. and Pearthree, E. (1999) 'The spread of the "Lapita People": a demographic simulation', *Journal of Artificial Societies and Social Simulation* 2: http://www.soc.surrey.ac.uk/JASSS/2/3/4.html

Doran, J. (1998) 'Simulating collective misbelief', *Journal of Artificial Societies and Social Simulation* 1: http://www.soc.surrey.ac.uk/JASSS/1/1/3.html

Downes, D. and Rock, P. (1998) *Understanding Deviance: A Guide to the Sociology of Crime and Rule Breaking* (third edition). Oxford: Oxford University Press.

Duncan, S. and Edwards, R. (1999) *Lone Mothers, Paid Work and Gendered Moral Rationalities*, London: Macmillan.

Dyke, B. (1981) 'Computer simulation in anthropology', *Annual Review of Anthropology* 10: 193–207.

Evans-Pritchard, E.E. (1937) *Witchcraft, Oracles and Magic among the Azande*, Oxford: Clarendon Press.

Finch, J. and Mason, J. (1993) *Negotiating Family Responsibilities*, London: Tavistock/Routledge.

Finger, S.C., Elliott, J.E. and Remer, R. (1993) 'Simulation as a tool in family therapy research', *Journal of Family Therapy* 15: 365–84.

Forward, S. (1990) *Toxic Parents: Overcoming the Legacy of Parental Abuse*, London: Bantam.

Gilbert, N. and Chattoe, E. (2001) 'Simulating the social construction of categories', in B. Schmidt and N. Saam (eds) *Co-operative Agents: Applications in the Social Sciences*, Dordrecht: Kluwer Academic.

Gilbert, N. and Troitzsch, K.G. (1999) *Simulation for the Social Scientist*, Milton Keynes: Open University Press.

Glover, J. (1983) 'Self-creation', *Proceedings of the British Academy* 69: 445–71.

Grabrucker, M. (1988) *There's a Good Girl, Gender Stereotyping in the First Three Years of Life: A Diary*, London: Women's Press.

Halpin, B. (1999) 'Simulation in sociology', *American Behavioral Scientist* 42: 1488–508.

Harding, A. (ed.) (1996) *Microsimulation and Public Policy*, Amsterdam: North-Holland.

Hegselmann R. and Flache A. (1998) 'Understanding complex social dynamics: a plea for cellular automata based modelling', *Journal of Artificial Societies and Social Simulation* 1: http://www.soc.surrey.ac.uk/JASSS/1/3/1.html

Hochschild, A.R. with Machung, A. (1990) *The Second Shift: Working Parents and the Revolution at Home*, London: Piatkus.

Jones, K. (1980) *Simulations: A Handbook for Teachers*, London: Kogan Page.

Klüver, J. and Schmidt, J. (1999) 'Social differentiation as the unfolding of dimensions of social systems', *Journal of Mathematical Sociology* 23: 309–25.

Malinowski, B. (1922) *Argonauts of the Western Pacific*, London: Routledge.

Mayers, S.D. (1995) 'Modelling the emergence of social complexity using distributed artificial intelligence', unpublished MSc thesis, Department of Computer Science, University of Essex.

Osmond, M.W. (1979) 'The use of simulation games in teaching family sociology', *Family Co-ordinator* 28: 205–16.

Redmond, G., Sutherland, H. and Wilson, M. (1998) *The Arithmetic of Tax and Social Security Reform: A User's Guide to Microsimulation Methods and Analysis*, Cambridge: Cambridge University Press.

Schelling, T.C. (1971) 'Dynamic models of segregation', *Journal of Mathematical Sociology* 1: 143–86.

Sharpe, S. (1984) *Double Identity: The Lives of Working Mothers*, Harmondsworth: Penguin.

Small, C. (1999) 'Finding an invisible history: a computer simulation experiment (in virtual Polynesia)', *Journal of Artificial Societies and Social Simulation* 2: http://www.soc.surrey.ac.uk/JASSS/2/3/6.html

Small, C. (2000) 'The political impact of marriage in a virtual Polynesian society', in T.A. Kohler and G.J. Gumerman (eds) (2000) *Dynamics in Human and Primate Societies: Agent-based Modelling of Social and Spatial Processes*, New York: Oxford University Press.

Smart, C. and Neale, B. (1999) *Family Fragments?* Cambridge: Polity Press.

van Imhoff, E. and Post, W. (1998) 'Microsimulation methods for population projection', *Population: An English Selection* 10: 97–138.

Walzer, M. (1983) *Spheres of Justice: A Defence of Pluralism and Equality*, Oxford: Martin Robertson.

PART V
Conclusion

15 Families, moralities, rationalities and social change

Graham Crow

Introduction

Contemporary social change is understood by a number of prominent social theorists in terms of certain overarching trends, among which individualisation, democratisation and globalisation have particular significance for the analysis of families, social change and the state. The accounts of the profoundly unsettling implications for family relationships of the unfolding trend of individualisation provided by Beck and Beck-Gernsheim (1995, 1996) and Beck-Gernsheim (1998) have been widely discussed, as have Giddens's (1998) thesis concerning the democratisation of traditional family life and his related (1999) ideas about the impact of globalisation on intimate relationships within and beyond the family. As a result, there is much discussion of whether what is being witnessed is nothing less than the emergence of 'the *new* family' (Silva and Smart 1999), 'brave new families' (Stacey 1998), 'the nuclear family' (Simpson 1998) or, more prosaically, 'the intertwining of change and continuity' (McRae 1999: 19) in the sphere of family and household arrangements.

Of equal importance are the related debates about what role the state can and should have in determining these unfolding futures. Rapid social change enhances the appeal in some quarters of traditional social arrangements, but it is an axiom of much of the social scientific literature in this field that many of the social changes currently underway are irreversible, or at least irreversible by governments. From such a point of view, the state's capacity to reshape family relationships is limited to interventions that mesh with the prevailing mood of the times (see Chapter 3 for instructive examples from family policy in Britain). In other words, there are very real limits to what the state *can* do, and in addition there are important differences of opinion about what the state *should* and *should not* do, rooted in competing understandings of whether collective provision saps individual responsibility and encourages dependency (as, for example, theorists of the New Right assert). It is against this background that the related notions of 'negotiation' and 'strategy' have come to have particular importance in the understanding of relationships between family (and household) members and between them and the various institutions and representatives of the state. The state may be able to modify the economic and social environment within which individuals make decisions about family relationships, but it is evident that people, in their family lives at least, do not respond simply as rational economic actors in pursuit of their self-interest. They are also guided by emotions and by moral notions, which are drawn upon creatively by individuals when it comes to putting them into practice (as many of this book's contributions amply demonstrate, but see in particular Chapters 5, 9 and 12). Governments can and do also appeal to moral notions such as altruism, but there is no guarantee that individuals will accept such exhortation uncritically as a guide to what they should do. The approach to 'the family' as a dependent variable that changes in predictable ways in response to altered economic and political signals carries with it very little explanatory promise. In an age in which individuals are prepared to question the appropriateness of the idea of uniform ways of doing things, even where these are sanctioned by authority or tradition, people's family lives are more diverse and nuanced than the dependent variable of conventional functionalist accounts (Allan and Crow 2001: 200; see also Chapter 7).

The mood of the times is unquestionably one of change and transformation, and it is incumbent on social scientists with an interest in people's family relationships to explore both the extent of change and the implications of the changes that are underway. Morgan has observed that the language of strategies and negotiations has been drawn upon with great frequency in recent analyses of domestic life, not least because 'this language emphasises process and change' (1999: 32) and can therefore capture the fluidity and diversity of family relationships more readily than conventional approaches were able to do. The language of strategies and negotiations also carries with it other associations, for example with individual rationality and calculation, as several authors including Morgan (1989) have noted. Such associations have obvious links to the idea that contemporary family relationships are being reshaped by the forces of individualisation and democratisation, but it remains to be established how much change there has been in this direction and what is driving it. There is, after all, an extensive literature in which family life in times past has been understood as the product of people's consciously adopted strategies, and this indicates the presence of important elements of continuity as well as change in this area (Hareven 2000: chapter 3). There is also a rather different body of research reports that has identified problems with the notion of 'choice' in the field of family relationships, exemplified in Burgoyne's critique of writers who argue 'that household structures and domestic lifestyles and strategies are individually and freely chosen' (1987: 85). The various agencies of the state that have a bearing on how people live as families are not a neutral influence in this respect. Recognition of their role in attempting to promote or foreclose particular patterns of family life needs to be included in any account of how and why change has taken place, albeit that the outcomes have by no means always been those intended by policy makers.

Studies of the history of public policy relating to families reveal the state to be powerful but not omnipotent. Hareven has usefully suggested that it is appropriate to regard 'the family's relationship to public agencies and bureaucracies as a dynamic process of interaction' (2000: 27), and there are numerous examples from different historical periods of how people have resisted attempts by state bodies to impose standardised conceptions of how family life should be organised. The general conclusion that can be drawn is that there are limits to how far the state can go in the direction of what Donzelot (1979) famously called 'the policing of families'. An equally important point is that the desire on the part of policy makers to oversee and regulate family life is historically variable. It is plausible to treat modern welfare states as the embodiment of a long-term tendency for intervention by public authorities in the sphere of family life to increase, but the suggestion that state bodies are currently moving towards less (or, at least, less direct) regulation of the private sphere is one that has to be taken seriously. To the extent that it has happened, the acceptance by policy makers of greater diversity in people's family patterns implies a retreat from the attempt to impose the particular set of norms and values associated with what commentators of an earlier generation took to be the conventional pattern and a recognition that social change has brought with it what Cheal refers to as the '*destandardisation* of the family' (1991: 133, italics in original). The extent to which such a shift has occurred or is likely to proceed in the future is the subject of extensive debate, as the previous chapters indicate (see Chapter 2 for an overall view of trends in Western Europe). There is, for example, plenty of evidence to support the view that policy initiatives have adopted a rhetoric of accepting diversity, at the same time shoring up the traditional family in a rather uncomfortable way (see Chapter 5). The discussions that these chapters contain also indicate that the implications of this unfolding trend towards destandardisation, if such it is, are profound and warrant further scrutiny.

Towards individualised and democratised families?

The argument that current trends are moving in the direction of family life becoming more individualised and democratised contains a number of strands. Beck's thesis is that the social foundations of the nuclear family have been dissolved by the development of welfare states in which traditional dependencies like those of full-time housewives on breadwinner husbands are made redundant. Beck, whose mode of analysis is necessarily speculative, describes the welfare state as an '*experimental arrangement for conditioning ego-centred ways of life*' (1997: 97, italics in original), suggesting that individuals have been emancipated from obligations rooted in dependency and that as a result they can exercise a greater degree of control over their lives. The implication of this process of individualisation for family relationships is that marriage is less binding than it was in the past, and that a range of possibilities are opened up as a consequence. The growth of single-person households can be interpreted as one expression of individualisation, as Beck and Beck-Gernsheim (1995: 9) note, but this is merely an illustration of the more general phenomenon whereby contemporary societies witness the emergence of 'the individual as *actor*, *designer*, *juggler*, and *stage director* of his own biography, identity, social networks, commitments and convictions' (Beck 1997: 95, italics in original). The other side of this trend is what Beck-Gernsheim refers to as the emergence of the 'post-familial family', an arrangement that embodies 'personally chosen togetherness'. She claims that this has been made possible by the loosening of the ties of obligation and permanence (1998: 61, 67), which she takes as a defining characteristic of traditional family relationships. Beck and Beck-Gernsheim's view that changes are ushering in 'the negotiated family' (1995: 2) is another expression of this perspective.

These ideas about individualisation are consistent with the thesis that contemporary family life is subject to a process of democratisation. According to Giddens:

> There is only one story to tell about the family today, and that is of democracy. The family is becoming more democratised, in ways which track processes of public democracy.
>
> 1998: 93

For Giddens, if contemporary families are to be durable they have to offer scope for their members to exercise individual choice and to be characterised by 'equality, mutual respect, autonomy, decision making through communication and freedom from violence' (*ibid.*). In its pure form, an intimate relationship (such as that between marriage partners) will not necessarily be founded on notions of long-term commitment but will rather, according to Giddens, 'be continued only in so far as it is thought by both parties to deliver enough satisfactions for each individual to stay within it' (1992: 58). In what Giddens calls 'the democratic family', the principle of equality extends beyond the relationship between parents and gives rights as well as obligations to children. As a matter of right, 'children can and should be able to answer back' (1999: 63), because they are also individuals who deserve a say in domestic decision making. Outcomes are negotiated in democratic families, and there is a requirement for 'flexibility and adaptability' (1998: 94) if relationships are to be sustainable. There are echoes here of Finch and Mason's argument that negotiation in family relationships is made possible and necessary by the fact that 'individuals do have some room for manoeuvre' (1993: 60) despite the fact that these authors attach greater importance than does Giddens to the structural constraints on people's range of options, as Finch (1989) herself had previously acknowledged. The recognition of the fact that individuals have room for manoeuvre is compatible with recognition that the extent of this room for manoeuvre will vary according to each individual's position in relation to social class, age, gender, ethnicity and other structural factors.

There are a number of points that can be made about the models of individualised and democratised families promulgated by Beck and Beck-Gernsheim and Giddens (see also Chapter 6). The first of these points is that there are strong similarities between the ideas on which they are based and the assessments offered by an earlier generation of family sociologists. To cite one example, as long ago as the early 1970s Fletcher was describing 'the contemporary British family' as 'entered into and maintained on a completely voluntary basis by partners of equal status, and therefore entailing a marital relationship based upon mutuality of consideration'. He also perceived it to be 'democratically managed, in that husband and wife (and frequently children) discuss family affairs together when decisions have to be taken' (1971: 128). The timing of Fletcher's claim matters, because it is precisely at this moment that Giddens argues that the transformation wrought by globalisation *began* to take hold. Other social scientists of the time were also anticipating elements of what are currently being presented as phenomena of a more recent provenance. Thus Beck's identification of globalisation as a force responsible for producing 'the unsettled, friable world in which we live' (2000: 52) bears more than a passing resemblance to Rosser and Harris's account of 'the transition from the "cohesive" to the mobile society' (1965: 299). A further reason for questioning the thesis that we are witnessing a radical break with the past is that family historians have found it useful to make sense of domestic relationships in previous generations (and, indeed, previous centuries) in terms of household strategies collectively arrived at but containing strong elements of individual rationality. Hareven's comment that 'Within the dictates of "collective" family strategies, individual members did not always succumb blindly to family demands' (2000: 98) was made with reference to the findings of studies from the early industrial period onwards, and it is clear from such data that the process of individualisation has deep historical roots. Pahl's (1984) analysis of household work strategies points towards the same conclusion.

A second general point regarding the thesis that contemporary family patterns are becoming more individualised and democratised is that these processes appear to have the potential to be taken much further than they have been so far. Jamieson's wide-ranging survey of the evidence that is available led her to the conclusion that 'The suggested shift to voluntary, equal, relationships of disclosing intimacy is … difficult to sustain' (1998: 161). Ribbens McCarthy and Edwards (see Chapter 10) also provide a critique of notions of individualisation as having different meanings in different spheres. Giddens's response to the objection that his theory does not fit the facts is to note that the democratised family is 'an ideal' and that it still makes sense to discuss an aspect of such an arrangement like co-parenting 'however far off this may be in current circumstances' (1998: 94, 96). This type of reasoning solves the problem only at the expense of creating another, because it invites consideration of what family relationships would be like if the forces that are said to be currently influential are allowed to run their course. Beck's remarks on this subject are instructive, given that the logic of individualisation will in the extreme produce a society made up of single individuals 'unhindered by a relationship, marriage or family' (1992: 116). Giddens rightly baulks at such a prospect when he discusses the challenge of identifying 'how family life might combine individual choice and social solidarity'. An example of the need for there to be some restraint on individuals pursuing their narrow self-interest in the realm of family relationships is provided by post-divorce arrangements, in which context Giddens speaks of parents having 'life-time responsibilities' (1998: 93, 95) that do not end with the termination of a marriage. Giddens goes on to argue that the democratic family means the acceptance of obligations, as well as rights sanctioned in law (1999: 64), and thereby identifies the existence of a potential tension between the forces of individualisation and democratisation.

A third general point that may be made about the notion of a movement towards individualised and democratised families is that these are not the only forces at work in contemporary societies, and this helps to explain why individualisation and democratisation have not been taken further. Beck and Beck-Gernsheim acknowledge this by noting that individualisation unfolds alongside 'considerable pressure to conform in a standardized way' (1995: 40) rather than ushering in greater diversity in any straightforward fashion. Beck-Gernsheim has gone on to argue that individualisation may also prompt resistance among people who express 'a longing for the opposite world of intimacy, security and closeness' (1998: 67). These comments help to make sense of the findings of research into step-families, such as that by Burgoyne and Clark (1984), that people seek to recreate 'ordinary' family life more often than they express a commitment to 'progressive' alternatives. It is also instructive that the term employed by Weeks and his colleagues (1999; see also Chapter 11) to describe non-heterosexual relationships is 'families of choice', or 'elective families'. Simpson's observation that the experience of divorce induces in those who go through it 'a quest for stability or "a peaceful life"'(1998: 3) is similarly open to interpretation as evidence of a reaction against individualisation. The complexity of the situation is captured in Beck and Beck-Gernsheim's delineation of a paradox, whereby 'we are under pressure simultaneously to become individuals and adopt standardized strategies' (1995: 40). They identify the commercialisation that has its roots in market forces as one of the strongest influences inducing standardisation, and in many ways this operates in opposition to the protection from market forces that the expansion of the welfare state afforded to individuals. There is also recognition in Beck's work that the role of the state can vary significantly, and that this will have a bearing on how far individualisation may proceed. Thus he remarks that 'It makes sense to distinguish between different contexts and forms of individualisation. In some states, particularly in Sweden, Switzerland and western Germany, we are dealing with a *comprehensively insured individualisation*' (1997: 101, italics in original), a situation that contrasts with societies in which welfare state commitments are less extensive. Beck's approach is at odds with prevailing opinion in debates on welfare state regime types in which the Scandinavian model is treated as distinctive (Crow 1997), but it remains the case that debates about different welfare state regimes and about supposed moves beyond the welfare state are highly pertinent to consideration of the question of whether it is appropriate to envisage further individualisation and democratisation of family relationships occurring (see Chapter 4 for the different 'type case' welfare states of Germany, Spain, Sweden and the USA).

A fourth point is that it is worthwhile considering in some detail what is understood by individuals as negotiators and strategists in the analyses of writers who adopt the broad approach of Beck and Beck-Gernsheim and Giddens. By framing analysis of individuals as 'reflexive selves', there is a danger that the contrasting structural positions of different groups of people will be overlooked. Smart and Neale have taken Giddens to task for the way in which his focus on individual choice leads to 'a certain glossing of class differences and inequalities' (1999: 11), and the same conclusion can be drawn about other key sociological variables such as gender, ethnicity, age and disability (see Chapter 10). Individuals vary systematically along these and other lines in the power that they have to negotiate with each other and with representatives of the state. It is equally vital to recognise that the households of which individuals are part also vary systematically in terms of the strategies that they are able to deploy. This is most obvious when contrasting middle- and working-class households (Anderson *et al.* 1994; Jordan *et al.* 1992, 1994), but the phenomenon is a more general one. For example, it also relates to the contrasting positions of lone parent and other household types, in the context of the more limited room for manoeuvre that the former tend to have (Rowlingson and McKay 1998). Klett-Davies' analysis of lone mothers draws the conclusion that the theory of individualisation 'does not sufficiently incorporate material circumstances … which can inhibit lifestyle changes' (1997: 189). It is therefore important that individuals are not treated as if they share a common capacity to shape their family relationships; the choices open to some are not as great as those available to others.

Negotiations, strategies and values

The policy implications of the issues discussed so far are, from some angles, relatively uncontroversial. There is wide agreement concerning the point made by Beck and Beck-Gernsheim and also by Giddens that social changes have been too far-reaching for a return to 'traditional' family patterns (which in themselves were historically created and variable) to be conceivable. Family diversity is here to stay, along with the basic structures of the welfare state and the modern labour market with which it is intimately connected. If this point is accepted, then the main task of policy makers is to facilitate the realisation of people's potential as individuals and as members of family groups, doing so by confronting some of the structural inequalities that lie behind unequal opportunities, for example. Of course, there are some writers who do not accept uncritically the growth of family diversity and who seek to place limits on the trend towards the proliferation of different family types. Communitarians such as Etzioni (1997) could be cited in this context, not least because they associate growing family diversity with the decline of the shared norms that they regard as crucial to the cohesion of communities. Etzioni's preference is for a two-parent family in which both fathers and mothers have the same rights and the same responsibilities (1997: 180), because in his view this is the arrangement that provides the most suitable context for the socialisation of children as moral agents who will act in appropriately other-regarding ways rather than narrowly individualistic ones. Communitarians like Etzioni are also suspicious of the extensive involvement of the state in family life because of the potential of such programmes to compromise individual responsibility, particularly in liberal welfare state regimes, in which the responsibilities of individuals are given particular prominence.

Communitarianism has a number of variants between which there are important disagreements, but what the broad perspective serves to highlight is the point that policy making in relation to the family involves something other than a morally neutral exercise of finding the most effective means of promoting what Giddens calls the individual's 'reflexive project of self' (1992: 198). Giddens's later work makes a more explicit acknowledgement of this issue by attaching greater prominence to the responsibility to others that the individual has.

In practice, neither the approach to understanding family relationships that has been put forward by theorists of individualisation and democratisation nor the alternative approach put forward by the communitarians offers a convincing analysis of contemporary change. To begin with, it can be noted that the social world is not composed of rational economic actors busily pursuing their self-interest through carefully calculated strategies and negotiations. Duncan and Edwards' (1999) study of lone mothers and how their relationship to the labour market is tempered by gendered moral rationalities provides a good illustration of this point (see also Chapter 5). The situation of childcare and maintenance following divorce also leads to the same conclusion. Bradshaw and his colleagues' research on non-resident fathers found the concept of negotiation to be of only limited value, because 'The moral duty on fathers (and all parents) to provide financially for dependent children is so strong that it is surely non-negotiable, a principle upheld by the Child Support Acts'. The majority of the non-residential fathers interviewed were motivated by more than narrow self-interest and conformity to the requirements of the law; rather, they were motivated by a concern for their children's welfare and wanted 'to fulfil all their parental obligations, social, emotional and financial' (1999: 205, 232). A comparable rejection of narrowly self-interested behaviour was found by Smart and Neale in their study of post-divorce parenting. Their comment that most of their respondents 'have not resisted the obligations imposed by the Children Act in principle, but they do find these obligations extremely hard to sustain in practice' (1999: 198; see also Chapter 9) reflects the fact that the best interests of the child require parents to compromise and accommodate rather than to press their individual agendas.

Many other examples could be cited of contemporary family relationships in which people refrain from the unbridled pursuit of individual advantage or even the calculation of what self-interested behaviour might involve. Commitment to the ideology of 'putting the family first' (Jordan *et al.* 1994), that is, to the idea that membership of families requires subordination of individual interest to the good of the group, is widespread, and research findings indicate that this is more than merely a rhetorical convenience. Women in dual-earner households who had returned to paid work after maternity leave reported to Brannen and Moss that they were motivated by the needs of the household, and they 'did not appear to want to calculate whether each partner was receiving fair and equal shares of household resources' (1991: 47). The more general point illustrated by such patterns of behaviour is that the emergence of new family forms 'does not mean that values of caring and obligation are abandoned' (Silva and Smart 1999: 7), only that people are finding different ways to express these values. As Wallman's (1984) classic study of diverse household types in Battersea demonstrated, the 'styles' according to which people live and the strategies that they develop cannot be read off from household composition in any deterministic way. Her account highlighted the need to pay heed to the local cultural context, and in particular the values embodied in that context. Duncan and Edwards' view of lone mothers' attitudes to labour market opportunities being 'negotiated socially within the context of social groups, social networks and neighbourhoods' (1999: 21) is a more recent statement of this important point, that the same family form may be consistent with a variety of different family practices. Nor should diversity of family forms necessarily be taken to entail diversity in the content of family relationships, at least in terms of their underlying rationality or morality.

It is instructive in the context of this discussion to remember that Finch's argument relating to the negotiation of family relationships has greater subtlety than the version of it found in the individualisation thesis. Finch's analysis acknowledges that relations between family members involve much more than negotiation, being as they are structured by 'the delicate balance between feelings of affection, moral imperatives of duty, and calculations about personal advantage and disadvantage' (1989: 77). Further qualifications concerning the openness to negotiation of family relationships might be made in connection with those situations in which negotiation is more apparent than real, such as the discussions between husbands and wives referred to by Dempsey as involving only 'token negotiation' (1997: 203), or the discussions between parents and teenage children analysed by Brannen *et al.* (1994: chapter 10), which in practice have a similarly closed character. Ungerson's (1987: 53) analysis of the development of caring arrangements provides a further instance of how 'negotiation' may be a euphemistic term to use when considering how families and wider kin networks actually operate. Carers in her study had not necessarily been involved in active negotiations to take on the role. Rather, it was the case that carers were 'selected ... according to dominant, normative, and gendered rules of kinship' (1987: 61) that it was very difficult to challenge or resist.

Negotiations take place within frameworks that include normative elements that are non-negotiable, ruling out certain courses of action as strategically unthinkable. The existence of room for manoeuvre should not be confused with freedom from constraint, including the constraints imposed by the local cultures in which people live. There is a partial endorsement of the communitarian position in this respect, but only a partial one because recognition of the importance of local culture or 'community' does not necessarily entail acceptance of the norms of behaviour that are contained therein. The two other parts of the equation are the broader policy framework provided by the state and the range of discourses available for people to draw upon in the construction of their 'family lives' (for the latter, see Chapter 10). The other side of communitarianism's emphasis on the importance of community values is the downgrading of the case for the state to provide the policy framework and the resources necessary to empower people in their pursuit of their chosen family objectives. This point has especial pertinence to people living in communities characterised by multiple deprivation. And both communitarians and individualisation theorists are found wanting with respect to the potential for conflict that exists over the policy issues to be addressed. The communitarian preference for one particular family form suffers from all the drawbacks of solutions imposed in a top-down fashion, not the least of which is that it goes against the wishes of those whose preference is to live differently (see Chapter 5). If patterns of family relationships need to be imposed, then they are likely to be resisted in the context of cultures in which social arrangements have legitimacy only if the people involved feel ownership of them (as James shows in his discussion of the ill-fated Family Law Act 1996 in Britain; see Chapter 3.2). At the same time, it needs to be recognised that the agenda of the individualisation theorists fails to acknowledge the complexities of the processes that have to be gone through if the opening up of choices to pursue different forms of family life is to avoid producing losers as well as winners. Unless the existence of inequalities along the lines of social class, age, gender, ethnicity and related dimensions between the people seeking to negotiate their preferred pattern of family relationships is addressed, and unless there is a challenge to the tendency of policy makers to reproduce the situation in which certain family practices are privileged while others are disadvantaged, the 'democratic family' will remain an elusive aspiration.

References

Allan, G. and Crow, G. (2001) *Families, Households and Society*, Basingstoke: Palgrave.

Anderson, M., Bechhofer, F. and Kendrick, S. (1994) 'Individual and household strategies', in M. Anderson, F. Bechhofer and J. Gershuny (eds) *The Political Economy of the Household*, Oxford: Oxford University Press.

Beck, U. (1992) *Risk Society: Towards a New Modernity*, London: Sage.

—— (1997) *The Reinvention of Politics: Rethinking Modernity in the Global Social Order*, Cambridge: Polity Press.

—— (2000) *What is Globalization?* Cambridge: Polity Press.

Beck, U. and Beck-Gernsheim, E. (1995) *The Normal Chaos of Love*, Cambridge: Polity Press.

—— (1996) 'Individualization and precarious freedoms: perspectives and controversies of a subject-oriented sociology', in P. Heelas, S. Lash and P. Morris (eds) *Detraditionalization: Critical Reflections on Authority and Identity*, Oxford: Basil Blackwell.

Beck-Gernsheim, E. (1998) 'On the way to a post-familial family: from a community of need to elective affinities', *Theory, Culture and Society* 15(3–4): 53–70.

Bradshaw, J., Stimson, C., Skinner, C. and Williams, J. (1999) *Absent Fathers?* London: Routledge.

Brannen, J., Dodd, K., Oakley, A. and Storey, P. (1994) *Young People, Health and Family Life*, Buckingham: Open University Press.

Brannen, J. and Moss, P. (1991) *Managing Mothers: Dual Earner Households after Maternity Leave*, London: Unwin Hyman.

Burgoyne, J. (1987) 'Rethinking the family life cycle', in A. Bryman, B. Bytheway, J. Burgoyne and D. Clark (eds) *Making a Go of It: A study of Stepfamilies in Sheffield*, London: Routledge & Kegan Paul.

Burgoyne, J. and Clark, D. (1984) *Making a Go of It: A Study of Stepfamilies in Sheffield*, London: Routledge & Kegan Paul.

Cheal, D. (1991) *Family and the State of Theory*, Hemel Hempstead: Harvester Wheatsheaf.

Crow, G. (1997) *Comparative Sociology and Social Theory: Beyond the Three Worlds*, Basingstoke: Macmillan.

Dempsey, K. (1997) *Inequalities in Marriage: Australia and Beyond*, Melbourne: Oxford University Press.

Donzelot. J. (1979) *The Policing of Families: Welfare versus the State*, London: Hutchinson.

Duncan, S. and Edwards, R. (1999) *Lone Mothers, Paid Work and Gendered Moral Rationalities*, Basingstoke: Macmillan.

Etzioni, A. (1997) *The New Golden Rule: Community and Morality in a Democratic Society*, London: Profile Books.

Finch, J. (1989) *Family Obligations and Social Change*, Cambridge: Polity Press.

Finch, J. and Mason, J. (1993) *Negotiating Family Responsibilities*, London: Routledge.

Fletcher, R. (1971) *The Family and Marriage in Britain: An Analysis and Moral Assessment.* Harmondsworth: Penguin.
Giddens, A. (1992) *The Transformation of Intimacy*, Cambridge: Polity Press.
—— (1998) *The Third Way: The Renewal of Social Democracy*, Cambridge: Polity Press.
—— (1999) *Runaway World: How Globalisation is Reshaping our Lives*, London: Profile Books.
Hareven, T. (2000) *Families, History and Social Change: Life-Course and Cross-cultural Perspectives* Boulder, Colo.: Westview Press.
Jamieson, L. (1998) *Intimacy: Personal Relationships in Modern Societies*, Cambridge: Polity Press.
Jordan, B., James, S., Kay, H. and Redley, M. (1992) *Trapped in Poverty? Labour-market decisions in low-income households*, London: Routledge.
Jordan, B., Redley, M. and James, S. (1994) *Putting the Family First: Identities, Decisions, Citizenship*, London: UCL Press.
Klett-Davies, M. (1997) 'Single mothers in Germany: supported mothers who work', in S. Duncan and R. Edwards (eds) *Single Mothers in an International Context*, London: UCL Press.
McRae, S. (1999) 'Introduction: family and household change in Britain', in S. McRae (ed.) *Changing Britain: Families and Households in the 1990s*, Oxford: Oxford University Press.
Morgan, D. (1989) 'Strategies and sociologists: a comment on Crow', *Sociology* 23(1): 25–9.
—— (1999) 'Gendering the household: some theoretical considerations' in L. McKie, S. Bowlby and S. Gregory (eds) *Gender, Power and the Household*, Basingstoke: Macmillan.
Pahl, R. (1984) *Divisions of Labour*, Oxford: Basil Blackwell.
Rosser, C. and Harris, C. (1965) *The Family and Social Change: A Study of Family and Kinship in a South Wales Town*, London: Routledge & Kegan Paul.
Rowlingson, K. and McKay, S. (1998) *The Growth of Lone Parenthood: Diversity and dynamics*, London: PSI.
Silva, E. and Smart, C. (1999) 'The new practices and politics of family life', in E. Silva and C. Smart (eds) *The New Family?* London: Sage.
Simpson, B. (1998) *Changing Families: An Ethnographic Approach to Divorce and Separation*, Oxford: Berg.
Smart, C. and Neale, B. (1999) *Family Fragments?* Cambridge: Polity Press.
Stacey, J. (1998) *Brave New Families: Stories of Domestic Upheaval in Late Twentieth-century America*, Berkeley: University of California Press.
Ungerson, C. (1987) *Policy is Personal: Sex, Gender and Informal Care*, London: Tavistock.
Wallman, S. (1984) *Eight London Households*, London: Tavistock.
Weeks, J., Heaphy, B. and Donovan, C. (1999) 'Families of choice: autonomy and mutuality in non-heterosexual relationships', in S. McRae (ed.) *Changing Britain: Families and Households in the 1990s*, Oxford: Oxford University Press.

Index

Page references for figures and tables are in italics; those for notes are followed by n.